Childbirth Without Fear

GRANTLY DICK-READ

Born in Britain in 1890, Grantly Dick-Read studied at Cambridge and at the London Hospital. He soon realised that there was something inherently wrong with the traditional methods of delivering babies, with their emphasis on intervention and the extensive use of anaesthetics.

The publication of *Childbirth without Fear* caused widespread controversy, but, encouraged by many women who had given birth using the 'Dick-Read method', Grantly Dick-Read dedicated his life to promoting natural childbirth. He died in 1959.

INA MAY GASKIN

Ina May Gaskin has been a midwife for more than forty years at The Farm Midwifery Center in Summertown, Tennessee. She is the only midwife after whom an obstetric manoevre has been named (Gaskin manoevre). She is the best-selling author of *Spiritual Midwifery, Ina May's Guide to Childbirth, Ina May's Guide to Breastfeeding* and *Birth Matters.*

PUBLISHER'S INTRODUCTION

This Pinter & Martin edition of *Childbirth without Fear* is true to the fourth, and last, edition Grantly Dick-Read completed in June 1959, the month of his death.

Grantly Dick-Read first published his revolutionary views on childbirth in 1933 as *Natural Childbirth*. He later expanded this work and in 1942, under the title *Revelations of Childbirth*, it became the first version of the book you now have before you.

Since the author's death, heavily edited versions of *Childbirth without Fear* have been produced. We hope this second Pinter & Martin edition will introduce a new generation of parents and health professionals to his work.

THE COVER PHOTOGRAPHS

The front and back cover photographs by Lynsey Stone are of the unassisted home birth of Phoenix, born April 14th 2009, to parents Gina and Cody Phillips. Gina: "8.23am His head delivers... My body tingles with joy. I begin to scream I LOVE YOU BABY! over and over again as his body delivers. I can't stop myself from saying it. I'm so overjoyed. I feel like a lion roaring these words. I feel ferocious and strong. I feel beautiful and powerful. I feel completely conscious and primitive. He is born into mine and Cody's eager hands and I bring him to me. There are no words... the perfect birth!"

Grantly Dick-Read

Childbirth Without Fear

The principles and practice of natural childbirth

Foreword by Ina May Gaskin

Childbirth without Fear
The Principles and Practice of Natural Childbirth

First published by Heinemann Medical Books 1942
Fourth edition first published by Heinemann Medical Books 1959

This second Pinter & Martin edition first published 2013

ISBN 978-1-78066-055-4
also available as ebook

British Library Cataloguing-in-Publication Data
A catalogue record for this book is available from the British Library

Set in Minion

Printed and bound in Great Britain by TJ Books Limited, Padstow, Cornwall

Pinter & Martin Ltd
6 Effra Parade
London SW2 1PS
www.pinterandmartin.com

Contents

To the memory of
Joseph B. De Lee, AM, MD
Late Professor of Obstetrics and Gynaecology,
Emeritus, University of Chicago, USA
this book is dedicated

For his kind interest in my work and
for his personal friendliness and appreciation
I shall always be sincerely grateful

Grantly Dick-Read

Foreword

Ina May Gaskin

I had no idea when I first read *Childbirth Without Fear* at the tender age of sixteen that the book would set the course of my life to an extent that is only obvious to me now. I found the book in the public library in my hometown and began what became a lifelong study of birth. Birth was a fascinating and mysterious subject at that time in my sheltered life, and this was the only book I could find about it. The edition I read had no photos, but it prepared me for birth and, amazingly, it prepared me to be a midwife in so many ways that it's hard to list them all.

Grantly Dick-Read's description of birth as a biological process, the functioning of which goes best when the labouring woman is calm and unafraid, made sense to me, because it matched all of the stories that I had overheard during the summer I spent at my aunt and uncle's farm when I was nine. In case you don't already know this, family farmers talk about birth a lot. My aunt took care to school me on the principles of mammalian birth, principles that my cousins had learned at a much earlier age. Even though I never had a chance to be around a labouring animal or see any kind of birth or pictorial representation of birth in any species, I quickly learned that it is inexcusable behaviour to frighten or bother a labouring female. I also learned how easy it is to unintentionally cause complications in birth in this way.

Never having been exposed to frightening birth stories when I read *Childbirth Without Fear* (my mother had assured me that giving birth was something that women could do), it wasn't hard for me to accept Dick-Read's message that approaching birth with a positive attitude of trust in one's body and in nature would enhance the spiritual experience that birth was meant to be. He made birth seem an exciting adventure that lay ahead, one that a man might even wish he could experience himself. What could be more encouraging to a young woman than to read a book by a doctor who described birth in this way?

What I didn't know when I was expecting my first baby in the mid-1960s was that hospital birth practices in most parts of the United States (including the place where I lived) were radically different from those which Dick-Read described in British hospitals (where a woman who chose a midwife might be able to successfully refuse routine medical intervention in a hospital if she chose to do so). The edition of *Childbirth Without Fear* that I had read at sixteen lacked the chapter "United States Tour".* Had I read that chapter before my first pregnancy, it would have warned me about the treatment I would encounter in a typical US hospital. That chapter recorded Dick-Read's astonishment at the degree of ignorance of the physiology of birth in healthy women and the practice of deliberate injury to women (on the excuse that this avoided worse injury) that characterized mainstream obstetrics when he toured many US hospitals over three months in the late 1950s: "It seemed there was no possibility of an emergency arising that could not be dealt with immediately," he wrote, "but there was no provision for the absence of emergency or abnormality. I was told it did not happen!"

As a gynaecologist, Dick-Read knew that many women who had had episiotomies suffered from gynaecological problems caused by the episiotomy itself, and that an episiotomy in a healthy woman often destroyed her enjoyment of further sexual contact with her husband. Knowing from his own experience that 90 per cent of healthy women attended by a competent obstetrician or midwife could give birth without episiotomy or other trauma, he asked several US obstetricians why every woman's perineum was deeply cut before the birth of the baby. Their answers amazed him. Episiotomies not only prevented tears, he was told, but they kept the baby's head from acting as a "battering ram" against the "rigid perineum" of the mother. In each hospital he visited, two-thirds to three-fourths of US babies were being pulled from their mothers' bodies with forceps, and episiotomies were mandatory because student doctors were taught it was dangerous for a baby to be born without first cutting through the mother's perineal muscles.

When he asked US obstetricians if they had ever seen a birth happen without episiotomy or tear and learned they hadn't, he realized he was encountering a peculiarly superstitious obstetrical practice that was more akin to religion than science. Seeing his skepticism and astonishment, one enthusiastic obstetrician assured him that in his part of the US, babies' heads were much bigger than they used to be and that there had been no reason to believe that the bodies of the women had grown proportionally larger at the "outlet". Dick-Read

---

* In the present edition this material appears in the Appendix, pp 318–30.

remarked, "I am not sure I could possibly provide evidence to show that you are wrong, but I have no evidence to persuade me that the youth of this great country become swollen-headed before they are born."

Since I hadn't been forewarned about the mandatory forceps operation that was in store for me because of my being American, I had to learn the hard way how deeply held US birth superstitions were. To my surprise and chagrin, I learned that no matter how quietly and uncomplainingly I behaved in labour until my cervix was fully dilated, the script had already been written. They were going to give me a caudal (a type of spinal anaesthesia that left so many women permanently disabled or paralysed that it is no longer used), whether I was in pain or not. Instead of being frightened of labour pain, I was frightened about the possibility of being unconscious or incapacitated because of medications that I didn't want or need. After many hours of unmedicated labour, a team of masked nurses and the obstetrician surrounded me, paralysed my lower body and then strapped my wrists and ankles to the delivery rack without any pleasantries or explanations why they were treating me this way. They did tell me afterwards that even after the anaesthesia wore off, I shouldn't try to lift my head even an inch for twelve hours if I didn't want to experience a spinal headache that could last for three months. For several hours, I lay alone in my hospital bed, wondering if I would remain paralysed. I didn't get to see my baby for twenty-four hours, and that separation greatly affected our early relationship.

What I didn't know in 1956, when I first read *Childbirth Without Fear*, was that even though it was a best-seller in the US in the 1950s as well as in Britain, Dick-Read was regarded as a heretic by those physicians whose minds were closed to his message and insights. It's clear from the first paragraph of his book that he knew how unpopular he would become by undertaking the "rather hazardous voyage" of daring to describe a new approach to obstetrics. He was fully aware that the science of obstetrics was young and immature. He knew that James Simpson had run afoul of the church for being the one who introduced the use of anaesthesia in birth in the 1840s, that Ignaz Semmelweis' success in saving women from dying from childbed fever by teaching doctors to wash their hands before vaginally examining women in labour brought him hostility and opposition by most obstetricians around the same time, and that Joseph Lister, who brought knowledge of antiseptics, had to ignore great ridicule and opposition from his colleagues for continuing to use them.

Because Dick-Read respected women of all ages and races so much and because he couldn't stand unnecessary fear and suffering, he took the lonely path of the pioneer and kept working to refine his message and bring it to women all over the world. I realize now that even though he knew this meant professional suicide for him personally, he tried as hard as he could to counteract the propaganda of the Middle Ages that superseded the earlier messages of Hippocrates, Soranus, and Aristotle, who focused not only on the body but on the mind and the body in their writings about midwifery.

Those who consider Dick-Read a heretic view women's bodies as defective machines and birth itself as inherently risky – a disaster waiting to happen. To them, women's emotions are completely irrelevant to the process of labour and birth. To Dick-Read, the mother's emotional state was everything: a prolonged state of fear could actually cause complications, while a state of relaxation during labour could lift the mother into a state of ecstasy and euphoria such as that I experienced before the caudal was forced upon me.

Today's heretics are those who are skilled at the art of assisting a breech or twin birth or at manually changing the position of a baby, or those who do not look with scorn on healthy women who prefer to give birth in the comfort of their own homes. The challenge birthing women face today is that in most parts of the world during what we can justly call the Age of the Caesarean, the most skilled practitioner can be called a heretic simply for making it obvious that the profession of obstetrics is losing the knowledge and skills that were once considered essential. Fortunately, I am meeting a growing number of physicians who are embracing heresy of the kind I am describing. I know they will gain much from reading Grantly Dick-Read's masterpiece.

When I first began attending births for the women in my community, I relied heavily on the insights I had gained from *Childbirth Without Fear*, and I still depend upon these today. I learned, for instance, how much it can help relaxation during labour for the labouring woman to slow down and deepen her breathing, how helpful it can be to ask her to relax the muscles of her forehead or to make low-pitched sounds instead of high, screechy ones. I learned that women will often be sleepy around the time of full dilatation of the cervix and that it can be good to maintain this restful state between rushes (contractions).

Dick-Read was such a good observer of labouring women that he didn't need to know the names of the "love hormones" of labour (oxytocin and neuroendorphins) and their protective functions in order to help women into the emotional states that facilitate their release.

Until I treated myself to a cover-to-cover reading of *Childbirth Without Fear* in preparation for writing this preface, I hadn't realized that I must also give Dick-Read credit for planting in my mind the concept that the vagina and cervix function in sphincter-like ways.

So thank you, Grantly Dick-Read. Some may still think of you as a heretic, but I thank you for teaching me about the beauty and sacredness of birth. You're my hero, and I hope that your book will some day be required reading for all obstetricians and midwives.

Preface to the First Edition

Grantly Dick-Read

Since the publication of *Natural Childbirth* in 1933, the significance of the emotional factors in the reproductive functions of women has continued to attract attention. Prior to that date, there were practically no monographs on the subject and very meagre, if any, reference was made to it in standard works of obstetrics.

General practitioners and midwives, particularly the latter, were not slow to appreciate the importance of this new light on midwifery.

With few exceptions, however, the teachers of obstetrics in the universities refrained from giving any real attention to the state of mind of the woman in childbirth. In 1936, Dr Francis J. Browne, Professor of Obstetrics at the University of London, published the first edition of *Antenatal and Postnatal Care*, in which he invited me to contribute a chapter on the 'Influence of the Emotions upon Pregnancy and Parturition', and in his third edition, published two years later, again asked me to amplify those observations because of the interest that the subject had awakened in the profession.

There is no doubt that his belief in the importance of this subject has been instrumental in bringing the attention of the academic schools of obstetrics to the possibilities which it presents. It is with the utmost sincerity then that I express my gratitude for the friendship and confidence that he has given me, particularly the privilege of lecturing from time to time to his students at University College Hospital.

In America, Professor Joseph de Lee, late Emeritus Professor of Obstetrics at the University of Chicago, although not accepting the immediate possibilities of the whole teaching, showed a most kindly appreciation by drawing attention to the value of its application under certain circumstances.

Today, writings upon the antenatal care of women and upon the conduct of labour very rarely omit some reference to the importance of the care of the emotional states of the woman. Perhaps it is no exaggeration to record that the mind, as a part of the mechanism of reproduction, is no longer overlooked by progressive obstetricians.

There is still, however, considerable misunderstanding in the method of application of this teaching. In a series of over fifty lectures that I have been invited to give upon the influence of the emotions upon labour, one fact is outstanding: those who have seriously applied themselves to the care of the mind have been enthusiastic about their results and both midwives and practitioners demand more knowledge in order to enable them to achieve the perfect labour.

It is, therefore, to those who have believed that I write again, not in academic dogma, but rather as one who records clinical observations.

It may be necessary here to justify certain lines of action in order to escape the criticism of wholesale experiment upon my patients. Actually there has been no wild experimenting. My work has been based upon the foundations of early scientific training I was happy enough to acquire. The elementary laws of biology were ingrained in me by Professors Shipley and Stanley Gardiner and by the writings of Professor J.S. Haldane. At the time when Langley and Anderson were demonstrating to the world their discoveries of the functions of the autonomic nervous system, they were my teachers. Whilst Sir Henry Head was still working upon eases of herpes zoster in order to perfect his theory of the zones of cutaneous hyperalgesia, I was his house physician. James Sherren, who cut the cutaneous nerves of Head's arm himself, so that they two between them could work out 'the consequences of injury to the peripheral nerves in man,' was my chief when I was house surgeon at the London Hospital.

Perhaps it is no exaggeration to say that the privilege of such association with great pioneers and teachers produces in the least receptive minds a desire for observation and an unwillingness to accept the truth as being necessarily the whole truth.

When, at length, I became resident accoucheur and saw midwifery in the mass amongst the mothers of Whitechapel, Poplar and Bethnal Green, I was convinced that something beyond the truths that we were taught held the secret of simpler and safer motherhood. I proceeded to write a long and detailed work on the modern conduct of labour, but discarded it because there was neither explanation of nor cure for so many occurrences that were contrary to the laws of nature.

Many years later, prompted by increasing experience, childbirth was examined as a natural function in the light of the foundations of my early training. I argued that if academic obstetric teaching could not explain these things, possibly light could be shed upon them by biology, physiology and neurology? The simple laws of maintenance and reproduction of the species, the profound influence of the sympathetic nervous system upon the activities of the viscera, the causes and interpretation of painful stimuli, the visceral reactions to emotional states, were the very subjects which my earliest teachers had presented to the scientific world in what has now become epoch-making literature. Gradually, their lessons dovetailed into my own study of normal labour; the truth of their views was put to the test; and although much remains to be done, there is sufficient evidence to suggest that many of the problems of midwifery will be solved.

It is my purpose, therefore, to present as simply as possible a theory of natural childbirth and its application both during pregnancy and parturition, based on my observations. For the style of my writing and for the manner of setting out my argument I ask indulgence, for surely the clinical observations of one whose professional career has in the main been that of a general practitioner are unlikely to be recorded with the perfection we expect from those whose calling has been professorial. This task has not been undertaken, therefore, for academic reasons, but rather as a further step towards proof of the philosophical principle that all progress, both moral and physical, ultimately depends upon the perfection of motherhood.

G. D-R – June 1942

Preface to the Fourth Edition

Grantly Dick-Read

It is not easy to go back year after year in order to rewrite an introduction to this work which has carried on a theme first written twenty-eight years ago.

In 1944 it was published in the United States of America and at first followed a course similar to the original publication in England twelve years previously. It brought new thoughts from an unknown pen and introduced theories upon the pain of labour that appeared at first sight to challenge the validity of much that was considered basic orthodoxy. It did not die, however, but survived in spite of small support from obstetric fields. Neither obstetric nor academic perspicacity gave it security. This came from women whose inborn faith in the goodness and greatness of motherhood was closely associated to spiritual forces and designs.

It may have delayed maturity of acceptance by those of us who sought to relieve suffering and to comfort the distressed before we knew why such physical and emotional discomforts should tarnish the glory of a woman's greatest hour, for still we as men are not near enough to the nature of women. We neither feel the magnitude of our responsibility nor plumb the depths of our compassion. We are frustrated by the yearning of a labouring woman for companionship we cannot give. She seeks to escape the threatening gestures of her most natural function and cries out to evade the consciousness of her incomparable achievement in motherhood.

We know how far apart this is from the design of nature. It is not in keeping with the creative genius of her construction or the brilliant mechanism of her component parts. There is a gulf between the limitation of science and the source of an omniscience which gives life and guides us in the usage of faculties beyond our comprehension.

Goaded on by the humiliation of woman's helplessness in distress, man hunted through the armoury of science to find some weapon he could wield in her protection and defence. The natural reaction of the male to such a situation is anger, destruction, obliteration, and annihilation of the aggressor. Since 1850 a hundred ways and means have been discovered and devised to rid our mothers of the pest of pain which invariably attacks them when they most deserve the natural joy of their supreme accomplishment in motherhood. Simpson, Semmelweis and Lister, Pasteur and Ballantyne were in the vanguard of the valiant company of knights who waged war upon the scourge of physical torment, mutilation, and death in childbirth.

The extent and magnificence of their victory during the last hundred years is beyond both praise and gratitude. The consciousness of woman's discomfort can now be dispelled, but only at a price, for with it goes the consciousness of birth and the sensations and emotions, not pains, which are the rock of experience upon which the stability and magnitude of motherliness have firm foundations. But that is not all – today we know the price of relief from pain devolves upon mothers and babies, husbands and homes. The cost is severe, but women must never be allowed to suffer discomfort in childbirth greater than they are willing to bear. The problem of our progress is no longer solved by physical interference, to secure general or local desensitisation. Throughout the ages the science of medicine has been hampered by the insoluble problem of pain. A close clinical study of natural childbirth has taught much about the cause and origin of nervous impulses which are not physiological. This modicum of knowledge has enabled us to prove the theory in application by preventing the development of these causes. Fear is a natural protective emotion without which few of us would survive. When through association or indoctrination there is fear of childbirth, it brings resistant actions and reactions to the mechanism of the organs of reproduction. This discord that disturbs the harmony or polarity of muscle action causes tension which in turn gives rise to nervous impulses, interpreted in the brain as pain. This is in keeping with the natural law of protection of the individual from abnormal or harmful activities in or about the body.

In 1919 I wrote a brochure upon childbirth. It was based upon observations made during the previous twelve years when, under the able tuition and teaching of Professors Shipley and Gardiner, Langley and Anderson at Cambridge, I revelled in zoology, biology, and physiology. Natural history was my hobby and companion in the isolation of a relatively asocial number six in a family of seven children. The notions and ideas upon the birth of the young of any phylum, class, or order that I saw filled me with wonder and curiosity. It was not inherent perspicacity that drew me to these ideas, but a resentment that the law of nature should be held responsible for such injustice to women.

I was senior resident accoucheur at the London Hospital at that time, but my immature and enthusiastic views upon childbirth were not received for publication but replaced among the copious notes that I had made. By 1929 evidences and experiences in homes and hospitals satisfied me and a large number of my patients that the effort to learn and follow the untarnished physiological pattern of normal childbirth was acceptable to nine out of ten women who knew there was such a procedure. Had but half that number found confidence and comfort from the teaching it would have made it more than worth the effort involved in learning what is called 'natural childbirth'.

In 1932 Heinemann Medical Books Ltd, through Dr Johnston Abraham, accepted my book called *Natural Childbirth* and published it with certain reservations in 1933. It was received with gentle kindliness, near to sympathy, by my colleagues in obstetrics. Ten years later a more mature book upon the practice and principles of natural childbirth was published. It was entitled *The Revelation of Childbirth* and was the first edition of this book for which I am now writing a combined preface for editions one to four.

Changes have been made in the text for different reasons; mounting experiences and disturbing misunderstandings require explanation and correction. Some emphasis is no longer considered necessary because the theory and theme of this work are so widely known, and paragraphs which in earlier editions have served their purpose have been deleted. A further effort has been made to simplify the principles and practice of natural childbirth because the majority of its readers and disciples have no medical education. I have deemed it wise to withdraw the jest or touch of jollity which I have shared refreshingly with friends and students of my generation at university and hospital. Time changes all of us, imperceptibly maybe but surely, and so the fashions of our time change in spite of our habitual pattern. In the last five years or so this book has reached a far wider circle than in the previous ten or twelve. Recently I have been surprised and disconcerted to learn that harmless banter and even gentle persiflage have no place in professional communications. There is much happiness in this book and here and there a kindly caricature has countered what might have been interpreted as melodrama at some unknown innocent's expense. I must make clear without apology for the customs of my era that nowhere has a word been written with intention to hurt the feelings of my readers. From this edition my friends 'Chief Holosombo' and the 'Urban District Icon' have gone. I shall miss them and many others who lightened for me the unaccustomed burden of authorship.

But their part is played, they have gone nobly on, unaltered and quietly smiling, both at appreciation and resentment.

Now there is no call for combat. Throughout the civilised world the lore of childbirth in the realm of nature stands unadorned and isolated in majesty beyond the comprehension of man. Today there is no need for further evidence or idle controversy to prove or doubt the overwhelming benefits it brings to man, woman, and child. In spite of hazards, and the absence of all aids from the modern brilliance of protective science, the apparatus and mechanism of human reproduction has enabled the numerical increase of man to be so rapid that the greatest natural menace to his survival is his immutable ability to breed.

The ascendancy of man throughout the ages of stern competitive evolution of mammalian life must speak well for the creative genius that planned and plotted his survival. If with culture and our way of life factors have arisen which we call faults, should we not search the era of precultural rusticity to find the antidote to such disease?

'To what has the welcome of this book been due?' I am often asked. There are many replies, but perhaps that which covers the widest ground was given before it was completed. Just on twenty years ago my wife Jessica found it, unfinished, discarded in the corner of my library. There were bombs and many deaths in those days; it may have been despondency or frustrating incredulity that men, so gloriously born, could be such fools that made me lose all faith in purpose. She placed the manuscript before me on my table and asked me rather pointed questions about myself and finished, 'Don't you realise? That is what women have been wanting for centuries.' So reluctantly, with her help, the book was finished. That may be why it has been so welcome to women and why, in so short a time, it has spread across the world. But that is not enough. Had those who put it to the test found failure, it would have died rapidly and justly, but the hope and comfort it has brought continues to increase the demand. Women themselves have been responsible for the teaching being made available to women – but now the normal cycle of acceptance is almost completed. It not only occurs in the medical profession but in all professions and many trades. I have recently heard the seven stages in the life of successful innovation (and the innovator) from a minister who was a close friend of Sir Halliday Croom, Professor of Midwifery in the University of Edinburgh. In short they are: 1. Amusement, 2. Opposition, 3. Hostility, 4. Vituperation, 5. Grudging acceptance, 6. Acquiescence, 7. Denigration. 'It is nothing new, we've been teaching it for years.'

I believe that a greater and more indestructible influence has made this simple truth so practical and so desirable to women. Childbirth is a physiological activity which is closely associated with emotions. In the natural state the emotional experience of childbirth raises a women to such delight and thankfulness that her mind turns to spiritual and metaphysical associations to satisfy her expressions of gratitude and joy. Whatever religion or gods are followed it is seen and spoken of by those who believe and many who have never previously believed.

In the Christian religion this is less publicised and more reluctantly expressed, but childbirth is fundamentally a spiritual as well as a physical achievement and throughout this book it must be read and understood that the birth of a child is the ultimate perfection of human love. In the Christian ethic we teach that God is love in which the blessing of sexual necessity and pleasure is but an essential part. Obstetrics must be approached as a science demanding the most profound respect. It must maintain the poise and dignity of those whose estimate of values finds a place for all types and variations of women. It demands cheerfulness without frivolity and sacrifice without reward, for of itself no guerdon could be greater than the gratitude of those whom we are privileged to serve.

I am persuaded from long years of experience amongst women of many nationalities that good midwifery is essential for the true happiness of motherhood – that good midwifery is the birth of a baby in a manner nearest to the natural law and design – and good midwifery, next to wise and healthy pregnancy, sets the pattern of the newborn infant and its relationship to its mother.

For this sequence a sound and stable philosophy is a basic necessity. Materialism and atheism are not included in the make-up of motherhood. Neither can a robot lead a blind man across the road.

G. D-R – June 1959

Introduction

Grantly Dick-Read

Reproduction of the species is one of the primary factors in nature; it is essential to the survival of all higher forms of life. The mention of the word 'motherhood' creates an atmosphere of reverence. Men, consciously and subconsciously, react with all the male instincts of preservation and protection when in its presence. A woman with child, or with her child, is beyond the law of conflict. Injury to mothers and their young is the basest form of cruelty. Tenderness is an emotion primarily designed by nature to protect the defenceless; it is an emotion only experienced by many men when in the presence of women.

Woman herself, however, is involved in a more complicated series of reactions. She knows that physically, physiologically and psychologically she is adapted primarily for the perfection of womanhood, which is, according to the law of nature, reproduction. All that is most beautiful in her life is associated with the emotions leading up to this ultimate function. Are there any joys in the life of the average woman comparable to the ever-increasing intensity of pleasurable feelings that are experienced during the successive phases of mating? We speak of it as being 'in love'; 'betrothal'; marriage; early married life; and finally, motherhood. The average woman associates all that is beautiful in her life with this series of events.

But, unfortunately, in the final perfection of these joys a large majority remember only the pain and anguish and even terror that they were called upon to endure at the birth of their first child. That is indeed a paradox. We have to ask ourselves the questions: does nature inveigle woman along the course of its essential purpose by bringing her first into contact with the irresistible demands of all that is beautiful? Is she led on and on from one joy to another by some force which intends to make her pay eventually the price of pain before she can achieve her objective? If this is in keeping with the law of nature, what can be its purpose? For generations, childbirth has been accepted as a dangerous and painful experience. Is woman expected to arrive at her perfection by the exhibition of beauty on the one hand and suffering on the other?

It is not suggested for one moment that by waving a magic wand over the heads of the community all children will suddenly be born according to the perfect law; but I hope that these pages will contain sufficient evidence to show that this is no dream, and that today there are methods of escorting women through pregnancy and parturition which will give these results.

From time to time pestilence and war sweep through nations, robbing them of much that is best in their stock. If we are to survive as a people, and as an empire, we must constantly be alert to improve our stock. The structure of society can only be erected upon the foundations of biological facts. The law of survival must remain the cornerstone of the temple of culture, however immense its scale or elaborate its external decoration. That law embodies only two principles: reproduction and maintenance.

The intricacies of maintenance of the species and in particular the freedom-loving peoples of the human race are revolutionising the thought and action of the world. Motherhood demands to be raised to its rightful position of pre-eminence in the affairs of state.

This book is presented, therefore, as an elementary step in the crusade to destroy some of the crudely medieval practices and beliefs that tarnish this glorious calling. Had the quiet strength and indomitable purpose of the natural forces of reproduction been heard in the councils of statesmen the world over, war amongst nations would have been stifled by stern emotional reactions which direct the human mind to fundamental truth and a greater understanding of the omnipotent but unseen forces of the universe.

1

The Science of Obstetrics

Before we embark upon this rather hazardous voyage – the description of a new approach to obstetrics – it may be well to outline briefly certain facts relating to childbirth during the later stages of civilisation.

There is a tendency in these days, when publication in the Press familiarises the man in the street with the most dramatic exploits in the laboratory, to accept each new discovery as 'the last word'. So wonderful do the revelations of science appear that the idea of introducing simplicity as a means of unearthing the even greater revelations of nature is not well received. But let us consider the position today compared with a hundred years ago, and with a thousand years ago. It will then become obvious that there is no reason to suppose that we have done any more in our time than add to our knowledge of childbirth. There is certainly no cause to consider that knowledge perfect.

Humanity has existed for a vast number of years. It is believed that the Neanderthal race lasted for more than two hundred thousand years. There is further evidence that men have lived and died in Europe for over a hundred thousand years. If we accept the Darwinian theory of evolution, the change from man-like apes to man himself is difficult to assign to any given period; but the essential fact remains that the function of reproduction of these species has not altered so far as the fundamental anatomical and physiological machinery is concerned. We still read that the pain of childbearing always has been the heritage of women because nothing in our modern teaching has enabled us to prevent it. It is believed because it has existed. Science of today can relieve women of their suffering, but only in recent years have the causes of pain in childbirth been explained. This has made it possible to prevent and avoid the unbearable discomfort of parturition. It is not without interest that the more civilised the people, the more the pain of labour appears to become intensified.

Since merciful relief of suffering is one of the greatest duties that physicians can perform, it has been easier to utilise the pain-relieving discoveries of science than to investigate its complicated causes. There can be no more horrible stigma upon civilisation than the history of childbirth. This is not a reference only to the unavoidable pains which accompany pathological states in reproduction, but to the most normal and natural parturition. The higher the civilisation of a country the more generally is pain accepted as a symptom of childbirth.

Efforts, of course, have been made to relieve this pain for many centuries. Old writings suggest that herbs and potions were used to relieve women in labour. Witchcraft was resorted to often very successfully. Three thousand years before Christ, the priests among the Egyptians were called to women in labour. In fact it may be said with some accuracy that amongst the most primitive people of which any record exists, help, according to the customs of the time, was given to women in labour. In the Book of Genesis, third chapter, sixteenth verse, 'The Lord God said to Eve – "I will greatly multiply thy sorrow and thy conception; in sorrow thou shalt bring forth children."' This translation of the holy book to the effect that a woman, because of her sin, was condemned to a multitude of sorrows and pains, particularly in the conception, bearing and bringing up of her children, has had a very considerable influence among Christian communities.

Even as late as the middle of the nineteenth century this was quoted by clerical and medical authorities as justification for opposition to any active relief of the sufferings of women in labour. In the fifth century before Christ, the great Hippocrates endeavoured to organise and instruct midwives. Their attentions bore little resemblance to those which are expected of midwives today, but according to their ideas of assistance so they practised.

In the second century after Christ, Soranus of Ephesus practised midwifery; it is recorded that he not only denied the power of spirits and superstitions, but that he actually considered the feelings of the woman herself (Howard Haggard, *Devils, Drugs and Doctors*, Heinemann, 1929).

In the Middle Ages, however, women appear to have been deserted once more. In many countries it was a crime for men to attend women in labour until the sixteenth century. Less than three hundred years ago, physicians commenced the practice of midwifery in Europe. It was not until the nineteenth century that the foundations of our present knowledge were laid. We must, therefore, realise how young and how immature is the science of obstetrics. Until the middle of the nineteenth century there was no anaesthesia; it had not been discovered. Until 1866 there was no knowledge of asepsis. It is difficult for people to visualise the state of affairs when limbs were amputated, abdomens opened, and caesarean sections performed without any anaesthesia and with an almost sure supervention of sepsis which gave rise to a high percentage of mortality in the simplest of operations.

In 1847, Simpson first used anaesthesia. On April 7th, 1853, John Snow anaesthetised Queen Victoria when Prince Leopold was born. For the use of anaesthetics for this purpose, Simpson was harshly criticised by the church. To prevent pain during childbirth, he was told, was contrary to religion and the express command of the scriptures; he had no right 'to rob God of the deep, earnest cries' of women in childbirth! But anaesthesia had come to stay. A year later, in 1854, Florence Nightingale was the first woman to make widely known that cleanliness and fresh air were fundamental necessities of nursing. It was largely because of her work during the Crimean War that the standard of both the training and the practice of nursing was raised. The gin-drinking reprobates who were found in great numbers both in hospitals and among midwives began to disappear. With their exodus, childbed fever less frequently occurred in midwives' cases. In the Maternity Hospital in Vienna, medical students' cases showed an average over a period of six years of ninety-nine deaths per thousand from puerperal fever. Semmelweis, who was physician at the hospital at the time (1858), believed the cause to be due to something arising within the hospital, and made his students wash their hands in a solution of chloride of lime. In one year the death rate in his wards tumbled from 18 per cent to 3 per cent, and soon after to 1 per cent. This success necessitated his facing opposition and hostility from those around him. But his work was done; he had laid a great foundation stone of safer childbirth. Although he did not fully understand the significance of the infection he realised that it was the physicians themselves who caused the deaths of their patients by transmitting it.

Probably all of us pause to think sometimes of how much harm we do in our efforts to do good; how much trouble we cause when conscientiously endeavouring to prevent it.

In 1866, Lister brought us the knowledge of antiseptics, which he continued to employ in spite of the opposition and ridicule of his colleagues.

So, gradually, truth has been discovered; the safety of women has been the object of investigation with results that would have been unbelievable when the mothers and grandmothers of many of us were born. But how short a time we have had – less than a hundred years, and man has been reproducing his kind for several thousands of years.

Now that many of the troubles and dangers have been overcome we must move on, not only to save more lives, but actually bring happiness to replace the agony of fear. We must bring a fuller life to women who are called upon to reproduce our species. The joy of new life must be the vision of motherhood, instead of the fear of death that has clouded it since civilisation developed.

It will be easier, therefore, in reading the succeeding chapters, to realise that they represent an effort to improve, an effort to construct new ways and means, not simply to destroy those which have done good service in the course of progress. Therefore, where there is obvious truth in this teaching, let it be augmented; and if any obvious fallacy is unmasked, assist in its burial.

When I wrote these words in 1940, my wildest and most ambitious hopes would not have allowed me to visualise what has actually happened in twelve years. No fallacies have been unmasked and no burial of a single tenet has taken place. This theory has not been found wanting and no criticism has been justified by experience. Vast numbers of women have found comfort and safety in this approach to childbirth. The sordid melancholy of prospective motherhood has been replaced by fearless and impatient longing for the moment of life's most satisfying achievement. No longer do the trembling hands of women stretch out to seek deliverance from the sorrows of death that compassed them. The science of obstetrics is on a new and higher plane. Motherhood offers all women who have the will and the courage to accept the holiest and happiest estate that can be attained by human beings. That we, as obstetricians, can help and guide them, is our greatest privilege, for with each succeeding generation we may establish the foundations of a new race of men with a clear vision of the future, that holds a practical philosophy and a purpose worthy of fulfilment.

2

Motherhood from Many Points of View

Let us digress for one moment from the science of pure obstetrics and consider the woman herself. Biologically motherhood is her desire and her ordained accomplishment but this apparently physical function goes far deeper and has greater importance than the purely mechanistic production of a child. A mother is a member of society with an intrinsic worth and she occupies a certain status in both the home and the community. If there is one characteristic more desirable to be maintained in communal life, it is the dignity of motherhood. Those of us who have known it from personal experience in our own homes, or from professional associations, visualise it in those calm, competent, and companionable women who live to a great age, acutely sensitive to, but unshakeable by either the cruelties or the rewards of having lived. Motherhood unfortunately does not receive the consideration that it deserves and is justified in expecting. It may be in the modern world that such thoughts are altruistic, but in the outpatient departments of hospitals and in clinics, mothers of families and young girls who are pregnant for the first time, are too often subjected to a surprisingly rigid discipline and impersonal regimentation. How sore or how submissive many of these responsive women become. They do not desire preference among their sisters who are not pregnant but they hope and many yearn for the companionship and comfort of a word of encouragement and confidence from those who in authority examine and dispose of them.

There is war between man and woman for the possession of motherhood. It is a prize of incalculable value for the church, politicians and the doctors.

The leaders of all manner of religious organisations, sects, and denominations recognise the holiness of motherhood and the basic value of the newborn child. We do not forget the significance of Christmas or the manger in the stable of the wayside inn.

Religious teaching calls for obedience to its codes, homage to the Creator, and loyalty to its spiritual and material purposes in the mother-child relationship. One factor knits in a common bond all the people of the world and that is motherhood. Apart from religion 90 per cent of all civilised countries profess to some form of religious persuasion. I am not persuaded that the communist ideology can destroy in so short a time the inborn devotion of a vast people to generations of motherliness and love of babies.

Five hundred million Roman Catholics revere the Madonna and Child and all that its divinity and dignity infers and implies to congregations and individuals alike. The millions of the followers of free churches in the USA all turn to the spiritual associations of childbirth and motherhood. In England, Germany, and western European Protestant communities the helpless, demanding individuality of a baby is accepted as natural social acquisition.

Politicians have long recognised the power of women in the home, particularly in this country since they obtained the vote. In their constituencies the children and especially the babies are centres of attraction at election times. The infants of wavering constituents are photographed in public being kissed by the prospective candidate. The big cry goes up 'Women and children first' in hopes that the boat will not sink after all. Childbirth and its agonies swept a bill through the British Parliament and carried the House, pregnant with (political) ambition to a painless delivery from party embarrassment. Men declared it to be an effective vote catcher that no woman should be conscious of the appalling experience of childbirth. The cry was 'anaesthesia for all' – women, however, knew better and so did experienced midwives who deliver more than 75 per cent of women in the British Isles and soon the reports from the provinces supplied the answer. Women preferred to do without it and so did the best of midwives.

Similar uses of childbirth have been observed in other countries. It has become a focus of political propaganda which gains easy and sympathetic entrance to the homes of the people. But with what result? Vast sums of money are expended on constructions and productions for economic prestige and sometimes profit. An increasing amount is voted by a political party for general education and repairs of the nation's stock which has not yet acquired the stamina to weather the storms of modern strains and stresses of living. But in this country a small and entirely inadequate amount of money represents the practical appreciation of the improvement of the stock of the nation. The equipment for childbirth is a disgrace to our ancient institution. When I was conducted proudly around the new Hospital Centre in Washington, DC, I did not envy but felt ashamed. Eight hundred beds cost 24 million dollars. Could not our Treasury be persuaded of the potential value of a turnout of 650,000 new lives into this small country each year? Given better equipment and teaching organisations of mothers, nurses and doctors, its quality could be improved and made competent to lead a new world to its yet undreamt-of possibilities. The standard of mind and body can be raised even before birth with our present-day knowledge. Where do politicians and industrialists look for the success of their major undertakings, in the production plants or in the repair depots? Where human beings are concerned repair depots of broken-down stock command enormous sentimental and financial support, but the production plants, which are the mothers of our nation, receive a small share only of the national purse, which must be interpreted as unpardonable ignorance and lack of foresight by those who invest for the future standard of progress of our own peoples.

The prestige of a satellite in orbit about the earth is infinitely greater than the prestige of a revolutionary approach to the breeding of better human stock, or the founding of homes and family units of happy and contented people. The uninhibited development of simple philosophy and sound physique which enables men and women to adjust themselves to an ever-changing world is allowed to occur where it may, if it will. Rockets and satellites, spaceships and hydrogen bombs absorb thousands of millions of the wealth of nations. The development of the human race to a higher standard of mental and physical efficiency is granted a niggardly and disgraceful pittance. We do not demand greater numbers – the objective must be the quality of the child. As the quality of the mother so the nature of the offspring will vary; the mother herself has been moulded by the manner of her birth and the environment in which she was influenced by her parents as a small child. The bondage or the freedom of her puberty claims the urges of her teenage years, which guide her to accept the father of her own children and so the cycle starts again in the birth of a baby. But no provision is made for this branch of education. The teenager is not taught the elementary rules of womanhood. Examinations of schools, colleges, and universities do not include in their curriculum the supremely important subject of motherhood.

Political influence cannot afford to take a long-term view. The survival of a party or a ruling combination is urgent and it must seize the vote power of today upon the promise of the immediate present. It must offer tangible rewards for loyalty to a hope and wield the power of words to support the fantasy of its invulnerability. But the potential

might of man's mind takes time to liberate, its rewards are not immediate, mutations are results of causes not the causes of results. So
politically childbirth appeals to those who seek party interests. They
seem to be blind to the obvious that childbirth is the entry into this
society of new life, yet this incomparable responsibility is not accepted
by the politicians, but handed over with grossly inadequate financial
support to a branch of an uncertain and immature science to lay the
foundation of our future.

Now let us see how the doctors who accept this responsibility for
the standard of our stock undertake the task.

Doctors are divided into many groups and subgroups, the largest
and most important of which has least influence upon the ethical
trend of its organisation. These may be termed Hippocratic doctors;
there are far more of them than is generally known. They work silently amongst the people, in their homes and in their hearts. They
are called *General Practitioners* and specialise in humanity, its troubles
and its weariness, its joys and successes, its well-being and its illnesses.
But when the strains and stresses of survival bring rare and unusual
disease, the *academic specialist* in that field takes charge and employs
his greater knowledge and experience of the single system or function upon which he concentrates his attentions. He does not treat the
person but the person's illness or disease. There is a trend in modern
medical science towards academic specialisation. It has advantages
– for here lies fame and fortune and sometimes these urges militate
against the Hippocratic standards of service and sacrifice; more often, however, the technical skill can restore to health and efficiency
the individual and enable her to resume life at its allotted level. And
there are the '*backroom boys*' of the medical profession, working in
laboratories or offices. They do not see the human being as such, but as
a specimen provider for the examination that may unravel the mystery
of health or disease. Finally, there are the *organisers* – those who have
attained seats in high places. Here we may find the truly great men
and women of the medical world, but in the era of pasteurisation and
emulsification it is not easy to discover the cream when suspended in
a medium that of itself would be very thin skimmed milk.

So motherhood, maternity and infant welfare it is called, is subjected
to a number of influences by different bodies within the medical profession. Unfortunately there is much dissension between the different
parties. Some want to look after their patients when they have babies
and some do not. Some think they are not safe and others don't think
much. Ideals and beliefs are subjected to committees formed for and by

those who have specific purposes apart from both beliefs and ideals. So motherhood becomes the shuttlecock and is beaten willy-nilly by strong persuasion into a permissive state. It sacrifices itself without the ability to resist the indoctrination of man – where I speak of man in this sense I include women doctors, a few of whom, unfortunately, have accepted the normal male attitude towards this supremely feminine function. It is difficult for those who believe in the maternal mind to understand how men dare to dictate to a woman a mechanistic routine for her maximum achievement in childbirth. The body is only a vehicle in which and from which a child is miraculously made and produced. It is the mind of woman that knows passion and desires the fulfilment of her biological purpose. It is the mind and its receptivity, its ability to integrate the fund of new thoughts and feeling that are physiological visitations of love and pregnancy, that moulds and fashions the child. It is the mind that, through understanding, resists the assaults of ignorance and fear and so reduces the strains of parturition to a bearable sensibility which avoids the harmful interference of man's routine and allows the consciousness of her achievement. It is the mind that bears the spiritual imprint of the newborn child and round it writes indelibly the mysterious circumscription of mother love.

We may well ask what factor is it in the human mind that assumes control and care of motherhood, yet exercises that responsibility with faint consideration for this major force that shapes the future of the home, the family, and the standard of our stock. It is not taught to students that mother love is a power that must be the centre of our work as obstetricians. Only those who have, through no fault of their own, been deprived of its security and protection whilst learning the necessities for survival, can wish to allocate the neonate to fosterage of the teat and bottle, the 'hired heart', or the expedient crèche. To me it is incredible that there is a tendency amongst modern civilised and even cultured women to discard, for one of many reasons exhibited as justification, the opportunity, given only to them, of implanting in the mind and body of their newborn infants the seeds of the fullest and richest possessions of life.

Does modern education of women include this elementary glorification of their inborn potentiality? No, but it appears to hide the science of living behind feigned expediency and leaves young women to the holocaust of maladjusted matrimony. Most incredible of all to mere man is the ready acceptance by women of the indoctrinations and demands of those whose guidance and care is sought in childbirth. Has the fear of childbirth robbed woman of the protective perspicacity of pregnancy and the astuteness of her mind at that time, so well known to all who practise midwifery? And yet, for some unaccountable reason she listens to the whisper of *the easy way*, and this is readily interpreted as a godsend to humanity, and the boon of modern science. She welcomes the soothing lullaby that calls her to the shadow of safety in obstetric desensitisation. She is comforted by the sirens whose song persuades her to turn aside from the course of nature which leads 95 per cent of women, at least, to motherhood without accident or injury to themselves or their babies. (This allegory must not be carried too far by those who know the Homeric myths.)

Fortunately there are courageous and wise women who have recognised the incongruity and the dangers of this intrusion upon their domains. They demand a fuller knowledge of the truth of their natural functions, not in the detail of scientific language but in elementary and understandable words that can be used effectively for accurate presentation of the subject. Thousands of women are learning every year, and in most countries every sizeable town has organised classes or schools for the education and preparation of women for childbirth.

It is almost incredible how rapidly women have seized the reins which guide their destiny as mothers of tomorrow's generation. In four months I was entertained by seventy different groups in the large cities and towns of America – Buffalo to New York, Washington to Jackson, Mississippi to New Orleans and to Denver, Colorado. From Santa Fe to the Western seaboard – San Francisco to Seattle, then Chicago and on to Milwaukee, Cleveland, and Cedar Rapids. Finally to Toronto, Ottawa, and Montreal in Canada.

Everywhere some organisation flourished for the childbirth education of women or natural childbirth education. The interest extended to the great universities – preparation for childbirth has come to stay and although it had not been accepted by some large hospitals, the demand of women for knowledge and understanding was not to be denied. The same conditions were found in Germany, Italy, France, and the Scandinavias, Spain and Portugal, and the great countries of South America. The immutable law of nature was sought and women prompted the search to success.

All praise and credit for those who are worthy in their efforts and ideals, but any doctor or nurse, midwife or health visitor who approaches the young woman pregnant or about to be, without tending first and caring for her mental processes, her emotions, and her hopes, qualifies for condemnation and severe criticism.

I cannot write too strongly of the cruelty that still exists in some hospitals and maternity organisations when the quality of kindliness is buried beneath the stern regimentation and routine of institutional efficiency. It sometimes seems that maternity hospitals are organised for the convenience of doctors and nurses to which the patients are subjected irrespective of their comforts and desires. There can be no excuse for this, from any point of view. If it occurred rarely, it might be forgiven as an exception 'that proves the rule', but close investigation strongly suggests that the mind of woman is not cared for or the sensitive feelings of women in labour given due respect and attention in many hospitals and maternity institutions throughout this country – and not this country only!

We realise that some senior gynaecologists who teach abnormal midwifery disagree with the antenatal instruction of women. 'It is better for us if they don't know anything about childbirth, and anyhow it is our job, not theirs,' I heard a senior congressional representative remark at an International Congress last year. That is the war I have referred to, of man against woman. There is a demand that women should be kept in ignorance of the truth of childbirth and that they should be unquestioningly submissive to the recommendations and demands of the orthodox obstetric profession. They do not know that this submission may expose them to routine interference and physical injury without any clinical indication that can justify such assaults upon their bodies.

I was proudly told by a gynaecologist before a gathering of colleagues that 75 per cent of his women were delivered with instruments. The labours of 85–95 per cent of his patients were surgically or medically induced to have their babies at a time convenient to all concerned. Also, he said that no woman was allowed to be either sensitive to the sensations of labour or conscious when her baby was born. 'No human being,' he exclaimed vehemently, 'should be allowed to suffer this appalling agony.' All women having their first babies were operated upon by having the outlet of the birth canal cut open to make it wider and he did not advise women to breast-feed their babies. It was an unnecessary call upon their time and it made them tired; social and domestic routine was disturbed and formula feeding gave better results.

He refused to listen to argument or discussion. 'I have used my methods for 25 years,' he said and 'I see no reason to alter my ideas.'

I asked him if he was interested in cerebral palsy. He was not – it was the pediatricians' business. Had he read the results of the recent wide-scale investigation and the report that medical authorities believe that over 70 per cent of these disabled children had been crippled by interference at birth? He replied that there was undoubtedly a lot of bad obstetrics, but what could be done about it? I pointed out that there were thirty thousand new cases every year in his country, the total was 1.25 million – did he not think that the natural or physiological method might be worth a trial in this fight against the tragedy of maimed babies?

He replied that with all respect he must tell me that there was no such thing as natural childbirth. It had ceased to be a physiological function; culture had seen to that and civilisation must be blamed for the diseases it brings with it.

Did he know that 10 per cent of all the children of low-grade mental development were in their sad plight because of meddlesome mid-wifery? He found the evidence difficult to accept and preferred to leave the cerebral trauma children, epileptics, and results of birth oxygen starvation to the experts. He was an obstetrician.

Had not the obstetrician a great responsibility to the nation as well as to the parents and homes? 'Yes, certainly, most important,' he said. And so the conversation finished.

But this is not, however, a true representation of modern obstetrics. There may still be many who practise midwifery in this way but there are others; those who seek to follow as closely as possible the natural law in childbirth. They practise on the basis of the *Fear-Tension-Pain Syndrome* and from the first visit of a pregnant woman every effort is made to allay her fears and give her confidence and courage by simple and truthful reiteration of the story of motherhood.

Pregnancy and its physical and mental changes, the baby and its nourishment and growth, the preparation of mind and body to the natural experience of childbirth are all a sensible part of her education. In some towns in England, hospital staffs organise classes for the education of women who have booked to be delivered in their care. Women seek this teaching and understanding because they have seen amongst their friends the happy and healthy results it brings, not only to the mothers, but also to husbands, families, and homes.

Never before in the history of man has he faced so great a power of militant women, exercised in a claim so justifiable and a demand so overwhelming. They are militant today in pursuit of their health and happiness in natural childbirth and the inborn beauty of the babies, who start life uninjured by interference, which could well have been avoided.

3

A Philosophy of Childbirth

I have often wondered if a woman in Whitechapel whose name I have long since forgotten has ever realised the far-reaching influence of a casual remark she made to me. For some reason or other the whole picture made an indelible impression upon my mind, although at the time I had no idea that it was the seed that would eventually alter the course of my life.

I had ploughed through mud and rain on my bicycle between two and three in the morning down Whitechapel Road, turned right and left, and innumerable rights and lefts before I came to a low hovel by the railway arches. Having groped and stumbled my way up a dark staircase, I opened the door of a room about ten feet square. There was a pool of water lying on the floor, the window was broken, rain was pouring in, the bed had no proper covering and was kept up at one end by a sugar box. My patient lay covered only with sacks and an old black skirt. The room was lit by one candle stuck in the top of a beer bottle on the mantelshelf. A neighbour had brought in a jug of water and a basin; I had to provide my own soap and towel. In spite of this setting – which even thirty years ago was a disgrace to any civilised country – I soon became conscious of a quiet kindliness in the atmosphere.

In due course, the baby was born. There was no fuss or noise. Everything seemed to have been carried out according to an ordered plan. There was only one slight dissension: I tried to persuade my patient to let me put the mask over her face and give her some chloroform when the head appeared and the dilatation of the passages was obvious. She, however, resented the suggestion and firmly but kindly refused to take this help. It was the first time in my short experience that I had ever been refused when offering chloroform. As I was about to leave some time later I asked her why it was that she would not use the mask. She did not answer at once, but looked from the old woman who had been assisting to the window through which was bursting the first light of dawn; and then shyly she turned to me and said: 'It didn't hurt. It wasn't meant to, was it, doctor?'

For weeks and months afterwards, as I sat with women in labour, women who appeared to be in the terror and agony of childbirth, that sentence came drumming back into my ears: 'It wasn't meant to, was it, doctor?' until finally, even through my orthodox and conservative mind, I began to see light. I began to realise that there was no law in nature and no design that could justify the pain of childbirth. Not many years afterwards the war took me to foreign lands. There I witnessed women having their babies in the most natural and apparently painless manner, but I also saw those who suffered pain and to whom the birth of their child was an experience horrible to remember. When eventually the war ceased and I was back at the London Hospital as resident accoucheur, the same problem occurred again. Most women seemed to suffer so much, but here and there I met the calm woman who neither wished for anaesthetic nor appeared to have any unbearable discomfort.

It was very difficult to explain why one should suffer and another be apparently free from pain. There did not seem to be much difference in the actual labours; they both had to work equally hard; the time factor was not markedly different one from the other. Perhaps those who suffered had slightly longer labours on an average than those who had less discomfort. In those days we did not know the mechanism of pain as we do today and a good deal was overlooked which certainly would not have passed unnoticed in the light of our present teaching. It slowly dawned on me, however, that it was the peacefulness of a relatively painless labour that distinguished it most clearly from the others. There was calm, it seemed almost faith, in the normal and natural outcome of childbirth.

So gradually my mind was influenced by these observations to investigate the part played by the emotions in the natural function of reproduction. Was the nature of labour responsible for the emotional state of the woman, or was the emotional state of the woman to a large extent responsible for the nature of the labour? Which was primary and which was secondary? Happily my own environment and the associations of my home had given me the privilege of knowing motherhood at its best. I had seen that unshakable faith in the power of love which met the tribulations and tragedies of life with a calm and courageous strength. As a young man motherhood was to me a holy estate, the mysteries of which were only shared by those who had endured. Perhaps nature designed a tenderness in man in order that he might protect the defenceless bearer of the young. The great painters of the past have searched for the reality of beauty, and have chosen to represent it in motherhood. Joshua Reynolds's pictures show the dignified pride of their accomplishment. Romney in his *Lady with a Child* has emphasised the peaceful delights of a mother as her small infant rests contented and fearless upon her lap. Memling and others of the Dutch school represented the satisfying possessiveness of motherhood, whereas Leonardo da Vinci laid stress upon its joys and happiness. But they all have one feature in common which is unmistakable: they depict an atmosphere of absolute peace. Perhaps in modern life this may represent a relatively unobtainable ideal, but even today, is there any happiness that can be compared with that of a woman with her small babies? Is there any love so unselfish and so inspiring as the love of a mother for her child? To healthy-minded women it is the realisation of their highest ambition, the fulfilment of their instinctive urge and the ultimate perfection of their bodily functions.

But we cannot think of motherhood only in terms of its satisfactory completion. We must look back into the life of a young woman and consider the thoughts and experiences which eventually lead her to become a mother. We need to delve into that experimental playground of psychologists which is popularly known as 'sex life.' We have only to recall the normal sequence of events that every healthy-minded girl and young woman of our time goes through. At an early age she learns all the happiness of love; it is an emotional development which radiates from a young girl. You will often find that in their untrained and undifferentiated affection life holds some joys too deep and too unfathomable for them to understand. This irresistible, nebulous urge to love is so mysterious that my daughter when fifteen years of age wrote to me from school: 'I wish you could explain to me why I feel as I do this term; it has never been like it before. I am so deliriously happy. There is no reason that I know of, but I am fond of everybody. I seem to see the good in them, and want to *think* lovely things, as if I were possessed of a heavenly spirit making me so much better than my real self.'

And so with every girl in varying degrees this power which will rule their lives begins to develop at an early age, until in due course they find themselves in love, and here the hotchpotch of their emotional life becomes concentrated, with all its thrills, its joys and its anxieties, upon one semi-divine individual. It is the spiritual refinement of her own ideal and in the normal course of events she becomes betrothed, but unwilling to believe that there are others who are equally fortunate, and blissfully ignorant of the fact that she is but an instrument in the design of nature. Eventually she marries and if all goes well, she conceives and prepares to bear her child.

The average woman associates all that is beautiful in her life with this series of events. It is the implementation of the power of life by the universal forces which govern all things to the end that the human race shall survive. From earliest girlhood, each forward step in this progression is made because of the desire for greater joy or fuller realisation of her dreams. The law of life does not drive a woman on by either fear or physical necessity, but attracts her to develop by the presentation of increasingly beautiful experiences, which she is not slow to grasp. Love may be beset by anxieties and doubts, but of itself it stimulates all the noblest and greatest qualities of which human nature is characterised at its best. It is the greatest power in the world and without it the races of mankind would finish in but a few generations.

We must ask ourselves: is it not possible that a force so fundamental may not be the motive power of life itself? When considering a metaphysical subject we must be neither bigoted nor impervious to the reasonings of others, for there are opinions sustained by evidences and arguments put forward by eminent people. Many mathematicians and physicists have discarded assumptions of both universal omnipotence and a divine omniscience; we cannot disregard their profound scientific knowledge and we learn nothing by denying ourselves the right of logical argument. I have been privileged to enjoy much discussion with my friends who are confirmed materialists. We are aware of the elementary principles of thermodynamics and the possibilities of phenomenal reactions in electromagnetic fields. We listen with admiration to deductions or presumptions based upon Carnot's exposition of the second law of thermodynamics.

In other spheres we join in the controversy that rages upon the subject of human intelligence and its relations to actions and thoughts. It is not necessary to differ or agree.

Myself when young did eagerly frequent
Doctor and Saint, and heard great Argument
About it and about: but evermore
Came out by the same Door as in I went.

My own personal and professional experience is sufficient to enable me to draw conclusions and to support them with apparently sound evidence. The value of a theory lies ultimately in the results obtained by its practical implementation.

It is my persuasion that the vast majority of women of the human race today have some form of religion and believe, although maybe in a very nebulous manner, that there is an omnipotent power ruling our lives, possibly designing purpose for each individual, and for that power the name 'God' is widely accepted.

It may be that in time scientists will be able to give such complete proof of the rightness of materialism that religion will become a weapon in the hands of the psychiatrists, and the church will be replaced by the clinic; but my close association with the birth of a child has led me to believe that there is a limitation to science and that the extending boundaries of human knowledge have only reached the foothills of the towering mountains of omniscience. This philosophy of childbirth is written, therefore, in terms of a belief in God, but at the same time I respect the arguments against this assumption, for in due course, they will either destroy or magnify our acceptance of divine power. Must we, however, paraphrase the simple dictum 'God is Love', or may we deduce with Euclidian accuracy the converse that 'Love is God'? At first sight this may appear to be a philosophical consideration not relevant to the argument, but if in a normal and healthy girlhood and womanhood before and after childbirth we find these outstanding qualities of beauty and greatness, what justification, what reason, or what presumption of truth can there be in the acceptance of an agonising ordeal as a normal accompaniment of fulfilment of the essential purpose of human love?

What manner of thing is this love that leads its most natural and perfect children to the green pastures of all that is beautiful in life, and urges them on by a series of ever-increasing delights until their ultimate goal is in sight, then suddenly and without mercy chastises and terrifies them before hurling them unconscious, injured and resentful in the new world of motherhood? I strongly suggest that there is only one answer – this is not the course of the power of love. This is not the purposeful design of creation. Somewhere, for some reason, an interloper has crept in, and must be eradicated. Something stands in the way which, through blindness and ignorance in the development of our civilisation, has been allowed to grow and impede the natural course of events.

Over thirty years ago I was persuaded of the truth that this aspect of childbirth held. The Whitechapel question still came back to me: 'It wasn't meant to, was it, doctor?' Then I knew, after years of apparently fruitless effort, that I had found a dogmatic answer, and that answer was: 'No, it was not meant to hurt.'

Unfortunately my colleagues had a very straightforward rejoinder to my 'noble' assumption, as they called it. 'Why, then, does it hurt?' This book is a record of the adventures and discoveries that I have made during the last thirty-five years in the uncharted waters of natural childbirth. Not only does it essay to explain the cause of pain in civilised labour, but also to demonstrate that those evil causes may to some extent be removed. It is obvious that my somewhat revolutionary teaching is not intended to be a panacea for all ills. The successful application of this theory is only possible in normal and uncomplicated parturition, but as that comprises probably over 96 per cent of all labours, unless made abnormal by attendant circumstances, its influence may be very considerable.

In outline, the theory of natural childbirth is as follows.

Superstition, civilisation and culture have brought influences to bear upon the minds of women which have introduced justifiable fears and anxieties concerning labour. The more cultured the races of the earth have become, so much the more positive have they been in pronouncing childbirth to be a painful and dangerous ordeal.

Thus fear and anticipation have given rise to natural protective tensions in the body, and such tensions are not of the mind only, for the mechanism of protective action by the body includes muscle tension. Unfortunately the natural tension produced by fear influences those muscles which close the womb and oppose the dilatation of the birth canal during labour. Therefore, fear inhibits; that is to say, gives rise to resistance at the outlet of the womb, when in the normal state those muscles should be relaxed and free from tension. This resistance gives rise to pain, because the uterus is supplied with sensitive nerve endings which record pain arising from excessive tension. Therefore, Fear, Tension and Pain are three evils opposed to the natural design, which have been introduced in the course of civilisation by the ignorance of those who have been concerned with preparations for and attendance at childbirth. If fear, tension and pain go hand in hand, then it must be necessary to relieve tension and to overcome fear in order to eliminate pain. The implementation of my theory demonstrates the methods by which fear may be overcome, tension may be eliminated and replaced by physical and mental relaxation.

When, in 1942, this book was first published, letters from mothers describing their labours were recorded as evidence of the absence of unbearable discomfort in natural childbirth. This was done lest the observations of an enthusiastic obstetrician should be waived aside as the vapourings of an encomiast. Many thousands of similar letters now swell my files. In a few short years the validity of these tenets has been established throughout the civilised world. The method has done all and more for the comfort and safety of mothers and their babies than was originally claimed or indeed expected; the truth and simplicity of this approach to childbirth have been judged by the results of practical experience in its usage. It is not only the relative freedom from pain that prompts the panegyrics of the grateful. They become conscious of a sense of exaltation and incomparable happiness as they watch the arrival of their child. Many women have described their experiences of childbirth as being associated with a spiritual uplifting, the power of which they have never previously been aware. I have witnessed this so often, and been profoundly impressed by the inexplicable trans-figuration of women at the moment of their baby's birth, that I have been led, as usual, to ask: why this? It is not sentimentality; it is not relief from suffering; it is not simply satisfaction of accomplishment. It is bigger than all those things. Can it be that the Creator intended to draw mothers nearest to Himself at the moment of love's fulfilment?

The natural reward of the physical achievement of pregnancy and parturition is not only a beloved possession, but an endowment of spiritual force enhancing the receptivity of divine guidance in moth-erhood. From this inestimable gift emerges the power of mother love, which forms the pattern of the infant's psyche as surely as mother's milk fashions its physique.

To such a woman childbirth is a monument of joy within her mem-ory. She turns to it in thought to seek again an ecstasy which passed too soon. The fearless woman advances to the dais of the Almighty to receive the prize for her accomplishment. She does not cringe in an-ticipation of admonition, but is proud and grateful for her just reward.

The philosophy of childbirth is in the reality of its spiritual manifestations and the incomprehensible miracle of its mechanism – familiarity with its natural performance directs our minds to a closer understanding of human nature and conduct.

As we strive to solve these problems by observing behaviour, men-tal processes and environmental and social influences, we are led, as if by logical deduction, to meditate upon the meaning of its mysteries – the supreme happiness of motherhood, in spite of its cares and respon-sibilities, is not the simple consequence of success. It is eudaemonism in its purest sense, the highest good that spans the gulf between ethics and metaphysics. The mother with her baby crosses this bridge and wanders blissfully in realms unknown to mortal man; neither logic nor psychology can trace the motive or the means of her translation.

For my own part, I stand in awe and utter humility before a woman with her newborn babe. There is so much to see and learn in her pres-ence, so much that I am unable to understand or to explain, so much that makes me aware of the limitations of my own ability. It may be that amongst my colleagues there are those who feel the same. Childbirth is not a physical function. The drama of the physical manifestations has blinded its observers to the truth – the birth of a child is the ultimate phenomenon of a series of spiritual experiences, from fantasy to fact and from fact to fruition.

The powers of physical destruction are established. If the peoples of this world are to survive, there will be a gigantic philosophical revolution. Armageddon is of the mind; ordnance of spiritual forces in the great conflict will emerge from childbirth and mother love. The full significance and magnitude of this supreme human function must not be neglected or belittled by the subjective materialism of modern science.

What change has time brought? Have we any reason to qualify or retract the thoughts and experiences of over thirty years ago? Far from it, for with a clearer understanding of the natural processes and designs of childbirth a change of attitude towards the science of obstetrics is discernible in all the civilised countries of the world.

Today the birth of a child is an emotional experience which brings with it all the noblest and most loveable qualities of men, women, and children. It unearths the fund of tenderness, companionship, and sympathetic understanding that smooths our social structure and brings confidence to replace suspicion. There is no greater joy than that of a woman who sees her baby born, hears its greeting, and holds it in her hands whilst it is still linked to her body by the avenue through which its lifeblood surged from the selective source within her womb.

The miracle by which new life is given to us has gained our highest respect, and we have seen, in awe, women pass from the physical to the spiritual comprehension of the magnitude of human love.

At the beginning of this book I state categorically that childbirth is a demonstration of the incomparable genius of a creative force. The gentle touch of its irresistible power and the violence of its tenderness in mother love has to be experienced, examined, and repeatedly observed to enable us to assess the true value of this inexplicable phenomenon. What creative force is, may be a matter of opinion.

We are all here to play our part in the great scheme from which an ultimate purpose will evolve, from that level the science of obstetrics must devolve. I find no place in the natural sciences for materialism, however brilliant its exposition, and however ardently the atheists ply their persuasions. We are small fry in this world but our numbers increase by 125,000 babies a day. 'Mere organs of the evolutionary process operating through society,' as Sir Julian Huxley put it. Can any science bear greater responsibility for the future than obstetrics?

I believe that our advance towards the ultimate perfection is of a divine agency, fashioned by a creative spirit, which is not, as we are, the outcome of evolution, but an immutable omniscience of which our development is but a progressive manifestation. Our evolution must develop on the psycho-social level, if at all, and, therefore, the science of obstetrics, in the teaching of natural childbirth, by the use of the natural or physiological equipment, by which we have attained our present relative pre-eminence, is more likely to preserve a progressive evolution than presumptuous interference and mutilation of the products of the original and successful design. Therefore its dignity and supreme importance must be maintained and fostered by all who are privileged to be associated with it, either actively or passively.

The care of the physical components of reproduction has for long constituted the main theme of obstetrics, but no matter how carefully and apparently successful this may be, the raising of the standard of the human mind cannot be accomplished unless men and women are guided by the creative and directive spirit.

A simple philosophy and a rational belief in a supreme and omnipresent mind beyond the limitations of science, are basic necessities for those who seek the full glory of motherhood.

As a branch of medical and social science, obstetrics in this country is not worthy of our high tradition. It has become entangled with surgical gynaecology and sociology, hypnotism, and deep anaesthesia. In places far apart we find a few brave men who make available for their pregnant women the ancient childbirth precaution of preparation for labour and try their best to carry out the procedures advised by those with thirty or more years' experience.

But prejudice denies women their wishes to be calm and courageously composed. The consciousness of the purposeful physical sensations, and the emotional reactions to those sensations is denied the modern wife. She is deprived of the full reward of childbirth, which is the realisation of her achievement in the birth of her child. Too many never know the deep glory of a woman's pride as the hungry child ceases its demanding whimper and draws the ready nipple to itself and snuggles in the soft, satisfying security of its mother's breast. Is this sensuous, sentimental, or scientific? I hope it's all three intensely and uninhibited – for if there is one thing I have ever envied woman, it is that perfect peace and alienated happiness she demonstrates in her movement, breathing, and facial expression when her baby lies contented and semiconscious at her breast. Can our male science willingly disregard these female experiences because it can never share them?

4

Anatomy and Physiology

I was talking to a nurse who attended cases with me until she herself was seven months pregnant. About a fortnight before, her baby was born, and I had an opportunity of asking her in detail what she thought about childbirth. Nurses are not always the best patients because they have a way of reviewing the abnormalities they have seen, and visualising them whilst they themselves are in labour. We discussed at length everything that had happened during her pregnancy and parturition. She had followed closely my teaching with which she had become familiar in the maternity home and gave as her final judgment that she could not understand why women should make such a fuss about having a baby. At one point only – and then for a very few contractions – was she in discomfort, but other than that the whole thing, as she put it, was an exciting and marvellous experience. She also made a suggestion to me that I should explain the development of a baby within the uterus, because so many women are ignorant of these elementary facts that anxieties and doubts arise in their minds which are difficult to overcome and cause much unnecessary trepidation.

I propose, therefore, to give a short note upon the ovum, fertilisation and the development of the baby in the uterus. This will answer many questions that I am asked by expectant mothers. During the last ten or twelve years, women have become more enquiring about the reproductive function; they wish to understand and the information they seek is evidence of a sensible interest in the natural activities of the human body in relation to childbirth.

Very shortly after the ovum is fertilised it starts to develop cells which are differentiated to form the various organs and structures of the body. Some of these are allocated in the great design to become the forerunners or mother cells of spermatozoa and ova and quite early in fetal life the sex of the child is determined. The complicated, fascinating and, to me, awe-inspiring science of embryology cannot be included in this synopsis of development. The causes and urges that marshal millions of individual living cells to take their allotted place in the vast community of the human body is incomprehensible to an ordinary mind. A number of theories have been evolved to explain these mysteries and scientists have carried out many experiments in test tubes to emulate the performance and procedures of the law of nature; but let us, as simple people, be satisfied to accept these wonders as the work of a power or influence beyond the boundaries of human perspicacity. This does not, of course, preclude a search for greater knowledge and understanding which is the foundation of true science.

We will accept the phenomenon of the formation of cells concerned with the reproduction of the human species. They are present in both the male and the female embryo and fetus during intra-uterine life.

The male child is born with testicles which, before birth, have moved down from the abdomen to the scrotum. In the vast ramification of minute tubules which form these organs there are the mother cells which produce spermatozoa, and there are also the cells of Sertoli which nurse and, it is believed, feed the developing sperms, which do not become active until puberty. It is estimated that each testicle has over one mile of sperm-producing tubules from the walls of which a healthy man may produce at each ejaculation over two hundred million spermatozoa.

In the female, ova-forming tissues are in the ovary of the fetus some months before birth. A large number of these so-called 'primordial follicles' lie just under the outer coat of the ovary. In the newborn child there are approximately seventy thousand of these follicles, five hundred of which are destined to become ripe ova at puberty in the female. One of these five hundred eggs ripens during the ovulation phase of the menstrual cycle each month; they are relatively large cells, being 0.2 millimetres in diameter and visible to the naked eye. Of these, an average of probably less than six are fertilised and less than four grow into human form; the others are cast from the body in the detritus of the menses.

These facts are wonderful examples of the prodigality of nature. Almost incalculable millions of spermatozoa and thousands of ova are wasted that one of each shall survive; but wasted is the wrong word, for if only one of each were provided by nature, the species would cease in a few generations. Possibly in the competition between so many, only the fittest may be victorious when their efforts are attended by good fortune. The union of the spermatozoon and the ovum is an essential factor in fertilisation.

The male element is ejaculated from the penis into the vagina of the female at the culmination of coitus. The mature sperm cell has a long, thin tail which, by waving in a compatible medium, enables it to move towards the opening in the neck or cervix of the uterus. It travels at the rate of about one inch in ten minutes, but there are many factors which influence its speed and motility. Considerable numbers find their way into the uterus and engage in what might be described as a race for the ovum.

The ovum escapes from the ovary by the rupturing of a sac known as the Graafian follicle in which it develops, and it is liberated into the peritoneal cavity. It is attracted in some way which is not clearly understood to the funnel-shaped end of the Fallopian tube, and is conveyed by small hairs, or ciliae, which wave it along its course towards the uterus.

In the tube it is discovered by the searching spermatozoa, one of which penetrates it and makes it fertile. The ovum undergoes an immediate change which prevents any further penetration of its outer wall by the spermatozoa which gather about it. In this newly fertilised condition, it passes into the uterus where it becomes embedded. From the outer wall of the egg, processes are extruded known as chorionic villi, which invade and merge with the cells of the inner layer of the uterus. From these villi, the placenta, through which the mother nourishes her child, is formed. The placental site rapidly expands, and the blood vessels and nerve fibrils bring vitality to the egg and the growth of the fetus becomes established.

Development of the Human Egg

At the end of the first month it is 4 millimetres long and lies in a fluid-like sac about the size of a pigeon's egg. At the end of the second month, it is 3 centimetres in length; arms, legs and head are clearly distinguishable. It is now fed through its navel by a cord which is attached to the placenta. This structure is firmly fused to the inner wall of the uterus and takes from the mother's blood the things necessary for the nourishment of the baby. At the end of the third month the foetus is 9 centimetres long, weighs about 5 grams, and the whole egg is about the size of a goose's egg. At the end of the fourth month the fetus has grown rapidly to 18 centimetres in length and weighs 120 grams; its heart can be heard beating strongly and it is possible to tell the sex of the child should it be born at this age. At the fifth month it is 25 centimetres long and weighs about 650 grams (or about 1.25lb). Occasionally one reads in medical literature of babies of this age having been born and surviving. By the end of the seventh month – that is, twenty-eight weeks old – the child is perfected, although not fully grown or fully nourished, but many twenty-eight week children have been born and survived perfectly happily. At the eighth month the child is 43 centimetres long and stands a very good chance of healthy survival. At the ninth month, or thirty-six weeks, the average weight is 5–5.5lb. Its organs and functions are all well developed, and although these children possibly require more care than a full-time child, they should survive perfectly well if born at this age. At the tenth month, that is, forty weeks – which is about the average time that a child takes to develop – it should weigh about 7–7.5lb, and be 48–50 centimetres in length, and it is in that condition that natural birth takes place. As the infant grows, so the womb or uterus grows round it, increasing in size.

Progressive Changes in the Size of the Uterus during Pregnancy

After two months, the pregnant uterus is about the size of a large hen's egg. At the third month it can just be felt in a thin woman above the pubic bone (the bone bridging across the lower abdomen). At the fourth month, it is halfway between the pubic bone and the navel. At five and a half months, or twenty-two to twenty-three weeks, it is up to the navel. At seven months, two to three inches above the navel. At eight months, about halfway between the navel and the lower end of the breast bone. At nine and a half months, or thirty-eight weeks, it reaches its highest point in the abdomen. At full term, or forty weeks, it has dropped back one to two inches.

The actual size of the uterus varies according to the amount of water in it and the size of the baby; but the levels in the abdomen at certain weeks of development do not vary very much in different women. With these facts in mind, we can consider the structure of the uterus when the baby is ready to be born.

At term – that is, when the baby is ready to be born – the uterus is a muscular bag about fourteen inches in length and approximately just under half an inch in thickness. It is well supplied with nerves which stimulate the muscle contraction, and it also has a copious blood supply, which is necessary to take fresh blood to the uterus and carry away all the waste products of muscular activity.

The Muscle Layers of the Uterus

There are three layers in the uterine wall: the outside layer consists of longitudinal fibres which spread up over the front of the uterus, or fundus, and down the back or posterior wall. They are, in the main, distributed so that by contraction they shorten the uterus. The middle layer is composed of fibres which run in all directions, matted closely together; the most important fibres are entwined in 'figures of eight' formation and whorls round the large blood vessels. The inner layer consists of fibres, most of which pass round the body of the uterus. There are very few of these fibres in the upper part, or fundus, of the organ; they are concentrated in the lower uterine segment – that is, the lower half of the uterus, and near the neck or outlet. The distribution of these various fibres should be carefully noted, as it is important to understand what is likely to occur when each group contracts. In practice, it is difficult to separate one group from another and in the dissecting room practically impossible to find a clear line of demarcation between the longitudinal fibres, the middle layer and the internal circular fibres. But broadly speaking, the outside, or long, fibres, when contracting, are expulsive – that is to say, tend to empty the uterus; the middle layer constricts the blood vessels when it contracts and by relaxing allows a free flow of blood through the venous channels; whereas the circular, or inner, layer, by contracting, tends to close the outlet of the uterus, and to hold up, or inhibit, the activity of the uterus during labour.

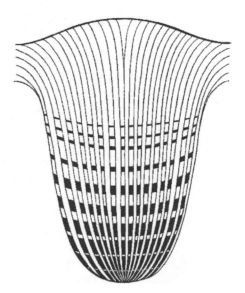

Showing diagrammatically the relative distribution of longitudinal and circular muscle fibres in the uterus at full term.

Nerves of the Uterus

Contraction of these muscles depends, of course, upon nerve supplies and there are three sources of nervous impulse to the uterus which send stimuli to these muscles. The circular fibres are supplied by what is known as the sympathetic nervous system. These same nerves supply most of the muscle tissue forming whorls or figures of eight round the large blood vessels in the middle layer. The longitudinal fibres have two sources of nerve supply: one from the parasympathetic group, and the other a local innervation from ganglia within the muscle of the uterus itself, which is not associated in any way with the spinal cord or the sympathetic nervous system. The importance of this local innervation will be seen when the question is studied in detail and when the harmony of interaction of the uterine muscles is discussed.

We may summarise this under four headings:

1. The local innervation, which is responsible for expulsive contractions.
2. The parasympathetic nerve supply, which stimulates the muscles of expulsion.
3. The sympathetic nerves, which inhibit expulsion.
4. The sympathetic nerves, which cause the muscle fibres around the large vessels of the middle layer to contract.

A further explanation of the normal interaction of these nerves is required before we can fully understand the difference between natural childbirth and childbirth subjected to outside and unnatural influences.

Harmony of Muscle Contractions

We have all over the body groups of muscles whose actions are opposed to each other. A simple example is the action of the biceps and the triceps: if we wish to bend the arm at the elbow, the biceps contracts and the triceps, which normally opposes it, relaxes. If, on the other hand, we wish to straighten our arm, the triceps contracts and the biceps at the same time relaxes. If both these muscles function at the same time, the arm goes into a state of rigidity. If the contractions are strong enough, the whole arm quivers, and in a very short time there is considerable pain in the limb. The same convenient harmony of muscle action may be seen in the bowel and the urinary bladder: when the bowel is emptied, the muscles which are brought into play in order to expel its contents are not opposed by the ring of muscles, or the sphincter, at the outlet, which normally holds the bowel tightly closed. When an expulsive effort is made, the outlet is relaxed. The same applies to the urinary apparatus: until it is convenient to micturate, the muscle at the neck of the bladder remains firmly contracted, thereby retaining its contents. When the muscle at the outlet is relaxed, the contractile wall of the bladder forces the urine out through the urethra. Both the mechanisms may give rise to acute pain if spasmodic contraction at the outlet occurs and resists the efforts of the expulsive muscles. The condition called fissure of the anus, which is extremely painful, may cause a spasm of the sphincter muscle so that it will not relax. The two opposing muscles, acting at the same time, combine to produce acute pain from abnormal pressure. When there is inflammation or irritation of the urethra, it is painful to pass urine, and spasm of the urethra may occur; the muscles of expulsion are unable to force the urine out, and acute pain results from increased tension.

This same harmony of muscle action is seen in the uterus during childbirth. The longitudinal muscle fibres contract and their action is expulsive, and in normal conditions the circular muscle fibres are relaxed and flaccid, allowing dilatation of the outlet to the womb and free passage of the child.

From the general principles of the construction of the uterus we deduce that labour without tension or injury depends upon:

1. Expulsive muscle activity without resistance from constricting muscles.
2. Expulsive nerve impulses active and constrictor nerve impulses inactive.
3. Elasticity of structures around arteries and veins between expulsive contractions so that a full supply of fresh blood may be maintained and the waste products of muscle action freely removed.

This short comment upon the physiology of childbirth is made in order to clarify the objects of this book. It is not the place to discuss the large variety of neurophysiological concepts which necessitate a close understanding of the recent work of Lord Adrian, Wilder Penfield and John H. Fulton and others. This fascinating and rewarding field of investigation carries us out of the domain of clinical obstetrics.

The validity of the physiological principles assigned to natural childbirth has been questioned. Neurophysiology is fertile ground for speculative adventures in the promising unknown. It is difficult to contradict many apparently authoritative statements because no one knows the answers and only those who know most are willing to admit that. Professor T.N.A. Jeffcoate wrote of my physiology as 'wishful thinking' and 'scientists point out that my views are unsound'. A serious enquiry that I made for more detailed information about such comments resulted in a letter from Professor Nixon of University College, London, in which he replies, '... I doubt whether anyone has studied the subject more than you, and for this reason I do not think they are able honestly to criticise.' Neither of these diametrically opposed comments have any practical value. The worth of the physiological thesis is estimated upon the *clinical* results obtained by its implementation. If a hundred professors denounced these tenets of the physiology of reproduction without offering any alternative which makes childbirth happier and safer for mothers, and babies, who could take serious notice? Beyond a certain level of comprehension we recognise the limitations of science and are grateful for the service rendered by any of our empirical presumptions.

The natural childbirth procedures have proved themselves to have contributed health and happiness to women of all civilised nations. Its influence upon the minds of husbands, wives, and children in social groups has been accepted by sociologists as a proven fact – beyond controversy. Evidence in many languages can be found in international and national libraries of the diminution of the fear of childbirth. We await, hopefully, for someone to expound the physiology of reproduction which will enable us to improve upon the present practice of natural childbirth. Till then we emphasise that this book has been written to the glory of motherhood, not for the establishment of names in 'halls of fame'. We cannot, therefore, be seriously interested in the ambitions of individuals, political ideologies, or prejudice in academic colleges.

We believe that motherhood is the highest form of manifestation of the genius of the creative spirit of nature. Its enemies are those who are blind to the dignity of motherhood and the spiritual potential of her primary purpose. They worship the golden calf of science and so seek a national hero to whom they may ascribe the works of God.

5

The Pain of Labour

The actual birth of a child is known as labour or parturition. When we speak of normal, natural or uncomplicated labour we infer that the child is the right size and in the correct position to pass through the pelvic canal without undue strain of injury to the surrounding parts. In the majority of labours everything appears to be perfect: the muscles contract well, there is no disproportion between the baby and the birth canal. Yet in spite of every favourable sign and symptom, childbirth has, for hundreds of years, been associated with pain. Therefore pain must be discussed so that we may try to find its cause and the means of preventing its occurrence in labour.

This is perhaps ground upon which angels would fear to tread; it is a subject which has claimed the attention of scientists and philosophers for centuries. A large part of all medical literature is concerned with the significance of painful sensations in disease and health. In 1915 Richard Behan published a book called *Pain*. At the end of this considerable tome he compiled no less than sixty-five pages of the names of scientists and their writings upon this theme. He also gave a long list of those who had attempted to define pain; they not only included physiologists and anatomists, but Schopenhauer, Spinosa, Cicero and many of the old philosophers. One of our greatest authorities upon this subject, Sir Thomas Lewis, commences the preface of the latest edition of his book *Pain*: 'Reflection tells me that I am so far from being able satisfactorily to define pain that the attempt would serve no useful purpose.'

This phenomenon has been evolved with a definite design. It is so general among all the higher forms of animal life that it is probably beneficial and not of itself harmful. It is an important device employed by nature to protect the individual from injury or the results of injury. The reaction to irritation is movement, which is demonstrated by the amoeba, the simplest unicellular form of animal life; if we place minute granules of methylene blue in contact with its surface, the response is movement in order to escape from or rid itself of the irritating particle.

As we ascend the scale to the higher mammals, awareness to stimulation increases. Whether reaction is associated with volition is open to discussion, and we must presume that in the absence of consciousness, defence movements are purely tissue reflexes. We can learn very little about pain from experiments upon animals, our knowledge must accrue from observation upon conscious human beings; they alone are able to describe their feelings. If we remove the consciousness, by any means, there is no pain appreciation and therefore vital resistance to pain is absent.

The Biological Purpose of Pain

The biological purpose of pain interpretation is protective, and it results in muscular activity to the end that the individual may either defend himself or escape from impending danger. For instance, if a finger is accidentally put on a hot stove, almost before there is any conscious mental interpretation of what has happened, it has been removed; the muscular activity of protection has been immediately employed by lifting the finger from the injurious stimulus. Pain also instructs us, lest its horrors should be repeated through our carelessness. The creation of such association and experience is exemplified by the small boy who withdraws his hand as the master's cane descends.

There are, however, pains from which we cannot escape so easily, arising from the internal organs and known as visceral pains. The uterus and the pelvic organs are viscera and therefore in this discussion we are primarily concerned with visceral pain. It must be borne in mind, also, that we are not concerned with disease but with healthy women carrying out a normal and natural function. *There is no physiological function in the body which gives rise to pain in the normal course of health.* When the natural urges to perform are uncomfortable, it usually indicates that the physiological balance is being strained. Excessive hunger may be considered a pain; acute thirst is certainly a pain. When the bladder should be emptied or when there is a strong desire to defaecate, these urges may be described as visceral pains, but they are protective and are demands which, in the natural state, would be satiated before discomfort arose. Once again we must ask the same question: how is it that normal childbirth should so consistently be associated with pain in the minds of cultured and civilised races?

How Pain is Felt

Over the surface of the body and upon various internal organs and structures, there are minute nerve endings which we know as pain receivers for which the scientific word is 'nociceptors'. The distribution of these nociceptors was developed when man lived in primaeval animal communities. They have persisted and are found in those positions upon the body and within the body which are exposed to injury from primitive assault. In the pristine eras of human development we were exposed to attack by tooth and claw; therefore the greatest profusion of nociceptors are found over the vulnerable areas of the body where injury would have most serious consequences. The sides of the neck, under the arms, the abdomen and the chest are all extremely sensitive places, for, if engaged in combat, it would be here that tooth and claw would inflict damage and cause the physical shock which places a fighter at the mercy of his foe. If we watch kittens, puppies or young bears at play, we can see where nociceptors are liberally distributed. There are definite areas which each endeavours to claw or bite – they roll, feint and jump to shield these places. They are playing, but unwittingly practising the more serious art of attack and defence.

But we need not discuss the pain receivers of the body surface, for we are interested in those within the abdominal cavity. The intestines, the internal organs and in particular the uterus, are not affected by external cold or heat; and the abdominal wall has to be severely injured or ripped open before they can be damaged; but they are well supplied with pain receptors which detect *excessive tension* or *laceration of the tissues*. No other nociceptors have been demonstrated within the abdomen – the intestines and the uterus can be burnt, cauterised, handled and moved without any sensation of discomfort to the patient, but if either of these structures is stretched or torn, considerable pain and shock results.

All nociceptors are specific, that is to say, they react to only one form of pain stimulation. It follows thus that the only pain stimulus that the uterus can record is excessive tension or actual tearing of tissues.* The pain of labour, whether referred or otherwise, must result from one, or both, of these specific stimuli. So we must ask ourselves: does nature intend that childbirth should be accompanied by laceration and injurious tension? If it does, why has not this important

---

*I have been persuaded from experiment and experience that specificity is a constant phenomenon in both conditioned reflexes and sensory receptors. *Vide* Pavlov and Sherrington.

structure adapted itself to its function, according to the law of Professor Julius Wolfe, which was, in short: 'Structure is adapted to function'? If nature does not intend this laceration and injury, then those pain receivers are there to respond only to stimuli other than normal. We must enquire: against what is the uterus protecting itself by giving pain sensations in carrying out a perfectly natural function? The physiological perfection of the human body knows no greater paradox than pain in normal parturition.

Before any further effort to explain the nervous mechanism of pain is offered it must be clearly understood that no one, least of all myself, knows all the answers to this complicated problem. My thesis was evolved from observations made by the bedside, not in the laboratory; it has been tried by clinical application to human beings who appeared to be suffering discomforts in childbirth. I do not wish to present this teaching as a dogma but rather, as I have said previously, for the contemplation of those who may be interested; and neither have I the effrontery to suggest that anyone who does not agree with me is necessarily wrong. Professor H. Hartridge wrote concerning the function of the receptors in the brain: 'At the moment the whole subject is full of contradictory evidence, the inconsistencies in which will doubtless be cleared up as a result of further research.' The importance of my theory is that its implementation in obstetric practice results in the relief of pain. Frankly, if there is a whole series of academic flaws in my argument, I cannot be too seriously concerned, for its practical application shows clearly that 'it works' with considerable success. The details of how and why may be clarified, as Professor Hartridge suggests, by further research.

I emphasise this because some of my colleagues, for whose academic attainments I have great respect, argue: 'You assume too much; this is not proved; this is not strictly scientific. We disagree with your neurology and your psychiatry is misleading, therefore you must be wrong.' My reply is, with all humility: 'Yes, of course' and I return to the labour ward to be greeted by happy women with their newborn babies in their arms: 'How right you are, doctor, it is so much easier that way.' That is what really matters to the clinician. He should use the method that gives the best and safest result from all points of view until something better is discovered. However, some explication may be an aid to understanding the general principles of uterine pain and its relief.

A stimulus is received by the nerve endings in the uterus. It traverses the spinal cord to the brain in a manner comparable to a communication by telephone. The exact path taken by these sensory stimuli is a subject of considerable controversy. They arrive, however, at the area of integration and organisation of nervous activity in a part of the brain which is generally known as the thalamus, where there is a large collection of special operative centres concerned with different organs or functions of the body. Seventeen to twenty nuclei or centres have been described. Here stimuli are received, their nature and intensity is interpreted, and they are then relayed to the outer covering or cortex of the brain where they are balanced and qualified so that adequate motor activity may be initiated in response to thalamic demand. The nature of the cortical reaction depends upon the magnitude of the message from the thalamic centres. But the thalamus not only receives and interprets sensory stimuli, it is specifically concerned with emotional expression. The essential protective emotion is fear, which brings about the strongest and most efficiently reinforced of all motor responses. Its influence is diffused throughout the entire receptor mechanism and the urgency of the inborn sense of self-protection amplifies or distorts the interpretation of both facts or fantasies of the emotions. The exaggerated messages prompt the cortex to precipitate a state of emergency in preparation for offence or defence. In this way somatic or physical changes may occur as a direct result of psychological states and this phenomenon is the basis of a rapidly developing branch of science – psychosomatic medicine. This vast and fascinating subject can only be referred to inasmuch as it concerns the pain of childbirth. In a paper published in the *British Medical Journal* by Sir Henry Head, one of the great pioneer neurologists, we read: 'The mental state of the patient has a notoriously profound influence over the pains originating in the pelvic viscera.' In other words, the interpretation of sensations arising from the uterus may be influenced in most astonishing ways by the mental condition of the woman concerned.

Pain is the interpretation of stimulus and varies as the intensity of emotional influences, concerning which I postulate this law: *A stimulus of fixed magnitude applied to any specific sensory receptor produces a motor response commensurate with the integrity of its interpretation.*

It is extremely important that this should be recognised in normal and uncomplicated labour, for a stimulus of fixed magnitude may be to Mrs Jones nothing that matters, but to Mrs Smith an agony of great intensity, whereas Mrs Brown may consider it a reasonably bearable discomfort. These variations depend entirely upon the condition of the mental attitude towards that stimulus of Mrs Jones, Mrs Smith and Mrs Brown at the time of labour. Now, since theoretically nature made no provision for parturition to be painful let us consider more in detail what actually happens.

A woman about to start her first labour has been told to expect certain sensations; if she has been instructed wisely her expectations have not necessarily been associated with pain but rather with a series of changing physical strains and stresses of which she has no reason to be afraid. The contraction of the uterus will be a new experience to her. If, however, fear has increased the intensity, and disturbed the integrity, of her interpretation of these new sensations, they will almost invariably be represented as pain. Should that be so, the thalamus in conjunction with the cortex, immediately sets up protective mechanism. Now the great protective mechanism of the body is innervated by the sympathetic nervous system, which overrides, by its powerful influences, all other nerve stimuli throughout the body. It activates the machinery for either fight or flight; it creates a state of tension throughout the individual which provides for an increase of muscular power. No one can run faster or fight more violently than when thoroughly frightened, particularly if their alarm is justified by discomfort. The branches which supply the circular or inhibitory muscle fibres of the uterus are amongst those which are stimulated by the general reaction of the sympathetic nervous system. Their contractions create a condition of rigidity in the lower segment and outlet of the organ. This introduces resistance to the efforts of the longitudinal muscle fibres. We have pointed out that the expulsive contractions of the uterus continue even if the autonomic innervation is cut off. Therefore we have two groups of muscles acting in opposition to each other, the powerful longitudinal fibres struggling to dilate the cervix and expel the child, whilst the fear-stimulated circular fibres render the lower uterine segment and the outlet resistant to dilatation. This rapidly produces tension greater than normal within the walls and cavity of the uterus. Excessive tension is recorded by the nociceptors specific for that form of stimulation and is correctly interpreted as pain.

The Fear-Tension-Pain Syndrome

The fear of pain actually produces true pain through the medium of pathological tension. This is known as the Fear-Tension-Pain Syndrome and once it is established a vicious circle demonstrating a crescendo of events will be observed, for with the true pain fear is justified, and with mounting fear resistance is strengthened. *The most important contributory cause of pain in otherwise normal labour is fear.*

But the circulation of the blood to and from the uterus is also affected, for persisting tension of the uterine musculature prevents complete relaxation between contractions. The great blood sinuses of the uterus are deprived of full expansion and the venous blood, replete with metabolites or waste products of muscular action, are unable to discard their contents as freely as they should. And further, stimulation of the sympathetic nervous system results in constriction of the arterial blood vessels bringing fresh fuel to the contracting muscles. As a medical student at Cambridge, I watched Professors Langley and Anderson stimulate the sympathetic nerves to the uterus. In a short time the organ appeared pallid, firm and bloodless, but when the stimulation was removed it rapidly filled with blood and became an elastic deep pink uterus. This phenomenon was first published many years before I witnessed it (Langley and Anderson, *Journal of Physiology*, 1893–1894). I have seen, on more than one occasion, what is known as a white or ischaemic uterus. Because of urgent fetal distress, caesarean section had been performed. Labour had been inhibited by strong but ineffective contractions. The women in these cases had no anatomical obstruction, but uncontrollable fear had caused, through the resistance of the circular muscles, such tension within and ischaemia of the uterine muscles that the baby, through excessive intra-uterine pressure and restricted oxygen supply, was unable to survive a protracted labour and vaginal delivery. The white uterus persisted in spite of surgical anaesthesia, which demonstrated the depth of fear within the psyche of the conditioned individual.

Sir Thomas Lewis (*Archives of Internal Medicine*, vol XLIX, page 713, May, 1932) described the results of experiments upon muscle pain when the circulation was partially restricted. He suggested that an impairment of circulation is a cause of pain because the blood flow is too small to dispose of metabolites. These substances, which may be crystalline in form, when in high concentration irritate by laceration of the inner walls of the blood sinuses and smaller vessels within the muscle fibres. Restricted circulation or relative ischaemia can give rise to severe pain in muscle tissue. Not infrequently I have observed in the prolonged labour of frightened women a tenderness of the uterus; even gentle palpation of the womb through the abdominal wall gives rise to acute pain; I have seen this pain disappear when fear has been allayed or when demeral, that is, pethidine, or a light analgesic has induced a state of mental relaxation. A labour without disproportion or malpresentation of the baby is long because it is painful, not painful because it is long.

I do not refer in detail to the chemical changes or the internal secretory activities that accompany the Fear-Tension-Pain Syndrome; under its influence the physiological processes of parturition are disturbed and the well-being of both mother and child seriously impaired. This disrupting emotion of fear, and the concomitant pain, not only alters the course of labour but is directly or indirectly responsible for interference, haemorrhage, tissue injury and psychopathies in the mother as well as anoxaemia, respiratory failure and exhaustion in the newborn infant. By these misfortunes not only the early progress of the child but its physical and psychological development may be delayed or permanently damaged. Therefore the pain of labour and its initiating cause, fear, extend their evil influence into the very roots of our social structure. It corrupts the minds and bodies of successive generations and brings distress and calamity where happiness and prosperity are the natural reward of a simple physiological performance.

Summary

Pain in an otherwise uncomplicated labour arises from the activation of the sympathetic nervous system by the emotion of fear.

Fear produces within the uterus excessive tension which causes pain and is rightly interpreted as such by the integrating nuclei of the thalamic area.

Fear induces restriction of the circulation of the blood through the uterus, thereby limiting in many ways the efficiency of the mechanism of parturition, adding to its discomforts the exquisite muscle tenderness of ischaemia.

The *Fear-Tension-Pain Syndrome* not only explains the origin of the discomforts of normal labour but has led to the discovery of a simple method of avoiding severe pain for, by removing fear, tension is reduced and pain is minimised.

6

Factors Predisposing to Low Threshold of Pain Interpretation

There are certain conditions of body and of mind which must be treated or avoided both during pregnancy and labour, because they intensify pain sensibility. These maladies or states of mind may influence the course of labour if they are allowed to persist and they should therefore receive serious consideration and attention from doctor, nurse and patient.

Anaemia. It may not appear at first sight to be the place to discuss blood conditions in pregnancy, but it is a subject which, in my opinion, is not generally given the attention its importance demands. I have rarely seen a good example of natural labour in a woman whose haemoglobin has been allowed to remain below 70 per cent from thirty-three to thirty-four weeks onwards. I do not mean that their babies arrive with difficulty, but not infrequently labour is long, exhausting and painful, with a slow recovery during the puerperium. I do not refer to severe cases of macrocytic and microcytic anaemia or the 'blood diseases,' but to women who are short of iron apart from the gross blood cell changes. The 'physiological anaemia' of pregnancy – that is, the plasma increasing in proportion to the number of red blood cells – should be compatible with good health, if it is accepted as a normal and natural state. The anaemias of pregnancy are fully discussed in *Antenatal and Postnatal Care* (Browne, 1939), but the clinical aspect in relation to pain interpretation deserves some attention.

The percentage of haemoglobin should be estimated at antenatal visits as a routine; it is simple to do and takes very little time. If it is low, but follows, during pregnancy, the normal curve of variation – that is, falling slightly at about twenty-eight to thirty-two weeks and then picking up – it does not require special treatment. But if increasing tiredness, exhaustion after normal activities, breathlessness without reasonable cause, depression and an absence of desire for meals are complained of, treatment is indicated. It is not suggested that the woman feels ill, but she may say, as many do: 'Feeling fairly well, but get so tired.' The exhibition of Blaud's 90 grains a day, or Ferri et Ammon Cit up to 120 grains a day, or one of the newer preparations of iron, often works like a charm and with the rising haemoglobin she will find new strength, spirits and appetite and quite likely tell you she has never felt so well in her life. The method of treatment will depend upon the diagnosis and judgment of the medical attendant.

In *Certain Aspects of Pain* Henry Head wrote: 'Anaemia is another cause of diminished general resistance to painful impressions.' Many of its symptoms in pregnancy are those factors which during labour lower the threshold of pain interpretation.

Let us think for a moment of a woman who, tired in mind and body, short of haemoglobin and forced to eat unsuitable food, bravely faces what she has previously endured, or what she believes she must endure. Labour commences – soon she is in pain, a weary, weeping woman. Whether she was tired before she started labour or whether because of the expenditure of nervous and physical energy at the time, is of no consequence.

Tiredness of body intensifies pain. An ache becomes a severe pain; the mind is worn out and seeks only peace.

Weariness of mind intensifies pain. In labour, the atmosphere of peace is a reinforcement to a well-nigh broken resistance.

How many nurses and doctors realise the agony of conversation, often about ill-chosen topics? There are awful people who try to cheer their patients by bright remarks. The mind should be rested, and some measure of pain will be spared.

As I sit with women in labour, I not infrequently remember those dark days in 1915 when I arrived from Gallipoli at the Blue Sisters Convent, Malta, blind in one eye and with clouded vision in the other, almost completely paralysed below the waist, longing to live, yet wishing that I could escape from life. I recall the horror of those sympathetic visitors who brought me flowers I could not see, told me to cheer up, I should soon be home. 'Remember how lucky you are to be alive' was their parting comfort. It made my whole body burn with agonising tension; my head throbbed and uncontrollable twitchings came into my legs; my spine felt as if it were torn in two at its fractured vertebra. I perspired and had I been able would have yelled in a wild mixture of pain and fury. One of the sisters came in after they had gone and saw me alone in my trouble. I had been given a room to myself. She was a tall, stern-looking woman of some fifty years, whose features I could not clearly define. She took my hand in hers and stood silently beside me. After a time she knelt beside my bed and in broken English said, 'I will stay with you. We will be peaceful, you in your way and I in mine.'

Can I ever forget the miracle of that understanding? My back relaxed and ceased to torture me; the uncontrollable spasms left my legs; my clouded eye seemed to clear and before I sank into my first long sleep for weeks, I saw her head bowed and her eyes closed as she sought in her own way the peace that swept over me. We may all have our own way of bringing peace to women in labour, but it is produced in the end by bringing restfulness to a tired mind – a mind which has no energy to withstand the irritations that intensify its discomforts.

Depression and disappointment are potent pain intensifiers. In labour, when the long first stage seems unending, when there is no reason to believe the contractions are any good, women are liable to become depressed and acutely disappointed. The sameness of the cycle of events, the uselessness of self-control, wears down their fortitude. There is no relief but in tears, no comfort in protracted hope. Each contraction becomes more uncomfortable; it is awaited with fearful anticipation; the recurring phases of expectant tension hold memories of recent discomfort as persistent pain impressions and the inevitable contraction adds 'fuel to the fire.' The misery of labour when depression and disappointment overcome the patient's courage is a picture of which all obstetricians should be ashamed. It is not infrequently initiated by the two great faults in the care of women: loneliness and ignorance.

There is no greater loneliness in the life of a human being than being alone with one's own suffering; and no suffering is greater than the mental torture of impending agony from which there is no escape and of which there is no understanding.

Do we remember these inner workings of a woman's mind when the hand is flung out to us and we are challenged with: 'Can't you do something for me?' How often companionship and sympathetic information, made practical by instruction, will change the scene and re-fortify the forces of consciousness that she wishes to retain – but how often the physician himself has only drugs and anaesthetics to offer.

Loss of control allows all stimuli to run riot. The slightest discomfort will become an unbearable agony and all the wiles and violence of animal nature are utilised in the effort to be freed from torment. It results from various causes and in hysterical women whose lack of balance is enhanced by pregnancy and labour, there is no rule-of-thumb treatment. Care must be taken during pregnancy; all influences likely to intensify her pain producing stimuli must be removed so far as possible. But remember the value of sleep; as Henry Head used to say: 'Sleep, that most salutary means of increasing central control.'

But the state should be considered pathological and require special consideration in a work not primarily concerned with normal and natural labour. At the same time we must recognise that loss of control is due to a breakdown of cortico-thalamic function and as such should concern the obstetrician who aims at harmonious neuromuscular mechanism in labour.

The centralization of thoughts upon new sensations, upon their causes and results, intensifies the reactions to stimuli which normally would never reach the consciousness. Would it help my readers to know how to make a uterine contraction hurt during labour? Inquire of the woman before it starts where the last one hurt her; agree that it was a bad pain; put your hand on the uterus and feel it beginning to contract, then say briskly: 'Now it's going to hurt. Try to tell me when the pain is at its height. Grip my hand; set your teeth; concentrate on your pain; close your eyes and suffer'! Then you will see a woman having pain. That appears to be Professor Chassar Moir's line of thought by which he has endeavored to investigate the immediate cause of pain in labour. He described it in the paper 'The Nature of Pain in Labour' at the Edinburgh Congress, in 1939. He said:

> In order to obtain exact knowledge of the relation of a uterine contraction to the time of onset and duration of the pain experienced by a patient, I have recorded in graphic form the waves of intrauterine pressure as registered by a small balloon (5cc capacity) inserted high in the uterus above the presenting part. The patient was given a bag to hold in her hand, and told to tighten and relax her grip with a rapidity proportional to her suffering. The bag was connected to a tambour which registered on the moving drum directly above the uterine tracing. This method has given valuable information, but it must be remembered that the accuracy of the record is entirely dependent on the patient's intelligent co-operation, and that a period of great physical suffering is not the time when accuracy of judgment and coordination of movement is best displayed.

He continues to describe many other interesting phenomena deduced from his pain-producing experiment. Would it not have been more interesting to have distracted her attention from the pain, relaxed her mind and body, instead of introducing concentration on pain and intensifying muscular movements? We cannot help wondering what result Professor Chassar Moir would have obtained from a natural labour. Contrast this with the following experience:

Mrs D (age 30; weight of baby at birth 8lb; previous baby stillborn – she could not tell me why or how this occurred) wrote to me as follows:

'Having recently had a stillborn child after a very painful labour, I was doubtful of the possibility of producing a live baby and quite incredulous at having a baby without pain or anaesthetics. ... I found I was able to relax during the contractions and was even able to sleep and doze during a good part of the time. This made an immense difference to the amount of pain felt. The peacefulness was very helpful and contributed in a large measure to the beauty of the whole experience. To be allowed to lie quietly on one's bed with no one bustling about and continually enquiring as to the pain or otherwise ... left one free to produce one's baby.'

I have many similar reports upon treatment which – amongst other things – assists in decentralising the thoughts from the focus of activity and so inhibiting the intensification of normal stimuli.

But this brings us within sight of the influence of suggestion. It might be said that the recording experiment was conducted under the influence of strong suggestion that pain must essentially be present, whereas Mrs D was influenced by auto-suggestion that very little, if any, pain was present. 'Yet this is not new,' writes Behan (*Pain*, 1915), 'for physicians have made use of this principle even as far back as the time of Pharaoh.'

In labour, however, AUTOSUGGESTION does play a definite part in pain production. As the result of impressions stored up in the memory centres, either from past experience, hearsay or mental imagery, subjective pain stimuli may arise from vivid reconstruction or some closely associated factor. As will be shown later, such memory impressions are present in the vast majority – probably all women – at the commencement of labour. As MacDonald Critchley writes in *Observations on Pain* (Lang Fox Memorial Lecture), 'The conception of psychogenic pain is closely bound up with such questions as the memory and the mental imagery of pain.'

This is profoundly important in labour, for muscle sensibility can so easily be felt even in the absence of pain, and autosuggestion occurs from the muscle sensation influenced by past experiences either of the human species or the individual. Thus, uterine contractions may be responsible for strong autosuggestion. The nature of uterine contractions is especially likely to produce this state; the weak beginning working up to a climax and passing into a decline. At the acme of a contraction – and often before – there is a definite sense of impending agony, which, under strong autosuggestion, firmly convinces the woman of the imminence of torture. She loses control in anticipation of that which she believes and fears to be inevitable and, like all frightened people, she does not hesitate to 'yell before she is hit'. When control is maintained, it is quickly realised that the sense of impending pain experienced at the acme of uterine contraction does not materialise. Demonstrations of escape and resistance, therefore, do not appear necessary. This is another cause and intensifier of pain perception which can be eliminated by education and treatment.

But one source of discomfort more difficult to deal with is SUGGESTION. Quite apart from pain sensations recalled from the memory centres is the suggestion of pain consciously or unconsciously conveyed to the woman in labour by people and things about her. Every clinician knows that pain can be produced by suggestion; it is indeed easy to convey strong suggestion to a woman who believes in the necessity for pain. Her whole sensory receptor mechanism is attuned to exaggerated stimuli and can perceive, in collaboration with her receptor centres, only those stimuli which are ripe for interpretation as painful. Thus, suggestion of pain is conveyed by the atmosphere of the labour room; it emanates from doctors, nurses and relations. They all believe in pain; subconsciously or consciously they suggest, expect and even presume pain. Upon the sensitive mind of a woman in labour, such authoritative suggestion, though only demonstrated by facial expression, actions for the relief of suffering, preparations for pain prevention, surgical precautions *ostentatiously* observed for the protection against the danger of sepsis, are a powerful adjuvant to painful sensations.

'Be brave, darling,' said by the mother as she leaves the room with a tense, pallid look of sympathy, is an excellent pain producer.

'Don't worry; now, don't worry; plenty of anaesthetic when it gets too bad. Not yet, of course; you must put up with it as long as you can,' from the cheerful medical man is confirmation of pain.

Wonderful heterosuggestion, so that neither she nor they are 'ignorant' enough to expect anything but the tortures of the damned.

We must learn to appreciate that a high percentage of pregnant women are acutely, sometimes illogically, sensitive. Every care that can be devised by a knowledge of human nature and a desire for its comfort should be exercised. In some famous hospitals, medical men who attend confinements are elected to the staff as 'Obstetric Surgeons'.

This implies to women interference – the word 'surgeon' means 'hand-work' – and in association with the science of medicine, it indicates manual activity in order to preserve or restore health, usually by the use of instruments. That is how the lay mind accepts this term, and this title has caused apprehension to many women because it is adopted by men of high standing in our profession.

Time and experience have shown that no normal labour subjects a well-trained woman to any discomfort that makes her wish to be anaesthetised, or suffer interference; but if women are not well-prepared and if their attendants have not learnt the power of anxiety and doubt, these two combine to destroy the natural peace of parturition.

7

Fear

The importance of the influence of the emotions upon pregnancy and parturition has been recognised during the last few years. The value of protecting women from fear is frequently referred to in writings and discussions upon antenatal care.

I think, therefore, that it will be helpful to some readers of this book who have not inquired into the nature of fear, if a short outline is given of the natural uses and the acquired misuses of this emotion.

Let us ask first: what is fear? It is an emotion which arises from the primary instinct of flight. In its earliest form it is an alertness to the presence of danger. It is the natural protective agent which enables the individual to escape from danger. In spite of its importance in the preservation of the species, in its most primitive form it is said to be roused by only two types of stimulus. A newborn babe is said to react only to falling, and to sudden, sharp noises. From my own experience I have found that within a few hours of birth a baby will start at a loud noise near to it such as a shrill whistle, the dropping of an enamel dish or the slamming of a door. It is, however, with some difficulty – possibly with considerable doubt – that I accept as proven the instinctive fear of falling. A baby is frightened, unquestionably, when it falls, but I am inclined to believe that it is not alarmed until it has fallen. There is a difference between the fear of falling and fear when falling or having fallen. If a baby appears to be frightened because it is nearly dropped by someone who is carrying it, it is subjected to sudden and unnatural movements which are made in order to prevent its falling. In the absence of the muscle-sense of support, it may or may not appear to clutch or stretch out its limbs in a manner which has been described as 'trying to hold on.' Newborn babes, however, do not hold on to things consciously, although reflexly their fingers may close if the palm of the hand is stimulated. Even this I have not found to be invariable.

Another important factor must be remembered: an adult who nearly drops a baby suffers from acute alarm, which is transferred to the infant and finally, if the infant is actually dropped, or falls, it feels considerable discomfort from the experience. When these factors are taken into account it is not unreasonable to deduce that the so-called fear of falling is in reality similar to all other fears in one respect – it is acquired.

The accepted teaching that we are born with a fear of sudden noises is also debatable. The auditory sense of a newborn child is untried. It is difficult to know how much a newborn babe can hear or, in fact, if it can record what we may term ordinary noises at all. A tuning fork brought to the ear and taken away again does not appear to create any impression. There is obviously no interpretation of the nature of sounds, even though it may be conscious of different tones. My own opinion is that both the hearing and the sight are collectors of impressions without any interpretation of those impressions being made. If, however, violent wave motion is set up in the proximity of the ear by loud and sudden noises, it is not frightening to the child, but actually painful. It is through the association with the painful impressions that fear is acquired.

For many years I took for granted the accepted teaching of the two inborn fears, but upon investigation I am inclined to believe that babies are born entirely free from any instinctive fears.

The human body is constructed in such a manner that it is not only adequate for the developmental life of infancy and childhood, but also for the exigencies and emergencies that may arise during that period. The protective machinery necessary for the child under the conditions in which it will live is supplied and ready to be used when required. There is no more reason for a child to be born with inherent fear than with any other emotion. The necessity for protection from injury and harm calls into use the machinery provided for that purpose when experience or association sets it in motion. All fear, therefore, in the human being is acquired either by suggestion or association. It is entirely a protective mechanism and is activated by apparatus which has been efficiently developed for that purpose by the phylogenetic experience of the species. Ontogenetic fear is, therefore, dependent for its development upon the receptor and perceptor organs built by nature upon the experiences of the past.

Professor Sir Walter Langdon Brown, in a paper on 'Fear and Pain' (*Lancet*, October 13th, 1935, pp 911 and 912), writes: 'What is the genesis of fear? Fear is the exaggeration and sometimes the perversion of that alertness to the presence of danger which is such a valuable defensive mechanism.'

Professor Crile, in *The Origin and Nature of the Emotions* (Saunders, 1915), writes: 'Fear arose from injury and is one of the oldest and surely the strongest emotion. By the slow process of vast empiricism nature has evolved the wonderful defence motor mechanism of many animals and of man. The stimulation of this mechanism, leading to a physical struggle, is action, and the stimulation of this mechanism without action is emotion. We may say, therefore, that fear is a phylogenetic fight or flight.'

Sadler, in *The Mind at Mischief* (Funk and Wagnall, 1929), states: 'Fear is the emotion associated with the inherent instinct of flight.'

Certain animals which have been provided by nature with other means of defence do not exhibit the emotion of fear. The skunk relies largely for its protection upon the production of nauseating odours. The porcupine, and probably the hedgehog, defend themselves from attack by exhibiting a mass of dangerous weapons to the assailant. The armadillo, the tortoise and the turtle present impenetrable fortifications into which they retire for safety. The oyster closes its shell, but the trout dashes to its hiding place. Protective apparatus may be found in all species, suitably developed to afford relative safety from hereditary foes. It is the arrival of new enemies with implements and means of attack which are the real danger to life. The ingenuity of culture has circumvented the defensive armament of phylogeny. Fight with or flight from the primitive aggressor was successfully conducted about and within the fortifications of primitive man. The disposition of the defensive forces and the system of warnings enabled the fighters to man the battlements and those who fled were protected by the ancient moat and portcullis when within the walls of the castle. Fear had adequate sublimation. It was replaced by action in fight or flight and thereby it served its protective purpose. When danger had been avoided, there was no longer fear; when the fight had been successful, this emotion had no purpose. It is equally true that however great the danger, if the inhabitants of the castle had complete faith in its indestructibility and the fighters advanced in the sure knowledge of victory, there was no fear.

From this it follows that faith eliminates fear. I must emphasise this statement because of its significance when discussing this emotion in relation to pregnancy and labour.

But we must visualise a different picture. Civilisation has broken down the edifice of primitive protection. It is no longer a question of physical survival or even of physical injury. Humanity is in the open; the unseen forces of culture which assail the human mind appear in battle array armed with weapons against which we have no provision. It is impossible to escape their devastating effects. The subtlety of the attack is such that time, place and method are ever-changing. The human mind is as helpless under the ravages of civilisation as the primitive fighter is against modern methods of warfare.

The work of readjusting the minds of women occupied in the primitive function of childbirth requires as much skill, precision and foresight on the part of those who are concerned with it as the countermeasures against bombs from aeroplanes, gas attacks, magnetic and acoustic mines, submarines and all the innovations of modern warfare demand from those whose business it is to understand these things. It does not seem to be fully recognised that civilisation calls for ever-increasing resourcefulness, not only if the species is to be maintained, but also if the human kind is to be effectively reproduced. Modern armaments against man, cultural associations against woman, reinforce the foes of natural survival. We can no more afford to disregard the one than the other. Fear is the strongest weapon in the hand of the enemy of motherhood. Its development in our everyday life is insidious. Like an evil propaganda, its destructive influence pervades the forces of human life. Were the man in the street to know the truth, its ravages would sound incredible. For my own part, after thirty years of close association with physical and mental derangements of health I am persuaded without a shadow of doubt that, with the exception of unforeseen accidents, the origin of every form of disease, both surgical and medical, whether hereditary or not, can be traced by careful investigation to the influence of fear upon the human mechanism. In particular I would stress that through its influence upon childbirth, fear has for many generations had an increasingly deleterious effect upon civilised people of the world.

We must be careful to understand that fear is an emotion of variable intensity. I have noticed many times that to suggest the possibility of fears being present in a woman's mind has been accepted by her as being an aspersion upon her moral courage. Fear is not necessarily abnormal; it is a natural protective state and has no relation to funk, cowardice or chicken-heartedness. In the presence of danger, fear engendered by knowledge is the stimulus which prompts to escape and, according to that which threatens, so the method of avoiding it is adopted in the light of past experience. If a wasp settles on the hand, we know that it may sting; most people, therefore, will either shake or brush it away. That is protection prompted by fear. We slow down, if we are wise, when passing over dangerous crossroads; we look in the direction of oncoming traffic before stepping into the road; the first spoonful of soup is taken gently; we test the temperature of the bath before getting into it. In innumerable small actions during every moment of our everyday life we take precautions or we act with caution. This is the ordinary, normal protective activity of the emotion of fear which preserves us from a host of dangers. These actions have become what we call second nature; they are compatible with normal human behaviour.

There is, however, an exaggerated state of caution. From the beginning of the war we were all asked to have our gas masks ready for use lest they might be required; that was a reasonable precaution prompted by the fear of enemy action, but I knew a man who, from the day war was declared, arranged the domestic matters of his home each morning before he left it on the assumption that he would not return; he proceeded to his business with a steel helmet, a gas mask, mackintosh clothing to protect him against chemicals and a revolver in his pocket. That, we will agree, under the circumstances was being a little over-careful.

As students at the university, we heard many stories about the 'height of precaution', and if we look around us, it will not be difficult to find people living under its influence, like the decrepit old gentleman who always wore the armour of a first-class wicketkeeper when he went out to play croquet.

It is probable that in primitive life most fears were based upon the experience of material danger, but with the development of the mind so the visualisation of the possibility of danger has increased. We may go further than that, for the laws of civilisation, the rules for safety, and the organisations to prevent personal injury are so highly developed around us that the fear of attack in the primitive sense is practically non-existent. We are much more concerned with maintenance, the economic structure of society, the stability of the social status of the individual, the relationship of persons one to another, and the pride of personal accomplishments, appearance and possessions – all these things are the foundations upon which anxiety states are built. In the absence of freedom of both thought and action, principles of doubt and associations of danger are conveyed by overanxious parents and nurses to children from the earliest age of understanding. The speed of modern life, the grim struggle for survival and the close competitive relationships of men demand an expenditure of nervous energy out of all proportion to its physical sublimation. To a large extent the primitive machinery is obsolete. The action prompted by fear was dependent for its efficiency upon neuromuscular fitness, whereas today the emotion which arises from the inability to survive by physical action must be effectively sublimated or depletion of nervous energy results. Those who have the understanding, the ability or the philosophy to sublimate satisfactorily this cultural counterfeit of primitive action are few and far between. Anxieties and doubts are prevalent in the minds of the vast majority; they may amount to obsessions, to phobias and perversions of mental activity which undermine emotional stability and physical health. This condition of constant strain, whether it arises within occupational, social or domestic environment, produces through the nervous system changes in the activation of the endocrine glands resulting in imbalance and discord where harmony is alone compatible with health. From this derangement, the chemical rectitude of metabolism is seriously disturbed, thereby producing a condition which increases mental strain, further depletes the nervous energy and so completes the inevitable vicious circle. No faculty or function of the human mechanism is safe from the aggressive inroads of the insidious fears of civilised existence.

The Mechanism of Fear

We have discussed fear in general, giving examples of its occurrence and definitions given by various writers upon the subject, but we have not answered the obvious question: what is fear? That is to say, what are the signs and symptoms of its presence and what effect has the mind, in a state of fear, upon the body?

We can describe two types of fear: that which is sudden and acute and that which is ever-present in varying degrees which may be termed chronic anxiety.

It is rare today to meet acute fear in obstetrics although thirty years ago it was by no means infrequent. The manifestations of fear vary from terror to alarm, dread, dismay and scare and purposeful attention. The intensification of these manifestations depends largely upon the nature of the stimulus and the nervous condition of the individual. Charles Darwin's book *The Expression of the Emotions in Man and Animals* describes this phenomenon so vividly and with such comprehensive accuracy that the condition can easily be visualised or recognised when seen:

'The eyes are widely open by the raising of the eyelids and the pupils are dilated. Hearing is finely attuned to sounds which normally pass unnoticed. The sense of smell is such that odours associated with the source of danger are instantly recognised. The skin becomes pale;

cold perspiration exudes from its glands. It is extremely sensitive to unexpected touch. The hairs upon the skin stand erect by the contraction of the small muscles which raise them and the thin layer of muscles beneath the skin may cause tremors or rigid spasm, particularly around the mouth and the fibres under the skin of the neck and shoulders which are called platysma myoides. The mouth and lips become dry and the salivary glands cease to secrete.'

Before I enumerate other signs of fear, attention must be drawn to the fact that all these I have mentioned are due to the activity of the sympathetic nerves supplying the structures which show these changes. From time to time these indications of alarm have been recognised in women who are frightened by some inadvertency in the conduct of their labours and it is possible that the high degree of sensitiveness that I have mentioned before, may, in reality, be due to an inborn alertness to danger, although the parturient woman appears to be quite calm. We should be aware of this when attending women in labour, for this evidence of anxiety, however courageously suppressed, may forewarn us of special care required in a particular case.

More generally, we notice that the heart beats strongly and often rapidly, breathing is quicker and sometimes irregular, being interspersed by a series of deep sighing respirations. The nostrils may be widely dilated to facilitate the intake of air, and not infrequently the mouth is slightly open for the same reason.

The digestive functions are inhibited and the muscles of the stomach which normally urge its contents into the bowel are quiescent and there is no secretion of the digestive glands. The peristaltic activity of the bowel also ceases with the possible exception of the lower colon which has a different nerve supply. In the early stages of acute fear that part of the large bowel may become relaxed and involuntary evacuation occur. The same applies to the muscles at the outlet of the bladder which control urination.

All cerebral functions are suspended except those immediately associated with the source of fear and the response demands for self-protection. The general or skeletal muscular system is in a state of tension unless the reaction to terror is so great that relaxation, collapse and unconsciousness, induced by severe shock, supervenes.

All these physical manifestations of the emotion of fear are purposeful and if we recall that the response to such stimulus is fight or flight with the greatest and most persistent energy, we will understand more closely the significance of these changes.

Functional activity that can be of no assistance, in combat or in escape, is arrested, but the organs and structures concerned with self-defence are prepared for the fray with the utmost efficiency. Nature has prescribed that noncombatant functions are shut out, but the fighting forces are equipped and invigorated for the struggle. But this is not all. A sudden vast discharge and expenditure of nervous and muscular energy is required and from the peaceful resting state of the body this abrupt call could not be effectively answered unless there were means of organising both reinforcements and the supplies required. Blood and more blood is demanded by the muscles and organs engaged in defence, for it carries the fuel that enables them to sustain the battle. It brings oxygen and extra sugar necessary for their supreme effort, it circulates substances from the internal secretory glands which maintain activity and enables large quantities of energising substances to be used with the greatest possible efficiency. It is equally necessary to carry away the increased waste materials which are the metabolites of violent muscular activity. It is for this reason that the heart beats faster, blood vessels become dilated, the liver pours out its emergency supplies of sugar, the air intake of the lungs is increased by very rapid respiration enhancing the supply of oxygen to be absorbed by the augmented flow of blood. These changes in respiratory mechanism also facilitate the egress of the excess of carbon dioxide from the blood. This could not occur unless the respiratory and circulatory systems had the faculty of increasing enormously their turnover of essential supplies under the influence of emergency and stress.

It may well be asked: where does all this extra blood come from? Two areas of the body normally maintain in use a high percentage of the total blood. They are the brain and the abdominal organs. Nature prescribes, therefore, as I have already mentioned, that only the cerebral functions vital to self-defence remain active. This liberates from the large blood sinuses within the skull a considerable quantity of circulating blood for use in other parts of the body. The activity of the abdominal viscera, including the digestive and the pelvic organs, is arrested and the blood vessels become constricted so that relatively large quantities of blood which circulate throughout the visceral blood vessels are deviated from its habitual course to reinforce supplies to the muscular system, thereby giving maximum efficiency in an emergency.

This short outline of the brilliant economy of nature in the mechanism of self-defence will serve to demonstrate the purpose of the signs and symptoms of acute fear that have been described.

Let us apply this to the picture of a woman who suffers from uncontrollable fear during labour. In preparation for parturition, the uterus has developed blood vessels many times greater than in the non-pregnant state; the increased circulation is necessary for the efficient muscular actions of contraction and retraction. We know, both from clinical experience and experimental observation, that the sympathetic nervous system stimulated by fear causes restriction of the circulation of the blood to and from the uterus. It is possible to postulate that in the absence of adequate fuel and an effective means of disposing of waste products, no organ can carry out its function successfully. This is one of the most serious influences of fear upon the reproductive apparatus. It alters, in different ways, the physiological mechanism of childbirth; in fact it is directly responsible for many of the unpredictable complications of otherwise normal labour.

The influence of chronic anxiety upon pregnant and parturient women is too frequently overlooked and is one of the main indications for careful and efficient antenatal preparation, particularly the elimination of fear. The human body is not a series of individual organs carrying out their allotted task unaffected by their neighbours; our bodies are unified structures whose components exhibit the most perfect harmony that science has the privilege of investigating. Our organs and purposes are interdependent and the chronically anxious woman reflects the stresses and strains consequent upon her emotional state in a variety of physical manifestations. We are all equipped to accept, under modern conditions of living, frustration and worry up to a certain intensity. Civilisation has brought, under the banner of emancipation, a world of laws, restrictions and regulations. These are a necessary corollary to the development of cultural communal life, and in the main they are drawn up to prevent man from giving vent to his natural inclinations. He is not allowed to acquire by force those things he considers desirable; the regimentation of our actions has taken the place of freedom within certain limits. This not only applies to nations and communities, but to the individual, for, from the earliest moments of life, that refined infliction known as education rests heavily upon human society.

But there are those who are unable to adjust themselves to the demands of a manner of living which is contrary to their nature. The motor mechanism of frustration and resentment – which are closely allied to self-preservation – is activated by the mental stress from which they suffer. No physical strain beyond our ability can be sustained without circulatory or skeletal injury and no chronic fear or anxiety can be maintained in the human mind without the disruption of the normal physiological balance. Its manifestations may be either psychological or physical; nature rebels against intruders upon its ordered processes. When a woman whose nervous system has been invaded by incompatibilities becomes pregnant, there is considerable risk of her focusing her half-buried anxieties upon childbirth. Such complaints of pregnancy as persistent nausea, sickness, constipation, desire for unusual foods, excessive salivation, headaches, backaches and the weariness of general malaise, should draw the attention of every clinician to the possibility of her condition having a psychological basis. As pregnancy progresses, if these physical manifestations of her fear are inaccurately diagnosed and allowed to remain untreated, they may be intensified by the added strain of childbirth. This is of far-reaching importance for, apart from the heritage of characteristics, the individual's emotional make-up begins at the moment of impregnation of the ovum from which he develops. I do not suggest that we are entirely dependent upon our parental genes and oocytes, those mysterious constituents, the mutations of which within the primitive cell, fashion our ultimate variations.

Out of all proportion to the skeletal growth of the baby is the development of its brain substances. Although an infant is frequently born with an unmistakable physical resemblance to one or other of its parents, this is purely superficial hereditary association, far less important than that which affects the psyche of the infant. It is within the brain itself that the heritage of parental influence is most readily discovered. It is the mother and the nature of the influence that she contributes to her baby's mental development, as well as the chemical substances that percolate through her placenta, that mould to a large extent, the future of the child. The maternal mental processes during gestation build within her the structure of an offspring after her own form and function. It is unreasonable to suppose that all babies are born with common potentiality, or that Mrs Jones will produce a baby after the physical and mental pattern of Mrs Smith. In AD 100, in Juvenal, Sat VI, 'Scolicet expectas ut tradat mater honestos atque alios mores quam quos habet?'

> 'Do you expect, indeed, that a mother will hand down to her children principles which differ from her own?'

From the earliest weeks of fertilisation of the ovum, brain substance is present in the embryo. At three-and-a-half weeks it can be differentiated into its three main divisions, and between three and five months it develops integrative cerebral function. One month before it is born its brain is perfected. Is it not reasonable to enquire: 'do mothers influence its growth and development according to the stresses and strains to which they are subjected during pregnancy?' There can be no greater urge, both from the point of view of the mother, the infant, the family unit and ultimately the social structure, than to persevere in the preparation of the woman's mind during the early weeks of pregnancy. By the inculcation of truth and confidence, anxiety states may be replaced by a sense of well-being through the receptive months of gestation without deep psychoanalysis but with intelligent and sympathetic education.

This antenatal preparation of the mind will be observed to have a close association with her physical condition. Many of her persistent anxieties will be removed by a psychological shift from her introvert self to the inborn child, particularly after she feels it moving within her. If her fears are allayed during pregnancy and kept at bay throughout her labour, the birth of her child takes place in full consciousness of the magnificence of her achievement. Her psychological constitution is reformed and recourse to a carefree state of mind will take the place of anxiety tension to which she has been subjected for many years prior to childbirth.

These elementary observations are but a synopsis of a far-reaching and important subject, but they suffice to draw attention to the urgent necessity for the elimination of the fear of childbirth. It not only concerns mothers and babies, but families and communities. It is one of the foundations of the progressive development and philosophical stability of the future races of man.

8

Imagery and the Conditioning of the Mind

Sir Francis Galton wrote much that has been overlooked in the modern teaching of medicine. In 1883 (*Enquiries into Human Faculty*) he discusses the importance of mental imagery. His investigations emphasise the vividness with which images, based upon thought and association, can be reproduced in the mind.

In 1910 I spent considerable time in collecting varieties of colour associations and the visual patterns of numerals. This was especially interesting to me, as I have (among other peculiarities) a certain form of colour blindness. Later I persuaded some of my musical friends to record the forms and colours connected with sound. We found that with practice definite types of colour pattern were consistently associated with the characteristic works of different musicians – Beethoven's defiant independence; Mendelssohn's pure refinement; the aggressive genius of Wagner and the spontaneous optimism of Mozart, all found expression in visualisation. Here, in works, we discovered the mind of the creative genius not only conveyed to us by sensuous auditory paths, but imprinted on our memories as clear and unmistakable pictures which, when reproduced in mental imagery behind closed eyes, woke up again the patterns, airs and harmonics that they represented. Dvořák has painted the simple pathos of the negro slave; Tchaikovsky has unveiled the panorama of tragedy and woe; Handel has opened our eyes to a great celestial choir massed upon white cumuli beneath the azure dome of heaven, flinging its song of praise across the amphitheatre of illimitable space. Thus, we find sights, sounds and associations, real and imaginary, imprint themselves upon the human mind to mould and influence its reactions to past experience.

Is it unreasonable that we should pause to consider the mental image of labour within the mind of a woman? Is it not essential that we should create by education and instruction the true and natural happiness of motherhood within the vision of her mind? The mental picture of her anticipated experience should be the image of all that is beautiful in the fulfilment of her love.

A woman who had feared, because of all the accepted causes, the arrival of her child, thus gained confidence and understanding before her baby was due; she had a natural and happy birth. Towards the end of the labour that produced her second, and much larger, child, she worked with tireless energy. 'How many more' she asked me excitedly, as she rested between the contractions. 'It will soon be here,' I replied. 'Why do you ask so anxiously? I hope you are not too weary.' 'No, no, not that; but this brings back to me so clearly John's arrival: I can hear his cry and see his fat pink body in my hands. I'm longing for that heavenly feeling again; I simply can't describe it to you. It won't be long now, will it?'

Could we wish to blot out the mental imagery of her first experience? It was a physiological device to prompt repeated reproduction. But how often in years gone by had we to meet in labour defence reactions, arising not only from fear and doubt, but from an imagery of semiconscious torture justifiably reproduced to urge escape from another such experience. Surely we cannot continue to overlook the importance of these natural phenomena when preparing women for pregnancy and parturition.

If, by association, imagination or lack of education, the first labour has been marred by the devastating influence of pain-producing fear, the mental image of that event becomes the pattern of parturition in a woman's mind, and preordains her misery in repeated childbirth.

This is one of the many factors which make the first birth so very important in the lives of both the mother and the child. We realise that the first baby arrives rather more slowly than others and also that it entails possibly more hard work in the second stage of labour; but there is no necessity for any more discomfort and certainly no reason to be more afraid of the arrival of the eldest child than of the birth of its brothers and sisters. We must emphasise, therefore, that primiparae should receive very careful attention; their minds, in particular, should be prepared to know the truth of childbirth; and they should be attended by those who are willing to assist them to have their babies in the happiest and most natural manner possible. It is not only that we require, as obstetricians, an easy labour, without risk of injury to the mother or the child; we must go further.

Every woman we attend should be enabled to appreciate the personal triumph of motherhood. Our work must be conducted in cheerful, optimistic, yet serious concentration, so that the birth becomes a culmination of the mother's own effort. It is rewarded by that elation which is the normal sequel of successful achievement.

The sight and touch of her child provides the natural thrill that accompanies the reality of possessing a coveted prize; its greeting cry imprints such joy upon her consciousness that for all time she can return to that sweet music and live again the crowning moment of her life. No woman ever forgets the first scream of her baby – it demands so much, it is vehement and appealing and yet the infant is so helpless of itself to survive. It is a call that vitalises mother love and the maternal sense awakens to protect, comfort and care for the child.

These are but a few incidents in the series of experiences and emotions that sweep the memory of effort or discomfort from the woman's mind. Her associations with childbirth are established upon the conscious knowledge of her happiness. The mental image of these moments, refulgent with relief and pride in ultimate success, becomes the mother's positive pattern of childbirth for all time. It is free from negative associations that might restrain her from embarking again and yet again upon this great and glorious adventure.

As her child grows older she sees upon the canvas of the past the tiny hands and outstretched arms appearing from the vault of her own body – she hears again the sound that brought tears and laughter to her joy. She reverences this monument of motherhood as a shrine at which to worship in her daydreams whilst the infant sleeps upon her knee.

How widely different from the images of those who were allowed to labour, afraid and uninformed and, when their fears brought discomfort and the anticipation of pain, were made unconscious of the true sensations of birth. Having been anaesthetised in a state of fear, they waken without the knowledge of their reward. They recall only the dread that filled their minds as they were carried Lethewards by drugs and anaesthesia. They have known only the unhappy things which are magnified in the returning consciousness by gratitude that science has the means of protecting them from the suffering they believed to be unavoidable! This tragic counterfeit is not the fault of women. They are learning it is a counterfeit. The dawn is rapidly breaking; the light of truth will soon enable all women to demand the inestimable gifts that every naturally born baby brings to mothers, homes and families.

The imagery of childbirth will no longer be clouded by mystery and anguish. The adolescent girl will not whisper disturbing hearsay to her friends, but seek to value, fashion and protect her mind and body so that she may, in the fullness of time, be fitted and untarnished to take her place with serenity and pride amongst the chosen women of her time.

Possibly the greatest pleasure that I have been privileged to enjoy since this book was first published has been brought to me in the letters sent by women, most of whom are strangers in far-distant lands. They have written, 'And now I look forward with joy to my second child's arrival,' or, 'Now I long for more children – as many as my husband's income will allow.' In other words, the same thought is conveyed – fearless desire to repeat the experience of childbirth.

Thirty years ago I used to hear, 'I suppose I must have another child to keep this one company, but I do dislike the whole business.' That attitude is gone, forgotten because of the change in the outlook and approach towards childbirth.

But there are other influences of which few women are aware that infiltrate the consciousness insidiously and antagonise the natural desire to bear children. They are reactions to a wide variety of stimuli upon all or any of our special senses – smell, taste, sight, hearing and touch.

There are two types: the first, known as unconditioned reflexes, are largely hereditary and are not acquired by experience in life. Some physiologists refer to them as 'inborn' and they are part of our nature, probably representing much that is loosely assigned to 'instinct' – we produce saliva when we eat, our pupils contract or we close our eyes to sudden bright light, our lower leg jumps if tapped sharply below the knee – a duck swims, apparently without tuition, a puppy walks, a bird flies. We are subjected to a natural inborn factor which the species has acquired without association or instruction. There are innumerable examples of these inborn reflexes and by acting and reacting upon each other in a complicated way they produce results of such variety that fundamentally no two people are alike. Indeed it may be that within this field of investigation we come near to the basis of individuality and personality. Here and there throughout the ages, two persons have given birth to one, who with another chosen almost at random produces a third generation, and so from the host of possibilities our forebears have mated and bred until we ultimately arrive on earth ourselves, each of us the fantastically problematical product of the union of pieces picked willy-nilly from the vast mosaic of our predecessors.

Professor Bradley M. Patten (*Human Embryology*) goes far to summarise the profound significance of, but also 'the luck of the draw' in, heredity. He wrote, 'That child must be most fortunate who has "selected his ancestors" with the greatest number of good traits to take after.' We must not, therefore, expect all women to be equally good at childbearing. The strain or stock of one may be compounded of such inborn reflexes that mind and body are well-equipped for childbirth and motherhood; another may be lacking much that fosters the reproductive faculties. But though some women have babies more easily than others, the deeply rooted urge and ability is present in all but very few. One, therefore, needs care and personal attention whilst another can retire into a thicket by the trail and give birth to her baby without discomfort or dismay.

It was mainly the work of Ivan Petrovitch Pavlov that brought to light the importance of conditioned reflexes. In 1927 he pointed out that things that give greatest pleasure may become conditioned causes of acute fear and hatred if continually offered with a terrifying accompaniment. There is a tremendous amount of good common sense, as well as brilliant scientific observation, in his work. His experiments to demonstrate his theory were made upon dogs and the process of salivation was selected as it presented an easy method of observing the various results and reactions of stimulation. Food was brought to the dogs but heralded by a light which, for each dog, was always the same colour and intensity. He found that after relatively few meals (about thirty) the light produced salivation before the food arrived though there was no sight or smell of an appetising meal. Many hues were used for different dogs, but each dog salivated only when the tint to which it had become conditioned was shown. Sounds of a definite pitch were used instead of colours and the same results obtained. Similar reactions were achieved by strong smells.

Other experiments were made with pain instead of salivation. The dog was struck with a whip after a light, different from that which caused salivation, had been exhibited. In a short time the light alone, with neither whip nor person visible, caused the dog to whimper and cower in the corner of the room. The conditioning to a reflex manifestation of fear was obtained with no difficulty by a variety of stimuli.

This phenomenon is responsible for many variations of behaviour. It is a personal and not a racial characteristic. Some people are born with a predisposition to these reflexes and others are not. Many young women from the age of puberty, and even before, have enquiring minds, particularly in relation to childbirth. Few hear much that is encouraging from girls of their own age. The temptation to seek information is not curbed but again and again, drawn as if by sirens, they satiate their greed for knowledge by listening to voices that entrance but utterly distort or destroy the truth. This series of events is frequently the origin, not only of an inherent fear of childbirth, but of physical manifestations of that fear. Women have asked me if it is right to marry the man they have fallen in love with, knowing that they could never submit to pregnancy.

I recall the visit of one woman in particular, about twenty-six years old, favoured in so many ways by the hand of fortune, attractive, accomplished and of noble and wealthy heritage. She was secretary of a well-known social organisation and during the Blitz was a motorcycle dispatch rider in London, a duty requiring superlative courage. She came seeking my advice. A man, who appeared to be suited to her in every way, had asked her to marry him; she became worried when I enquired of her if she felt confident about the intimate side of marriage. She rose from her chair, her hands clenched and her face pale: 'I could never go through it. That awful business. Women seem to talk of nothing else. When they bring their troubles to me I hate my office and feel desperately ill when I hear the word.' 'What word do you refer to?' I asked her, and she stared at me and whispered: 'Labour.' It was not difficult to destroy this reflex to which she had become conditioned by changing her environment and substituting a fresh approach to the subject of motherhood. Had this state of mind and its physical reactions persisted, she might have refused the offer of marriage whereas she is now a happy mother of three children.

There are those in whom the coloured light of their own visualisation destroys the harmony of their homes. Every act that leads, in the normal sequence of events, to the possibility of pregnancy becomes inhibited by the urge to escape. The chill of fear creeps into the warmth of love, the kiss becomes a peck upon the cheek, the passion that was possessive and overpowering ceases to bind life partners in the harmony of marriage. Coitus becomes an unjustifiable risk, bereft of all the joys of freedom and romance. Its pleasures fade and disappear before the fear of impregnation. And soon the conflict between the demands of nature and the fear-conditioned mind sets up physical complaint, backache or headache, dyspepsia or constipation, listlessness and muscular apathy, depression or weariness of mind and body. Menstruation is prolonged and painful and for a few days prior to its onset irritability, sharp words and tears disturb the peace of the home. Happily nearly all such women can be cured of this affliction if the origin of their malaise is understood.

The light of truth replaces the red orb of warning that heralds only suffering or worse. They become pregnant and are moulded gradually throughout the months of gestation to a fuller understanding of childbirth. They have their babies well and themselves are born again.

This has been witnessed so many times that those who doubt are only those who have not seen.

The manner of a woman's approach to childbirth will tell us much of the stock from which she comes, the way in which she bears her children enables us to estimate the potentialities that she has at her disposal as a mother and as a wife. Whether they are used or not depends upon so many factors that we can only help and hope, but never prophesy.

9

The Fear of Childbirth

Part 1

Quite apart from the natural causes of apprehension and doubt in the ordinary human being, a woman about to have a baby is subjected to fear-producing factors peculiar to the stage of pregnancy and childbirth.

Professor Langdon Brown said he believed no patient ever entered his consulting room except in a state of fear. Professor Ryle says he has every reason to believe that no patient ever asked the opinion of a medical man without anxiety. It is not unnatural, therefore, to presume that very few, if any, women can set out upon this great adventure without having at least some misgivings as to its outcome. Let us therefore consider some of the influences which are responsible for the mental attitude that the average woman adopts towards childbirth.

Any of us about to undertake a new and important adventure would naturally weigh up the odds for and against success. In order to do this, careful consideration would be made of the experiences of other people who have embarked upon similar voyages into the unknown. First, we would wish to hear the opinions of those about us, the people whom we respected and whom we believed had no reason to exaggerate the facts or mislead us in any way by the expression of their ideas. Secondly, we would be particularly interested in the history of similar undertakings as related by those who had personal knowledge of their significance. We should probably gain great confidence or entertain severe misgivings from the stories they told us. We must include the influence of the husband in this group, for he has formed his opinions upon hearsay and exerts strong personal persuasion upon his wife both directly and indirectly. Thirdly, we should be unable to refrain from paying considerable attention to the public opinion concerning our proposed adventure. Fourthly, corroboration of this recently collected evidence, records handed down from writers and historians from the past, especially if these records were hundreds and maybe

thousands of years old, would appeal to us as of considerable importance; and finally, we should take careful notice of the activities of the
experts about us as they prepared for our care and for the success of
our enterprise. There may be other influences, but these five sources
are probably the most important.

Now, how does this apply to the girl who is about to have her first
baby? The past experiences of women of mature years who have been
associated either socially, environmentally or professionally with
childbirth are an extremely important source of influence upon which
the psychological attitude of a young mother is formulated. We must
accept the fact that even today a large number of women speak of this
natural function with bated breath, an air of mystery or insinuation of
its inflictions. A few, more kindly disposed, may essay a word of sympathy by suggesting that, after all, most women seem to come through
it all right.

From a very early age, however, girls become aware of the accepted
teaching that to have a baby is a dangerous and painful procedure. This
was brought home very closely to me when one of my own daughters,
at the age of seventeen, made these remarks in her weekly newsreel to
me:

'Jenny's mother is going to have another baby; she is terribly upset
about it and awfully worried because her mother told her it was absolute hell. Isn't it too frightful for her?' It was near the end of term, so I
did not reply in any controversial manner, neither did I waste any time
at the beginning of the holidays in introducing my daughter to the
opinions of those who not only entirely disagreed with Jenny's mother,
but who would like to have told her of the infinite harm this effort to
gain the sympathy of her daughter had done, not only to her child
but to her children's children. To my own child this was an example
of the hearsay with which sooner or later all girls become familiar,
even in those schools where it is not a frequent subject of conversation
amongst the girls themselves.

We must realise that young women hear directly and first-hand
from their relations and others who have borne children. It is a very
strange thing that a high percentage of women delight in recalling
their own 'dreadful' experiences; they do not hesitate to exaggerate the
modesty of their story by such phrases as: 'Of course, finally they had
to take it away,' or even more frequently: 'My doctor said I was one of
the worst cases he had ever attended.'

I myself heard a woman of very considerable influence in London
society, who was a grandmother, state, 'After each of my children I

vowed I'd never go through that again, but then, my dear, you know what it is...' This was to her daughter-in-law whom I was about to attend, and was said with the strange idea of giving her courage. Wherever women are gathered together and the subject of childbirth arises, the general trend of the remarks is that childbirth is a martyrdom which, though probably best forgotten, is satisfactorily recalled with obvious pride. I am not infrequently amused myself by the abhorrence with which women relate the story of the arrival of their first-born, having prefaced their remarks by telling me that fortunately they knew practically nothing about it.

A man wrote to me: 'My poor wife was really very brave. I am glad to say that as soon as the pains started she was given a large dose of morphia. Our daughter had to be helped into this world with instruments. When I went in to see her about an hour afterwards, my wife was just coming out of the chloroform.' I have since understood that these two people do not intend to have any more children because of the agony it entails. I had previously understood that child was not intended. I have no doubt, however, that this is the sort of case which will spread fear to large numbers of sympathetic young friends, and which will materially increase the sale of contraceptives in at least one small section of London society.

Unfortunately, mothers, sisters and husbands are amongst the worst offenders. Have we not all known the mothers who have been brought near to nervous breakdowns by the anticipation of their daughter's ordeal. I can never forget a stern, country matron not only the mother, but the tyrannical empress, of a family of eight, who exercised her sway over half a county from the baronial mansion of her patient husband's ancestors. She led into my consulting room, literally by the hand, a fat, red-faced young woman of twenty-four, placed her in the chair by my desk, drew herself up to about five feet ten, pulled down her Norfolk jacket with a jerk, shook her neck a little further out of a stiff collar, and without greeting me, opened the conversation in a low, dramatic voice:

'I have brought my daughter to you; I am afraid she has conceived.'

I took a hurried glance at the girl's left hand, and was relieved to see she wore a wedding ring. She then went on to explain that she had told her daughter all about it and hoped, when her time came, she would conduct herself with courage in keeping with the family tradition, that she would not flinch in the face of danger nor cringe before the necessity of pain. I did not enquire what she had told her daughter; it was with the greatest possible difficulty I persuaded myself to undertake to look after her at all. In their country home some two months later, the girl had a miscarriage. Two years afterwards I heard she was being treated for acute alcoholism. I have since heard that she is divorced from her husband.

Can any of us doubt that the agony of fear through which this girl was led was at the root of all her trouble? Can we imagine what her four sisters went through when they had their children? This may have been an exaggerated case, but is it any worse than many others?

On one occasion I had spent three hours with a girl of nineteen and just at the beginning of the second stage of labour she assured me that everything was fine. She had learnt how to conduct herself and her labour and was going extremely well when her mother tiptoed into the room. She wore an agonised expression on her face; she went to the other side of the bed and took her daughter's hand, stood whilst she had the next contraction, then with tears rolling down her cheeks whispered: 'Darling, if only I could bear some of your agony for you.' Fortunately, by that time my patient had transferred her confidence to me, because she smiled at her mother and said: 'Yes, it must be painful for you to watch. Now please go.' I regret to say I added in a stage whisper: 'Yes, please go.'

Husbands are sometimes extremely sensible and understanding people, but some, unfortunately, are serious menaces. That a man should be anxious whilst his wife is in labour is only right and quite reasonable. I was found reading the daily paper, apparently calmly, when my first child arrived, except that the paper was upside down! This, I regret to say, was true, for every obstetric abnormality that I had ever seen was, to my knowledge, occurring upstairs. This condition is infectious, and on three occasions I have had husbands work themselves up into such a frenzy of anxiety that they have telephoned for other doctors to come and assist in the last stages of the confinement. Such an emotional state is communicated to the wife, even in the most normal labours and not infrequently increases the difficulty of controlling the patient and thereby assisting her to maintain control over herself.

Both during pregnancy and labour the influence of the husband is important. Most men know very little about childbirth, except it is something which they have been led to understand is frightful. It is quite natural that many of them should fear for their wife's safety and sincerely sympathise with her in what they believe to be her 'ordeal'. Are we not frequently told by women how worried the husband is about the arrival of their child? Few and far between are those who urge their wives to realise that childbirth is a natural function and not to be feared.

This state of anxiety from which the large majority of husbands suffer is so frequently met with that there was, perhaps, more than humour in the remark made by the doctor to a husband quoted in *Punch* to the effect that he had seen many hundreds of babies into the world and he had 'never lost a husband yet'!

Such emotional tension in a home during pregnancy and labour cannot fail to be communicated in some form or other to the woman about whom it is centred.

Similarly, we recognise that very few daughters learn much which is likely to be helpful from their mothers. The days of large families have passed. We still meet those happy girls who are members of families of from ten to sixteen children; in most cases they have the easiest labours. Only recently a girl who was tenth in a family of fifteen gave birth to an 8lb child. She herself was eighteen years old. There were so few signs of labour that she persuaded the nurse only with difficulty that her baby was about to arrive. She explained afterwards her mother had had fifteen children without any trouble; she had been brought up to believe there was nothing in it and certainly nothing whatever to be afraid of. 'What mother can do fifteen times and be as well as she is, I can do,' and it was her inborn attitude towards childbirth. This, we will agree, is a very rare occurrence today. It is more usual for mothers to refrain from discussing the subject with their daughters; there is a tendency for women to look upon their daughters, up to the age of twenty-two or three, as children; their virgin simplicity is assiduously guarded against the horrors of *truth!* The facts of childbirth are withheld because the experiences of the mother have been such that she has no wish to communicate them to the child whom she believes to be about to suffer. If, in a moment of confidence, any information is given, it is more likely to be fear-producing than a stimulus to courage.

Only too frequently, however, married women come into my consulting room entirely ignorant of the most elementary facts concerning childbirth and ask me to tell them about it, since it is a subject they could not dream of mentioning to their own mother. Unfortunately, we still have to accept the fact that the influence of too many mothers upon their daughters, either through subtlety of their information or through the mystery of their silence, is a serious factor amongst the fear-producing elements in childbirth.

We must remember, also, the friends of those who are about to have a baby. If, in a party of women, one were to state boldly that she had enjoyed every moment of her pregnancy and the happiness of her labour was quite indescribable, most of those in the room – if they had had children – would either think she was mad or being funny or, more usually, not speaking the truth. So firmly rooted throughout society is the belief that childbirth is a painful and frightful affair, that even those who can state quite honestly, from their own personal experience, it is not so, are disbelieved and even laughed at. Several of my patients have told me they would like to spread the gospel of natural childbirth, but, having given their opinions once or twice, they recoil from the criticisms and incredulous jeers of their friends.

It must not be overlooked that those who have suffered are justified in believing in suffering; neither must it be forgotten that the weight of opinion in this matter is entirely on the side of those who accept the agony of labour as a natural and essential ordeal through which a mother must pass. There is no blame to be laid upon those who are honest in their opinions, neither was it their fault they suffered. It does not, however, mitigate in any way the crime of their propaganda, for to produce alarm can never assist in the accomplishment of a task, however unimportant.

Mothers, husbands and friends must therefore be recognised as agencies for the production of fear in the minds of the vast majority of young married women.

I have decided, in re-editing, neither to delete nor alter the above twenty to twenty-five lines. They were written nearly twenty years ago and are a fair description of the attitude towards childbirth prevailing at that time and which is still all too prevalent today. They call attention to the salutary and almost dramatic change since this book was first published, for an ever-increasing multitude of women approach this subject with more tolerance and less introversion. The overwhelming mass of evidence has stemmed the wild whirl of thoughtless condemnation. Mothers say quietly they wish it had been so in their time – they envy rather than criticise. The word has gone forth and there are few who do not believe. The inborn sense of woman feels the truth – her hunch in these matters is more reliable than her deduction.

Thirdly, apart from the more intimate sources of information about childbirth, women cannot escape the influence of the general trend of public and popular opinion. They read books, study papers, listen to the broadcasts on the wireless, and see pictures at the cinema. These things comprise the modern foundations of both education and amusement. In and from all of them the same atmosphere is found: childbirth is an ordeal, essentially painful and dangerous to the life of the mother.

If the novelist of today finds it necessary to increase the interest of the story by describing the events which occurred when one of the chief characters of the book gave birth to a child, the incident is fraught with poignancy and tension, drama, suffering and possibly death. Such students of human nature well know that nothing is more likely to gain the attention of the reader; therefore, words are not minced and scenes are described with the maximum of detail likely to pass the censor. Do we often – or, in fact, have we ever – read of a normal character experiencing any happiness in childbirth? I think few of us are able to remember a maternity case described in fiction in such a manner that we could assume anything other than horrors attending this natural function.

A woman of twenty who had just had her first baby wrote to me after she had had a perfectly natural parturition, recalling all the influences of which she was conscious surrounding with mystery and apprehension the arrival of a baby. Going back to her later school days, she wrote: 'In the holidays, in casual reading, one occasionally encountered mystifying and terrifying descriptions of women in labour, which left a lasting impression. For example, *Honourable Estate* (Vera Brittain); *Mother India* (Kathleen Mayo); and Ernest Hemingway's *Farewell to Arms*.' Everyone who reads novels has, from time to time, been impressed by the drama of childbirth.

I do not suggest that authors of all books in which reference is made to the subject dramatise its supposed tribulations. Peter Freuchen, in *Arctic Adventure*, describes the birth of his son. His wife, Navarans, was delivered at 3am. She was up at 8am, cleaned the house and went for a walk with her baby on her back. She led the dancing at the ball held that night. He also mentions Tarpartee's wife, who asked her guests to leave for a few minutes as she was going to have a baby. They did and she did and in a short time the party continued. On the other hand, we have Sigrid Undset's heartrending description of Kristin's confinement in *Kristin Lavraansdatter*. We can only hope that this brilliant authoress was not recounting personal experience.

If, for the sake of information, scientific or partly scientific books have been perused by women who are about to, or hope to be about to, have children, there is very little comfort to be found there. Pain is the first essential; all our great obstetric writers preface the chapters on labour by some remark which conveys the fundamental truth that labour is recognised by its pain. It would serve no purpose to mention the individual authors who subscribe to this teaching for there is no exception. There are very few chapters written upon normal labour which do not assume from beginning to end that the contractions of the uterus give rise to severe physical pain. The whole act is described from the point of view of its mechanism; the impression we get is that the woman concerned, for the time being, becomes a machine, without either consciousness or volition; things happen in the reproductory mechanism; stages follow one upon another; the child is expressed from the uterus by a series of agonising contortions which cause it to rotate, extend and advance, according to plan. We never read of the thoughts of the woman during these hours of what is described as 'labour'. We are never told whether the mother is likely to have any views or whether the attendant obstetrician has any duties to perform at the upper end of the body as well as the lower. The consideration that the average student is taught to give to the woman herself is exemplified in *Midwifery* by Ten Teachers, published in 1920 (2nd edition). Little has been added in the textbooks of the last twenty years to that human advice in the chapter on the 'Management of Labour':

'If everything *is* found to be normal, the patient should be told all is going well. She is usually much relieved when she hears that all is *straightforward*.'

Those observations are, of course, correct; the italics are mine. I have felt many times when I have read similar remarks that an addition should be made in brackets after the word 'normal' – 'which is extremely unlikely'. It would be more in keeping with the depth of encouragement that such a generous communication holds. But still, we must admit that even a dry crust of bread is better than nothing to a starving woman. But here once more, in the year of our Lord, 1954, we discern a change of outlook. Authoritative textbooks upon obstetrics draw attention to the importance of eliminating fear, both in antenatal preparation and in the conduct of labour.

From books we are likely to gather very little that will encourage a young woman to seek motherhood cheerfully. It is not exaggeration to say that 'motherhood', maternity, childbirth and even birth of a child have become words which many women consider to be unpleasant. Not infrequently has it been heard, 'I do dislike the term "motherhood"' or 'Maternity is a dreadful word.' On several occasions after lectures women have bravely risen in the audience to ask whether they could not be called something other than midwives because to the lay mind it seemed to convey a displeasing atmosphere. It was suggested at one large centre that the term 'obstetric nurse' should be used.

These may have been the criticisms of over-sensitive women, but there is something in it and I am inclined to attribute the apparent dislike for these terms to the associations which they stir in the mind of the average person who hears them. There would be different replies if a series of women were asked which they would prefer to hear when being announced at a large public reception: 'Miss A, the well-known film star (and her fourth husband),' or 'Miss B, the well-known midwife (alone).' Perhaps a little imagination is needed to visualise the expressions upon the faces of those who turned to look; a little more imagination is necessary to answer the question: why? I suggest the answer is association that is largely gleaned from such influences as books, writings and hearsay.

We cannot blame the daily papers for seeking good copy; they are printed in order to be read. The story of a straightforward birth is not news, unless it occurred in a taxicab or a telephone kiosk. But the story of a mother's death when a child is born is almost worthy of headlines. The meeting of a learned society is rarely front page news, unless it is a discussion or report upon maternal mortality. The publication during the last few years of the records of maternal mortality, of its seriousness as a threat to national stability and the acute interest that has been afforded it by the leaders of both the scientific and the social life of our country, has exaggerated its incidence in the mind of every woman who is not familiar with the details of the subject. The reasons why one woman in a thousand dies are rarely stated. The causes of the abnormality or the responsibility of the organisation which, by its imperfections, indirectly allows of inadequate attention, are never mentioned. One great factor has been overlooked and that is the harm done by these publications. It is out of all proportion to the benefit obtained by their readers. The thousandth chance is a very definite one; millions will take a ticket in a sweepstake where their chances are much less than a thousand to one, but until the prizes are drawn they will continue to believe that fortune will favour them. How many women, therefore, who hear that one in a thousand dies in childbirth, can disregard the fact that they are likely to be the one? It has been said to me: 'Women do die in labour; can you promise me that I shall come through safely?'

And so we found in 1942 there was very little, if anything, that was read in the daily papers, the weekly magazines and the monthly journals that was likely to remove anxiety from the minds of girls about to have children. But in 1952, women's magazines, journals and digests published the truth – illustrated and often beautifully written. How great a change in ten short years – the gigantic colossus of the press had combined to overthrow the fear of childbirth.

In the life of today, cinemas have considerable influence upon the minds of people. From time to time pictures are shown which, after the manner of some novels, make a great point of the drama of childbirth. The silent fortitude of an agonised woman is insinuated, if not actually shown and the bleat of a newborn baby is heard from behind a screen. The tense anxiety of the husband gives the author a wonderful opportunity – a young man may be seen walking up and down the room wringing his hands, perhaps drinking innumerable whiskys and sodas, looking imploringly towards a closed door or dashing hysterically at a bearded doctor. The company in waiting registers (I think it is called) a series of 'expect-the-worst' expressions. Such films as *The Good Earth*, *Goodbye, Mr Chips*, and *The Citadel* demonstrate this play upon the emotions, although happily in some it is so exaggerated as to become laughable.

But the same general trend of thought about childbirth is found here as in other places. There seems to be a demand by those who produce such pictures to publish to the world the sufferings of women in labour. No girl who is pregnant can see these representations without becoming acutely conscious of the possibilities that may attend her own confinement.

And so it is that both in words and pictures those who have direct access to the emotions of the public make profit for themselves or their cause in horrifying presentations. Pain, illness and death wring tears and pennies from the people; falsehood and fear are dangled before their eyes; their hearts are expanded by benevolence. It does not matter how many women are terrified and who cares so long as it attracts the necessary attention and money rolls in. If childbirth were represented as easy and pleasing, it would not be good copy. There must be drama for publicity, tragedy for donations. Play on the tender spots in women's minds; it pays in the long run. Young women and girls who see and hear these things cannot face the facts of labour without fear; they have heard no comfort and seen no joy in childbirth, either from the moving pictures or from the appealing broadcast. What a wonderful opportunity these vast organisations are missing by withholding the truth of natural childbirth from those who are ready and waiting to accept it.

But these many causes of fear are rapidly being overcome by declaration of the truth and courageous testimony. The great organisations of the lay press have brought hope and comfort to hundreds of thousands of women. The author's hopes of some few years ago have been realised more fully than in his wildest dreams. For three successive years it was reported that over forty million people read journals in which natural childbirth was described by those who had experienced its benefits to mothers; but the thoughts and words I wrote long years ago still apply to far too many women. The effort must not weaken and the torch so bravely burning shall be handed on to those who carry this message from generation to generation.

Part 2

There are many historical writings from which the reader will be led to conclude that labour always has been painful. The most important of these writings are those which are most likely to be widely read. Many women read and study their Bible carefully – it is still the best seller in the world. A high percentage of women, particularly during pregnancy and childbirth, have a strong religious background to their lives and it is not unreasonable that those who have been brought up to accept its tenets and inferences, if not its analogies, should believe that childbirth is a grievous and painful experience. They read of its sorrows; we teach of its joys. They read of its pain; we teach that pain is avoidable.

Unfortunately, neither the Old nor the New Testament provides any cause for comfort, but rather gives them good reason to be afraid of childbirth. Genesis 3, v16 quotes the Lord God as having said to Eve: 'I will greatly multiply thy sorrow and thy conception; in sorrow thou shalt bring forth children.' This passage has been known as the 'curse of Eve' and the authority of the translators since the time of James I has not been questioned. There are many other passages which convey the same impression; misery, pain and sorrow:

Galatians 4, v27. 'Rejoice thou barren that bearest not; break forth and cry thou that travaileth not.'

Isaiah 66, v7. 'Before she travailed, she brought forth; before her pain came she was delivered of a man child.'

Isaiah 13, v8. 'They shall be in pain as a woman that travaileth.'

Isaiah 21, v3. 'Therefore are my loins filled with pain; pangs have taken hold of me as the pangs of a woman that travaileth. I was bowed down at the hearing of it; I was dismayed at the seeing of it and my heart panted; fearfulness affrighted me.'

Revelation 12, v2. 'And there appeared a great wonder in the heaven; a

woman clothed with the sun and the moon under her feet and upon
her head a crown of twelve stars. And she being with child cried,
travailing in birth and pained to be delivered'

Hosea 13, v13. 'The sorrows of a travailing woman shall come upon
him.'

And in other places in the Bible the same picture of pain, frightfulness and grief illustrate the accepted opinions of childbirth during
those hundreds of years represented by the historical writings.

There are a number of people who disbelieve in natural childbirth
because they are of the opinion that it is contrary to the teaching of the
Bible. This argument has frequently been brought forward as indeed it
was by the church when James Young Simpson first used chloroform
in order to relieve the pain of abnormal labour. If those who believe
the translators and others who compiled the various editions of the
Bible were under divine guidance no argument will be of any avail; but
if this work had divine inspiration it appears likely that the writers of
the original manuscripts were inspired and not the translators of the
various editions in different languages.

It is for these reasons that the Hebrew manuscripts, from which
much of the Bible was translated, have been examined. Being interested in this subject for many years, I have acquired in my library a
considerable collection of ancient Bibles and find that some of the
translations differ from the Authorised Version, the great work which
was started in 1604 and completed in 1611, in the reign of James I.

Take, for example, Isaiah 21, v3. I turned this up in my copy of the
Geneva Bible, first published in 1560, and find that the words 'pain'
and 'pangs' were not used, but 'sorrow' was repeated three times. In
my copy of the Bishop's Bible, however, first published in 1568, the
words 'pain' and 'pangs' appear and since the Authorised Version was
largely a revision of the Bishop's Bible and not the Geneva Bible, the
same terms have been repeated by the authors.

This matter was referred to Hebrew scholars, one of whom, the Rev
B.D. Glass, spent much time investigating this subject and wrote to me
as follows:

'One thing, however, that puzzled me was why the Bible referred
to childbirth as such a painful and dangerous ordeal. That is how I
was taught and later on taught my pupils. After studying your book
Childbirth without Fear (*Revelation of Childbirth*) I felt I had to search
the Bible more thoroughly to find the deeper meaning concerning

expressions about childbirth.

I was very pleased when I read the first sentence of Genesis 3, v16, where the Hebrew word "etzev", which is usually translated as sorrow and pain, has obviously been misconstrued. The words of pain in Hebrew are "ke-iv" (pain), "tzaar" (sorrow), "yesurim" (anguish).

At no time would any Hebrew scholar use the word "etzev" as an expression of pain. The meanings of "etzev" are manifold, ie, labour (*vide* Gen 5, v29, referring to Noah: "The same shall comfort us concerning our labour and toil of our hands").

In Proverbs 14, v13, "etzev" is used as expressing labour, eg, "that in all labour there is profit."

"Etzev" can also mean "concerned" or "anxious" as is mentioned in Genesis 6, v6, where the word "grieved" is not used in its proper sense – "displeased" or "concerned" would have been more in keeping.

In chapter 45, para 5, although "etzev" is again translated as "grieved," it is used in a wrong sense; "displeased" would have suited the expression better.

Again in I Kings, 1, v6, the correct translation of "etzev" is given, namely "displeased", "and his father had not displeased him", etc.

"Etzev" has yet another meaning: that "of being perturbed," as it is expressed in Samuel I, 20, v3. "Lest he be perturbed."

I find that throughout the Bible the word "etzev" is used approximately sixteen times and not once does it convey the meaning of pain as we are made to believe. "Etzev" can assume different shades of meaning regarding the sense in which it is used.

I think that is why the translators of the Bible in the olden times, believing in the ordeal of pain and anguish in connection with childbirth, translated the word "etzev" to imply such. None of the prophets ever used this word in their expressions regarding childbirth. They used the words "tzirim" (hinges) and "vchavalim" (threads) which mean hinges and threads, or nerves. Not being a medical man it is hard for me to explain these terms. I can, however, explain "vchavalim" which means the contractions or stretching of the muscles and fibres.

In all your quotations from the Bible, the above two words were expressed and they do not really signify pain. It is only because "yeloda", which means "a woman in childbirth," is always used in conjunction with these same two words in question that the translators added on their own behalf these words as meaning pain and travail.'

We should, therefore, consider more carefully the meaning conveyed by the earlier or original documents rather than accept as indisputable the translators' words. If we put ourselves in the place of those brilliant classical scholars of James I's time, that is from AD 1604–1611, the years occupied by them in completing this work, we may find justifiable reason for the thoughts that were expressed upon childbirth. During this era obstetrics was at a low ebb. Anaesthetics and antiseptics were not discovered until two hundred and fifty years later. The first English book on midwifery had been published only fifty years, and although several manuscripts appeared, mainly for private circulation, they demonstrated little advance upon the works of Soranus, who lived from AD 78–117. Women died in large numbers in maternity hospitals and the appalling conditions of the Hotel de Dieu in Paris were found to some extent in English institutions. Surely it was reasonable that the translators should give significance to words and phrases referring to childbirth, in keeping with the accepted belief and experience of their time. They used the word pain because they had no reason to believe any other term was applicable.

Many years later we find the introduction of the pain idea into biblical translations. An investigation by Herr Ernst Burkhardt, who translated this book into German, brought to my knowledge facts of considerable interest. Part of his comments to me reads:

'I enclose an article of mine, published recently by *Die Neue Zeitung*. Professor Joseph De Lee (in the preface of his *Principles and Practice of Obstetrics*, 1947 edition) says that since unthinkable times all races understood contractions in labour as a painful experience and accordingly spoke either of pains, dolores, dolori, douleurs and (in German) Wehen. There is no evidence for this assertion. On the contrary, it seems to be sure that these termini developed only with civilisation. Our German word "Wehen" cannot be traced beyond the Middle Ages. Our frequently used pain-suggesting word "Wehmutter," I found, had a definite artificial origin. Dr. Martin Luther invented it when translating the Bible. It does not exist before the year 1540.'

Dr Rudolf Hellmann of Hamburg in his paper *Schmerz oder Erlebnis der Entbindung* in January, 1959, gives additional consideration from Germany. Translated into English we read:

'Dick-Read maintains that the underlying Hebrew word "etzev" should not be translated as "pain" but as "toil, trouble, distress, and labour". It is all a question of a predominant psychic understanding. H Adler and other investigators I have questioned have moreover come to the conclusion that there is here no command of the Lord. Several years ago Dick-Read has shown that a confinement, as a natural event, need not be, and should not be associated with violent pains. He is convinced that it could not have been the will and intention of the Creator.

In the Bible we also find references to easy deliveries, just as today they are happening as "natural births". In the Second Book of Moses (Exodus) 1, v15, the King of Egypt commanded the Hebrew midwives Siphra and Pua to kill the sons immediately on the stools (here no doubt the reference is to the birth stools which were in use in Luther's times). The midwives referred, however, to the easy deliveries of the Hebrew women with the words: "They have been born before the arrival of the midwife." This expression is recognised as sound. Luther, who liked to associate the birth with pain, has probably invented the painful-sounding word "Mother of Woe", a translation which was only discarded after 1540.

When Graf Wittgenstein, in his book *Man Before Delivery*, translated after Gunkel: "Much will I prepare your toils and groans; in labour wilt thou bear children, your longing shall be for thy husband, but he shall be your master," so one should hope that this version will be widely known. Archaic, inaccurate explanations and translations were learnt, in good faith, by clerics and teachers, and by children and grown-ups true to the words of books and letters.'

He mentions in his excellent contribution that the Greeks called pain the 'barking watchdog of health' and that pain occupies an important place in the extensive system of warning and protection of the organs; '... it seems to us rather senseless that it should be the alarm signal of delivery as at the same time it hinders the mother in her activities.'

It is forgivable that the translators of three hundred years ago should interpret the Hebrew in a manner which was in keeping with the birth customs and beliefs of their era, but I find it difficult to understand how these obviously controversial translations should be accepted by modern scholars of the classics who have many more manuscripts and advantages from which to deduce the significance of the words. For instance my attention has been drawn to the Revised Standard American version (1952).

This translation is regarded as 'the last word' in accuracy but a study of these verses shows clearly that the minds of the scholars were dominated by the traditional attitude to childbirth and this warped their translation.

> 'Genesis 3, v16. "To the woman he said: I will greatly multiply your pain ("itstsabon") in childbearing; in pain ("etzev") shall you bring forth children."
> Genesis 3, v17. (To Adam) "Cursed is the ground because of you; in toil ("itstsabon") shall you eat of it all the days of our life."
> Genesis 5, v29. (Regarding Noah) "Out of the ground which the Lord hath cursed, this one shall bring us relief from our work and the toil ("itstsabon") of our hands."

Obviously 'toil' is the correct translation of 'itstsabon' in the case of the 'curse of Adam' and the prediction concerning Noah. Why, therefore, should it be translated 'pain' in the case of the 'curse of Eve'? Obviously because the translators came to their work with the preconceived idea that childbirth for a woman meant not toil or labour but pain. But the Bible really says 'labour'. Why in translation, make it say something that it does not say?

Also, since in Genesis 3, v16 the two words 'etzev' and 'itstsabon' are used, according to the Hebrew idiom of repetition, as synonyms, surely here the word 'etzev' should also be translated not 'pain' but 'toil' or 'labour'.

Dr James Moffatt, 'A New Translation into Modern Speech':

> Genesis 3, v16. "I will make childbirth a sore pain ("itstsabon") for you. You shall have pangs ("etzev") in bearing."
> Genesis 3, v17. (To Adam) "Cursed is the ground on your account. You shall win food from it with suffering ("itstsabon") all your life."
> Genesis 5, v29. "Lamek called his son Noah saying: Now we shall know a relief from our labour and from our toil ("itstsabon") on the ground that the Eternal cursed."

Not considering Genesis 3, v16 – having translated 'itstsabon' as 'sore pain', Dr Moffatt is compelled for the sake of consistency to translate the same word as 'suffering' in verse 17, although that is quite inappropriate as describing a man engaged in agriculture. A farmer may have to work very hard, but so long as he has an object in view and is getting results he would be very much surprised if you described his work as 'suffering'.

The fact is that the words 'hard work' appropriately describe both the strenuous labour involved in giving birth (in the case of the woman) and that involved in ploughing, digging, reaping, sowing, etc (in the case of the man).

A difference is that civilisation has largely alleviated the 'curse of Adam' by the application of labour-saving machinery; but it has done exactly the opposite in the case of the 'curse of Eve' by multiplying in her mind the suggestions of fear from innumerable sources ancient and modern, thus making her 'labour' infinitely harder than it need be.

Our contention is that in both cases there will always be hard work; notwithstanding all the labour-saving machinery, a farmer's life will always be hard, and a woman's childbirth labour will always be most strenuous – but it *need not be painful*.

During the next three or four years a new translation of the Bible is being made by the Churches in Britain from the original texts. It will be supplementary to the authorised version to help those who perhaps find the language of the Bible archaic, remote, and sometimes even unintelligible. We can only hope that this translation will remove once and for all the use of words and phrases which create a fear of childbirth, for we know that those words are intended to have different significance from pain and we know that unbearable pain is not an essential accompaniment of childbirth.

But that is not all, for a woman's fears are supported by the Prayer Book in which there has been no substantial alteration since 1662. There is a special service known as 'The Churching of Women', which is a thanksgiving after childbirth. It has remained over the years unabridged and unaltered. 'Forasmuch as it hath pleased Almighty God of his Goodness to give you safe deliverance and hath preserved you in the great danger of childbirth; you shall therefore give hearty thanks unto God and say...' 'The snares of death compassed me round about and the pains of hell gat hold upon me. I found trouble and heaviness, and I called upon the name of the Lord; ... I was in misery and He helped me. Thou hast delivered my soul from death.'

Although the Dilexi quoniam has several different translations, I have taken those passages from the prayer book of my grandmother, to whom this service was read many times. And finally, this thanksgiving finishes: 'Oh, Almighty God, we give Thee humble thanks for that thou hast vouchsafed to deliver this woman thy servant from the great pain and peril of childbirth.'

Are we still to expect women to believe childbirth can be painless, that it can be a moment of transcendental joy? I must repeat that the evidence will have to be very strong before we can hope to persuade women that the translation of the Bible and the compilation of the Prayer Book are misleading. And yet how many mothers are willing to deny that the arrival of their child was a moment of supreme happiness? When discussing this service with a girl of twenty-three she said: 'But you would not expect the most wonderful gift of God to come unpleasantly.'

Is the pride of possession and accomplishment that fills the heart of every young mother when she first sees her baby, unworthy to be recalled? Is a lame apology for gratitude adequate thanks to the Almighty for the gift of a child? This practical manifestation of the perfection of human love is not deemed worthy of mention when a woman kneels before the God of love. The church simply asks her to say: 'Thank you very much for having allowed *me* to come through all that frightfulness unscathed; it is so nice to be alive in spite of having performed the greatest of all natural functions for which You especially built me, although You did make it dangerous and painful for me.'

What a travesty of the truth! It is not for the escape from pain and danger that women thank God; in my experience mothers are not made like that. It is for their child. Women do not believe that the Lord of nature prescribed suffering and the fear of death as the cost price of their biological purpose in life. I have reason to believe that there are influential dignitaries of the church who favour the prayer that I have suggested to them, which has been formulated after discussion with many seriously minded women:

'Forasmuch as it hath pleased Almighty God of His goodness to entrust to your care and keeping this child, and to have raised you to the holy estate of motherhood, you shall give hearty thanks unto God and say...'

Then follows the alternative Psalm 127, *not* Psalm 116.

A Lord Bishop, closely associated with the Archbishop of Canterbury, wrote to me on the subject; he had been discussing it with his wife, who had borne him a family of fine boys:

'We both of us are entirely in sympathy with the idea that lies behind it: that motherhood is a holy estate, and that the thanksgiving after childbirth should be primarily for the gift of the child and the privilege of being entrusted with it.

I know that the Prayer Book is deficient here. ... I shall do what

I can to have that prayer included in the services and to counteract the old-fashioned emphasis on the peril and danger and the pains of hell. ...'

The vicar of a church in Cambridge had a pamphlet printed for his congregation entitled 'The Thanksgiving of Women after Childbirth, commonly called The Churching of Women'. In a beautifully worded service he emphasised in the prayers the blessing of the gift of a child and, 'Oh, God, by whose spirit knowledge is increased and the understanding of natural processes advanced, accept that thanksgiving of Thy servant ... for raising her to the holy estate of motherhood.'

If that sort of atmosphere could be created throughout society, one important cause of fear would be eliminated from childbirth. The church would be able to teach its beauty and to encourage confidence in normal, natural function. The influence of this change would be worldwide; childbirth would no longer be considered the great ordeal of womanhood. The shadow of injury and death would cease to mar its beauty, and motherhood, that human state nearer than any other to the divine, would be exalted to its true position of importance in our national life.

When we review the Bible and the teaching of the church, we find nothing that could give comfort or courage to women who are about to become mothers, but today a vast number of women know these ancient representations of childbirth are entirely fallacious. Their thanksgiving is for the happiness and the exultation of motherhood, and their gratitude is for the privilege of achieving this holy estate. It is difficult, therefore, to ask them to accept the teaching of the Bible when their own personal experience has made them critical of its truth. A large number do not attend the service of thanksgiving after a child is born because, as one woman wrote to me, she did not feel that her soul had been delivered from death, nor was she in misery. Another wrote about the church service: 'Mothers don't take any notice of the words.'

Whether or not these anachronisms will be rectified by the ecclesiastical authorities in their desire to remove the fear, and, therefore, the pain, of childbirth, can only be awaited with patience; in the meantime let us assume as historical necessity the teachings of the past, but let us also move forward with the advance of science that has overcome so much of the distress to which our forebears were subjected.

10

The Retreat of Fear

And, finally, when a woman becomes pregnant for the first time, she usually seeks medical advice. According to her social position, she either attends the outpatient department of a hospital, an antenatal clinic, or visits a doctor. In some country districts, the local midwife takes complete charge from the beginning. This of itself is evidence of anxiety; she wishes to know that all is well and to be in contact with some person from whom she can get advice upon matters relating to the birth of her child. From these sources she will arrange for the presence of a midwife or a doctor at her confinement and for a bed in a suitable maternity hospital if it is not convenient for her to have her baby at home.

We overlook, perhaps, the excitement which attends these preliminary arrangements and the disappointment when preparations cannot be made according to plan. During pregnancy, the average girl needs considerable support; she requires explanation of unfamiliar occurrences. From these people, who, in her eyes, are the experts on childbirth, she learns – the doctor, the nurse and the antenatal clinic are responsible for her attitude towards childbirth.

It would be expected, therefore, that a woman whose prenatal history is not marred by ill-health should not have any anxieties about labour or fears for herself and her child. It is obvious, however, that in spite of the close attention given to young mothers during their first pregnancy, fear is not completely eliminated.

We must examine this question from the point of view of the woman herself. Although there is no constant law, there are certain factors which the average girl thinks about. Some supply an adequate answer for themselves; others do not trouble to ask themselves or anyone else any questions. But we may perhaps enquire: what are some of the thoughts which predominate in the mind of a sensible girl who is pregnant for the first time? I suggest that most of them feel that they have embarked upon a rather risky adventure; they have the courage to see it through, of course, but cannot help thinking about it sometimes, and even wondering what will be the outcome.

Many of them consider that it is only right and proper that they should suffer certain discomforts. I find that very few women are willing to believe that sickness and nausea are not necessary for pregnancy, and some even consider it their duty to be either sick in the early morning or the late afternoon. There are vast numbers of women who have had large families who have felt neither sickness nor nausea during pregnancy and yet it appears to be an accepted fact that, if pregnant, there is sickness, and sometimes if there is sickness, it is presumed to be pregnancy. This association was so fundamental to two people who came to see me that the woman, who was about thirty years of age and very large, confided to me before her husband that although they had only been married a few weeks she was afraid that she had fallen because her husband had been sick every morning for ten days. This was most seriously stated and with equal solemnity I had to point out I thought it more likely to be the husband who had fallen; he had the facies and physical appearance of a 'bottle a day' man! Morning sickness is one of the horrors of pregnancy to many women of all classes of society, although it frequently occurs at teatime! To women who are energetic or who have to earn their own living, the limitations of their habitual activities cause considerable distress. Many resent giving up those occupations which had meant pleasure, exercise or livelihood. It is not yet established as a teaching amongst women that all normal pursuits which do not demand any grossly unnatural performance are in keeping with healthy pregnancy and if a woman has to earn her living, she should be able to do so within a few weeks of the birth of her child. Expectant mothers do not give up housekeeping in the homes of our working classes until their babies actually commence to be born.

When a girl is very young her appearance, shape and gait are matters of serious importance. She is rightly proud of her figure; she demands to retain its beauty; she dislikes the ungainly spectacle of women whom she has seen in the later months of pregnancy; she fears swollen ankles, pigmented patches upon her face, white lines and stretch marks upon her abdomen and development of the breasts. Without attention to these matters, and explanation and care from one who shows obvious interest in her well-being, she may brood and become depressed until pregnancy itself is a menace to her most cherished possessions.

We have already pointed out that she will have good reason to believe that these discomforts will culminate in a painful experience of danger to herself and her baby. Even if all goes as well as it is possible to expect, she has got to suffer pain, and however bravely she may discard this ominous threat, she will find it difficult to compare favourably the state of childbearing to the physical freedom and spiritual buoyancy that were her delight during the first few weeks of marriage.

Do doctors, nurses and antenatal clinics delve into the thoughts of women who appeal to them for help? Do they realise the profoundly important influence of these most intimate considerations? Experience teaches us that here and there an understanding midwife or medical man, prompted by human sympathy and insight, will tactfully eliminate these causes of physical and mental disturbance. But the general teaching of experts is that antenatal care should be primarily scientific; the anatomy and the physiology of the woman should be investigated; the efficiency of machinery and metabolism should be determined and at all costs an abnormality or even a suspicion of abnormality should be recorded. Few women are interested in their own antenatal investigation beyond receiving a positive reply to their request: is everything all right? That indeed is some comfort in their suffering – a small mitigation of their sentence.

They have their pelvis measured; their blood pressure taken; their abdomens listened to and prodded; the urine is examined from time to time; blood is taken for grouping, rhesus factor and group listed; if all is well, a few hints as to exercise and diet echo in their ears as they pass out of the building, wending their way among those who anxiously await investigation. Perhaps one of their number exhibits an abnormality – there is a flutter in the dovecote; contracted pelvis, albumen in the urine, a breech? Whispers are heard – she is too small; her kidneys are wrong; the baby's upside down. The reality of danger is imprinted upon the minds of all who become conscious of its presence in a neighbour.

It is not suggested for a moment that all antenatal clinics are organised in such a manner that this can happen, for gradually an increasing number are paying attention to the minds of their women patients, and every care is taken to maintain a cheerful confidence in the natural outcome of pregnancy. There used to be two kinds of antenatal clinic – one which laid great stress upon the obstetric care of women and the other which conducted obstetric examination but emphasised the art of mothercraft and personal health during pregnancy. Each was good in its way, but each lacked a feature which was essential. Today, these two aspects are combined in the best schools, with the result that mind and body receive adequate attention.

It is perhaps those attended by a private doctor who, in many cases, meet with the greatest difficulty. A doctor's wife who came to me, six-

and-a-half months pregnant with her second child, astonished me by remarking, when I took her blood pressure: 'I have never had that done before.' Knowing that her first child had been seen into the world by an obstetrician of high repute, I suggested that perhaps my blood pressure instrument was different from those previously used, but she said: 'I have never had my blood pressure taken before.'

She complained of great lethargy and tiredness, and told me that she still had some nausea every day. I asked her if she had ever had any advice upon her diet. Her reply was, 'No. I have been told to eat normally.' I took a drop of blood from the lobe of her ear and found that her haemoglobin was under the 60 per cent mark. I inquired if she had ever been given iron during her previous pregnancy and she replied, 'No. I do not think I was suspected of anaemia.' She told me that at the time when either her third or fourth period was due after the first baby had started, she had considerable haemorrhage. She was put into a nursing home for some weeks, and it was suggested that a placenta praevia was present. She felt very ill for the rest of her pregnancy and was not allowed to take any exercise or do any exercises. She was in labour eighteen hours before her medical attendant arrived and told me that she suffered an agony of suspense and was conscious now of having resisted by every means at her command the progress of labour, lest the child should arrive before the doctor. When he arrived she was anaesthetised with chloroform on a mask and recovered consciousness about three hours later. She does not know how her baby arrived. I asked her if instruments were used and she said she had not been told.

Being suspicious, I inquired, 'Were you torn at all?' And I was amused to hear her say, 'Oh, it was only a scratch.' 'Did you have any stitches?' 'Yes. My nurse told me that only three were necessary; one inside and two outside.'

That was the story of the wife of a specialist, cared for by specialists, with every advantage and opportunity that science and skill can offer. And what was her final request to me as she left after that consultation? 'I want a baby that I know to be my own. My child is very sweet, but I have never really felt that he is mine. Can you make this baby part of me after it is born?' I could only reply that I would do my best.

Now, if that can happen to a woman who has the opportunity to receive the most highly perfected education and treatment during pregnancy and childbirth, what are we right in presuming of thousands of women who attend doctors who, although equally conscientious, are less well informed, less competent and less experienced in the arts and crafts of obstetrics?

Twenty years ago it would have been much easier for me to have described the fear-producing activities of a midwife. Since then, I have had the experience of lecturing to midwives in many countries, of answering their questions and discussing with them the difficulties and problems which arise in their daily practice.

Today it is generally recognised by members of Midwives' Associations, Maternity Centre Associations and their subsidiary branches that one of the first principles of good midwifery is to protect a woman in labour from fear-producing words and actions. I believe it to be true that in certain sections of society women have more confidence in the midwives who attend them than in medical men or women. But there is still much to be done; the obstetric nurse has to be present from the beginning of labour; she has to bear the brunt of the woman's emotional strains and stresses of the first stage of labour; it is her province to explain what is going on; to give confidence and maintain calm. In my opinion, the first stage of labour is not only the most important but the most difficult to conduct efficiently. How many doctors have, in their lives, been with a patient from the beginning of her first labour to the end? It is during this time, when the mind of woman is more acutely sensitive to impression than ever before, that a superlative degree of tact and understanding is required. Such things as the preparation of the room, the laying down of dust sheets, or maybe newspapers, sterilising bowls; drums and innumerable dressings; antiseptics; lotions, methylated spirits, etc, make women wonder: why? It is difficult to lie in bed, or even be up and walking about, whilst you are subjected to entirely new sensations in the early stages of what you believe to be a great event and to watch preparations going on about you for later stages of that event, the details of which are still mysterious. Possibly one of the greatest sins a midwife or nurse can commit is to exhibit the overefficient bustle of a woman who is determined to make her presence felt. It is a temptation to endeavour to gain the confidence of a patient by demonstrating the methodical perfection of preparation. It is also a great temptation to some nurses to establish their reputation by recounting previous experiences or by describing the abnormalities it has been their privilege to witness. I only wish to draw attention to the possibility of selfish thoughtlessness. Unfortunately even today we hear of women who have been told the most alarming things in order that they should be 'kept quiet'.

It seems strange, as I examine my notes and peruse records, that on the whole, and I believe it to be true, a much higher percentage of practising midwives appreciate the importance of fear in labour than is found amongst medical men. A Canadian member of the Midwives' Institute, who has been working for twenty years in one of the outposts of the Commonwealth, over forty miles from either a telephone or a doctor, wrote home to her teacher, who is now one of the senior officials of the Midwives' Institute in London: 'We must avoid as far as possible any tendency to fears that the prospective mother may have. Fear is infectious and we must guard against the malady ourselves or it will be reflected in our patients.'

Let us consider what happens to a girl in a maternity home for her first baby. She probably has every care and attention from the purely obstetric point of view, but is it often remembered that nothing is more terrifying to her during her first labour than being left alone? These rooms where women in the early stages of labour are taken 'to get on with it' until they are ready to be moved into the labour ward, constitute a considerable source of trouble. Two, three, or even four women lie together, some quietly bearing the unexplained sensations; some suffering pain; some crying out in sheer terror with each contraction. From time to time a nurse comes in; there may be a word of encouragement; it may be that the clothes are just turned back so that nurse can 'look'. But there are few words of explanation, little or no instruction and not infrequently they hear the moans of their neighbours in the labour ward as the door swings open. To me there is nothing more horrifying than the state of mind of a sensitive girl who has to go through the isolation and desolation of those waiting hours. At length, with her spirit almost broken by assaults of agonising doubts and fears, she is deemed ready for the final stages. If she is well enough, she puts on her dressing gown and shoes and walks or staggers to the labour ward, stopping for a while to hang on to the nurse's arm whilst another contraction comes and goes. She then finds herself being led into such a room as she has never seen before. In spite of her condition, she notices in the twinkling of an eye her surroundings; the nurses, and perhaps the doctor, draped in long white gowns, white caps and masks; she sees only their eyes and is therefore unable to be comforted by kindly expressions on the faces of those about her. In a small annexe, or even in the room itself, are sterilisers and large, bright, metal drums. She does not fail to notice the glass-fronted cupboard in which hangs a large collection of instruments; she has heard of instruments, but had no idea that they looked like that. On the table by her bed are bowls, dressings and towels; at the head of the bed, or somewhere nearby, are stands with cylinders of gas.

Then she climbs upon a high bed, harder and more uncomfortable than any she has ever known; she probably feels the chill of the mack-intosh sheet with only one thin covering over it. She lies in whatever position she is told.

I wonder if the average man can even imagine the thoughts that would go through his mind if he were subjected to a similar experience? Some, I know, would be unconcerned, particularly if they had been told what was going on, but it must be remembered that many young women even today do not know what lies ahead of them, for 'having a baby' means, to a primipara, what she has gleaned from other women; that is usually poor comfort.

And so she lies upon her side or upon her back, awaiting the next move. Possibly she is informed that when the pain becomes unbear-able she may have a whiff of chloroform or a breath of gas; she is not told why, neither is she given the opportunity to discuss the question; if she were, doctors would frequently hear something they would be unwilling to believe, for many women have stated frankly and openly that their cries were not in pain – they just could not help crying out; their demand to be put to sleep was not because of pain, but a means of escape from the fear of the unknown that possessed them. I hesitate to say how often women have demanded anaesthetic, not because they were in pain, but because they 'felt it was about to hurt'; not because of the pain they had, but because of the pain they believed must inevi-tably arrive.*

We must, to the best of our ability, examine closely every moment of the experience of parturition if we are to eliminate the pain-causing factors which are not only unnatural but unnecessary. I have discussed this aspect of labour with my friends who are in charge of obstetric units of large hospitals; the more experienced are willing to admit that it is a weak point in their organisation, but their invariable comment is, 'It's got to be like that. We have neither the time nor the skilled at-tendance available to give the personal and individual care that you suggest.' Unfortunately, the construction and organisation of our most modern hospitals show that little provision is made for the care of the mind of the woman in labour. Although this is still true of far too many hospitals, the organisation for the mental care of the patient is being rapidly acquired by progressive obstetricians. No new hospital

---

*Since this was written a change has been made in many of the great obstet-ric hospitals of the world. The ideal of natural childbirth is being sought and a much happier reception may be expected by young mothers. Their fears are allayed by the understanding of the nurses and doctors in attendance; the im-portance of the emotions in labour is recognised.

is being built without special attention to this important aspect of parturition.

Of the innumerable instances of the influence of such surroundings I will only quote one, but it is typical of many. She was a patient of mine, aged about twenty, in an extremely well-run maternity hospital. She was the wife of an army officer, and had had her first baby naturally. She took an interest in what was going on and assisted in the birth of her baby without any desire or demand for anaesthesia. My visits to her had been a great joy to me as she was what I considered to be an excellent example of the true happiness of motherhood; the atmosphere of her room was entirely carefree and refreshing to all who went to see her. Her baby was ten days old when I paid the visit that depressed me. It was my accustomed time when I opened the door of her room, expecting to see the sun shining in through her window, vases of flowers filling the room with colour and fragrance, her face wreathed in smiles of welcome and to hear her cheery greeting. I was surprised, therefore, to find the curtains drawn and the girl lying down, resting. When Sister let in the light, I saw my patient looking miserable and tired, and quite different from her usual, normal self. When I asked her what was the matter, she hesitated to tell me because, she explained, she was afraid I might think her rather silly. Sister, however, offered me an explanation. During the night a woman had had her baby in the hospital and she had made a frightful noise which started at about three o'clock in the morning and went on continuously until five-thirty. I was given to understand that someone was in charge of the case who was not familiar with the methods that are now practised there. It was the first time this girl had ever heard the sort of noise women can make when they lose control and are not looked after properly whilst their babies are coming. I offered her no explanation, but said I was very sorry she had such an alarming experience and assured her she must never associate it with a normal natural labour. But what interested me was the remark of this girl of twenty, who had been so completely controlled and so excellent throughout the whole of her own labour. She looked up at me with tears in her eyes and said: 'If I had heard that before my baby arrived I think I should have felt like dying when it started to come because I should have been terrified. I think it was the most awful noise I have ever heard in my life. It made me turn cold every time it happened.'

I replied that I was very glad she had not heard it before her own baby arrived and suggested the possibility of the other woman not having been instructed sufficiently about labour, or taught how to conduct herself, for had she learnt control and been given understanding, she would have had no reason to cry out and no desire to cause such a disturbance. My patient asked, 'Why was she not taught?' And in reply I handed her a small handkerchief from her bed table and smilingly suggested she should wipe a large tear from her cheek.

In the hospital in which I have to do most of my work this unhappy situation not infrequently arises. The Matron and the labour ward sisters are beyond reproach; they use, with exceptional ability, the procedures of natural childbirth, but many patients are sent in by their doctors without any antenatal preparation. Others arrive who have attended so-called prenatal classes at which they have learnt nothing from their inexperienced teachers which is of value to them in labour. There is nothing so disconcerting to a woman in labour as to find that she has been misinformed of the part she must take in the process of parturition. Untrue statements are worse than no teaching for they add to disappointment a complete loss of confidence in the attendants. It is not unusual for these unhappy women to lose self-control and make unnecessary noise, which is very disturbing to the equanimity of women in labour in adjacent wards.

Much damage can be done by this inadequate preparation. The good intentions are there, but one important factor is absent and that is the protective education of pregnant woman. A wonderful picture of positive painless achievement is repeated at each meeting or class. Surely any teacher of experience knows that no one has the right to imply without some qualifications an invariable course of labour.

A hundred variations of physical and emotional phenomena must be provided for in the mind of the good clinician and any that are harmful or threatening to the comfort or well-being of the mother or her child call for special attention and care.

Women trained and prepared for a natural birth have suffered severe frustration and disappointment when deviation from the absolutely normal is deemed best to be rectified by assistance. Others who suffered more discomfort than they were led to understand might occur have hesitated to ask for, and even been unwilling to receive, pain relief and thereby increase their babies' and their own troubles. Women improperly prepared believe that pain relief by injections, drugs, or analgesics is evidence of failure and become morbidly depressed. I have too many reports from others who blame themselves because salutary scientific interference has been clinically indicated and skilfully employed. This is not the woman's fault. Had she been properly and understandingly prepared she would have known the possibility that help might be advisable. In some way or other birth can be made easier for both mothers and babies in a certain number of cases. This easement of the mental or physical stresses or strains is correct in obstetrics as well as in the course of human kindliness, during pregnancy, parturition, and the puerperium, that is, before, during, and after labour.

No woman unprepared for the possibility of rectifiable difficulty has been taught the natural childbirth principles for in these it is strongly emphasised, in simple terms, which enables her to understand that modern science can help when in trouble. Such knowledge gives courage and confidence and not fear.

But however well prepared and confident in her ability to achieve a satisfactory and natural birth a woman may be, ultimately her success depends on each individual of the team of people to whose influence she has been subjected during the changing phases of her reproductive activity. A word, a thought, a look, or a gesture from nurse or doctor can wake up doubts and fears which not only assault her faith, but cause tensions and discomforts that may, in a flash, turn a happy progressive natural performance into a conflict of discomfort, disappointment, and distrust.

I cannot repeat too often the wide field of responsibility of nurses and doctors. It is not only the absence of irrational fear, but the positive emotions that must be encouraged and in truthful terms made a reality which justifies confidence. This is when the attendants must give, not take. They must appeal to gentle reason and firm common sense for rigid regimentation is of itself a one-way track to fear when the way is not familiar. This situation must arise until all women are properly prepared and their emotional changes during labour recognised by the attendants.

Although from the point of view of the medical attendant the strict avoidance of all possible causes of fear during labour will be emphasised when the conduct of labour is discussed, attention must be given to some of the more common errors of judgement that occur.

The obstetrician should be fully aware of the extreme sensitiveness to all forms of stimulus of the parturient woman. The keenness of her perception must be appreciated; every expression, movement and incident is observed; no word or action passes unnoticed; the occasion demands her fullest concentration. Nothing else matters, and everything of which the human mind may become conscious is gathered in by her alert receptors, either to increase or to decrease the tension of the moment. Any communication from those in attendance which can possibly be construed to disturb her peace is harmful. An excess of sympathy may be mistaken as foreboding trouble; a jocular demean-our does not help to dispel her fears. Exhortation to be brave, if crude-ly given, is as harmful as the suggestion of lack of courage.

Many obstetricians will remember having inquired if the pain was getting worse or where the pain was being felt. It is overlooked that such questions constitute strong suggestion to the end that sensations are intensified and their interpretation as pain becomes inevitable.

Women demand above all things complete confidence in the de-pendability, personal strength and skill of the man who is with them during labour. They do not want soft words and sob stuff but expla-nation, instruction and encouragement. They want to hear that all is going well, that the baby is well and that they are conducting their job in an admirable manner. If they are not told these things, they assume that all is not going well and become alarmed with each new, though normal, phenomenon of labour. Many women have been ter-rified when, at the height of a strong contraction, the membranes have ruptured; they have felt the flood of warm liquid of which they had not been warned. Many women have felt no discomfort, but have actually been interested in the hard work, until an officious attendant has asked them to say when the pain becomes unbearable as it is about time they had some anaesthetic. I have actually heard a man say in the labour room, 'You had better get my forceps boiled, nurse. I don't think I shall need them, but you had better have them ready; you never know.'

So many of these would-be kindly actions are prompted by igno-rance of the true meaning of the phenomena of labour. The groan with which the diaphragm is released after a strong second-stage con-traction is thought to be a moan of pain, demanding relief. It has no relation to pain. The tight grip of a woman's hand is not an indica-tion of her suffering; the call for anaesthetic is not necessarily a cry to be relieved of physical agony, but a demand to escape from some impending horror that her imagination has formulated in the absence of truthful instruction.

After I had lectured to the Gloucestershire Midwives' Association, a lady of the committee, commenting upon such observations as these that I had made, related the following story:

Her niece was in labour. Being a natural and healthy girl who be-lieved that parturition should be a simple and not a complicated act, she proceeded to play her part extremely well. Her attendant was a kindly and experienced physician. As the second stage progressed he was somewhat astonished at the calm and purposeful behaviour of his patient. As the violence of her contractions increased, he seemed to

share with her the agony that he believed she suffered, but she quietly
perservered. Peacefully unconscious of her surroundings between the
contractions, she was vigorously helpful when they occurred. Finally
it became too much for him; he could sit by no longer and watch such
torture, however courageously borne. He produced a mask from his
bag and a bottle of chloroform. 'Now, when the next pain comes, just
put your face in the mask.' With the next pain she buried her face in
the pillow. Somewhat surprised, he repeated his request, with the same
result. Feeling that she did not understand, he said, more loudly, 'Now,
with this pain, put your face in the mask, and I will give you a whiff.'
But she put her hands over her face instead, Possibly by this time his
dignity was disturbed, for quietly but very firmly, with the warning
of a contraction, he admonished her. 'You must do as I ask you; will
you please breathe in the chloroform. It will take away your pain.' She
avoided the mask however, and when the contraction had been well
and truly used and she had taken one or two deep breaths and had
again become relaxed, she turned her face up to him and, smiling politely, said, 'Oh, do please go away. Can't you see I'm busy?'

How many thousands of women have longed to say that, even less
politely, when they have been pestered by a surfeit of sympathy and
misunderstanding.

It is obviously impossible to protect women against the ravages of
fear if their mental processes remain a mystery to their attendants and
the phenomena of labour are misinterpreted.

But let us consider another aspect of this subject – what does the
doctor think of childbirth? How will he influence his patients by the
thoughts, unexpressed it may be, that formulate the attitude he adopts
towards his patients? Unfortunately, it is not yet recognised how the
opinion of the medical man is understood by the patient not only in
health but in disease, without any word to communicate his feelings.
There is an atmosphere; there is an unexpressed thought and apart
from that there are those psychological influences which are conveyed
from mind to mind by some mystic method of which we are at present unaware. There is, none the less, no doubt whatever that from one
person to another a very definite influence is conveyed. Confidence is
imparted or fear is awakened and although the patient may enter the
consulting room in a state of anxiety – as indeed all patients do to a
greater or less extent – it is that mystic something which the physician
conveys, not only in his manner, but in his personality, which formu-
lates the end result of the consultation. A cheerful voice, a glib remark
and a smiling face is never sufficient to hide the apprehension that the

physician may have for the well-being of his patient; neither is the bald expression of confidence sufficient camouflage to cover any anxieties that linger in the back of the physician's mind. An obstetrician of no little repute once remarked to me, 'When a girl comes into my consulting room and tells me she is going to have a baby, I often wonder how she will stand the pain and what the effect will be upon her body and her mind of the ordeal which she is so ignorantly undertaking.' I look upon that as one of the most pitiful remarks that a scientist can make. He presupposed from the beginning that that woman was going to suffer an agonising experience; he made no allowance whatever for the skill and the modern methods by which he could prevent that suffering. He knew that labour must be painful and therefore cogitated upon how she would stand the experience of pain. In that he was not alone. It may be that many obstetricians do not even consider how a woman will behave; they merely consider whether she will be within the range of normal, and whether the case will present to them difficulties which are likely to cause anxiety or necessitate interference.

It is generally believed in the medical profession that labour must essentially be a painful and trying ordeal to every woman. There are very few doctors who are willing to admit that they believe labour can be a pleasurable experience because there are very few who have the slightest reason for holding that belief and, further, most doctors today would scorn the idea that labour could be a happy experience. And why should they think that labour could be anything other than painful, dangerous and a time for anxieties both for the woman, her relations and the doctor himself? They have been educated to that outlook; their teachers have taught them that it is so. In the wards they saw women in pain; it was understood that women should have pain; they absorbed the belief that travail was the ordeal of motherhood and nothing in their experience had ever come along to disprove that belief. We cannot therefore cast a single aspersion upon medical men who are willing to accept this medieval attitude towards one of the greatest, or, I may say, the greatest, of all human functions.*

Our science has not considered the necessity for altering the views of medical men by discovering cause and reason for pain, so that the

*What a wonderful change since I wrote this twenty years ago. Practically every doctor of the younger school knows today that childbirth need not be unbearably painful. The approach to a parturient woman is one of confidence, not fear; it may be that the stereotype obstetrician still saturated in the teachings of three decades ago finds it difficult to alter his ways or his ideas, and so it is for a short time that with many the old order remains.

mind of the doctor may convey an honest persuasion of safety, peacefulness, happiness and success to the girl who enters his consulting room with the information that she is about to become a mother. What they think, they convey to their patients; as I have said before, they may try to maintain a cheerful attitude and discuss normality and nature, but always in the back of their minds is the corollary, '...and should there be pain, I assure you that anaesthetic will be given; you shall know nothing about it, and we will do our best to prevent you from suffering those things which women usually suffer.'

I would make it clear that this is no accusation, and that it is most certainly not a condemnation of my professional brethren. They look upon this thing called labour, childbirth, reproduction or whatever else you will, in much the same way that those who have gone before looked upon a variety of illnesses for which no cure had then been discovered; the wasting, neuritis, and the suffering of those who died in thousands from beriberi, was considered inevitable. The cause was unknown; the cure was unknown, until someone stepped forward to point out that owing to civilisation, the rice, the food of the people, was being polished, and the pericarp which nature had provided as the antidote to this disease, was being removed. Then it was understood why beriberi occurred. It is now not only avoidable but curable. The neuritis, the wastings and the horrors of that disease are no longer considered inevitable. We read that suppuration of wounds, particularly of amputations, was, by the old surgeons, looked upon as inevitable; it was part of the disease; nothing would prevent it until antiseptic surgery was discovered and used and until its demonstration proved that suppuration was not necessary. Now, suppuration after a clean amputation is looked upon as a surgical failure.

And so it is with innumerable conditions to which the human body appeared to be heir in generations that are past. Until the causes of conditions which were considered inevitable were discovered, no treatment was accepted as a cure until it had been successfully demonstrated. Each pioneer who has brought forward some means by which the cause and cure of one of these accepted tragedies have been made plain, has been subjected to stern criticism, to scorn, and even to the accusations of those about him. It is always the hardest possible thing to persuade our profession that this or that need not be.

And so it is with labour. It is my belief that there is not one feature from the beginning of pregnancy to the end of the puerperium which should in any way mar the health of a woman, but that it should on the other hand increase her happiness and her physical stability for all time. I am prepared to state that in the not very far distant future, inevitability of painful parturition will be a relic of the past. I believe most definitely that since the probable causes of pain have been investigated, and since certain theories have been promulgated and demonstrated with relative success, pain, and therefore fear, will be eliminated, not by anaesthetic, but at its source.

But for the moment we are dealing with the physician and with his belief and with, therefore, the direct influence that this belief has upon women about to undergo the perfecting of their own function of motherhood. Why, I may be asked, does this increase the fear that a woman has of childbirth? My reply is that the average medical man is unable to destroy or prevent the causes of fear that have been referred to previously in this chapter because he is unaware of the influence of fear and therefore there is nothing upon which his patient can place her entire confidence. Frequently fear and pain are initiated by the physician himself owing to his entire lack of understanding of the true significance of the phenomena of pregnancy and childbirth. It is difficult to give confidence when you have none; it is not easy to eliminate fear in another when you are apprehensive yourself. Confidence, understanding and fearlessness are essential factors in easy childbirth.

It is just over twenty years since I wrote the last four or five pages of the chapter upon the fear of childbirth. It was my intention to remove them in this edition and write more of the immediate present, but, as I read and reread, the lessons of those twenty years came vividly to my mind. What a wonderful change has come over the people; we no longer hear the constant terror story from the lady of the tea table or luncheon party. The fear of childbirth is no longer a dominant factor in the homes of the newly wed. The great multitude of young obstetricians of today had not started their medical curriculum when these pages were extracted from records and observations of over twenty-five years of attendance upon women, most of whom were fearful in childbirth.

In those early days women were not educated in affairs of motherhood. They were not seen in public places in the later months of pregnancy and before the First World War we did not discuss childbirth or maternity matters in mixed company.

But today how magnificently different. Motherhood and childbirth have become the proud privilege of woman in all classes of society and all civilised countries of the world have caught up with the ancient and cultured races in the religious and spiritual association of childbearing and mothering of their babies.

In Great Britain and throughout the Commonwealth women meet together to discuss frankly and openly the problems of pregnancy and labour. Trained and experienced teachers instruct and prepare them so that they understand much that was unspoken mystery to their own mothers. They know that healthy woman is not designed to suffer in childbearing; she is wonderfully constructed and equipped for this, her most desirable attainment. In these classes – women call them antenatal schools – the education is in natural childbirth. The law of nature, when understood in its simplest form, replaces fear with awe and respect for the creative spirit. Throughout the United States of America every city and sizeable town has its natural childbirth organisation. Some chose different names, but all the same basic teaching. And so it is in every country of Europe and in the countries of South America. The ancient fear of childbirth is rapidly fading from the cultural horizon and with it so much illness of the mind and body which today we know originates from injury to, or disturbance of, the physical plan by unnatural or exaggerated emotional states.

I have been given permission to quote a pamphlet from the Natural Childbirth Association of Milwaukee, USA, which is also used by La Leche League of Franklin Park, Illinois, USA. These are examples only of the approach to childbirth of hundreds of women's organisations which have been founded and prospered all over the world.

It is, in a way, an advertisement and if some women are persuaded by happy experience that they must give all women an opportunity of similar childbirth they have every right to use what methods they find most efficient for their purpose.

WHAT IS NATURAL CHILDBIRTH?
FACTS YOU SHOULD KNOW

Natural childbirth is
FEARLESS childbirth
TRAINED childbirth
RELAXED childbirth
EASIER childbirth
SATISFYING childbirth

especially if a mother is helped to GIVE *birth* to her baby
consciously without too much discomfort, instead of 'being
delivered' while unconscious.

TO PREVENT POSSIBLE MISUNDERSTANDING
HERE ARE SOME THINGS
NATURAL CHILDBIRTH IS *NOT*:

Natural childbirth is NOT necessarily painless childbirth.
Natural childbirth is NOT an endurance test. Anaesthesia is used if
needed or wanted.
Natural childbirth is NOT a failure if an anaesthetic used.
Natural childbirth is NOT a denial of the achievements of modern
obstetrics.
Natural childbirth is NOT a step backwards.
Natural childbirth is NOT a denial of the importance of the doctor
for physical care during pregnancy and labour, but a belief that
psychological care is also important.
Natural childbirth is NOT hypnosis.
Natural childbirth is NOT connected with 'birth control' or 'planned
parenthood'.
Natural childbirth is NOT a cult, nor does it have any religious,
political, or racial affiliation or bias.

The explanation of natural childbirth as herein expressed was prepared by the Natural Childbirth Association of Milwaukee and is
reprinted with their permission. It is offered as a service to mothers
by:

LA LECHE LEAGUE OF FRANKLIN PARK

THE PRINCIPLE OF NATURAL CHILDBIRTH
IS THAT CHILDBIRTH IS A
NATURAL – NORMAL – BODILY FUNCTION

and should not cause any discomfort that would be unwillingly
borne by a normal, happy mother...

WHO has the co-operation and encouragement of her husband,
WHO wants her baby and fearlessly and lovingly welcomes its birth,
WHO is healthy in mind and body,
WHO is prepared in mind and body for the great event of birth,
WHO understands what is happening to her and to her baby during
the process,
WHO knows how to relax during labour when this is needed,

WHO knows how to work with the forces of labour when this is
needed, and
WHO has kindly and understanding support and encourage-ment
from those who attend her in labour.

Anything new and important becomes the centre of controversy.

My first brochure upon the facts of childbirth was written in 1919, but it was not acceptable for publication. Forty years ago it was considered disputatious but in 1933 *Natural Childbirth* was published and not only did the subject become controversial but the author 'a controversial figure'! Today there is no longer any controversy. The influence of fear in childbirth is an accepted fact in universities and maternity hospitals of cultured communities. Neurophysiologists offer a variety of opinions upon the activities of nerve tissues in the psychosomatic manifestations. For obstetricians, however, the *Fear-Tension-Pain Syndrome* as a basis for clinical events gives excellent results in over 95 per cent of natural births.

But in so short a time, a change of this magnitude cannot sweep aside the orthodoxy of yesterday. There are those who have not learnt, those who do not wish to learn and those who have not been given the art of learning, but they retain the right to publish their unhappy experiences and derogations of principles they have never known!

It is from these groups that stimulating criticism comes and draws attention to the natural childbirth teaching, by high praise, faint praise, dull apathy, condemnation and active antagonism. The enthusiasm of the first two of these groups is the result of practical experience, defended and justified by results. Of the last three, none has accurately or repeatedly employed the full teaching of natural childbirth, or indeed read its precepts before offering stern, apparently authoritative, advice against this 'recent innovation'. The human race has survived and vastly grown for a quarter of a million or more years without any fundamental change in the biological pattern of woman's reproductive function. What is called a 'recent innovation' is in reality only the uncovering of the immutable law of nature. Only the mind, which has been granted the exercise of its own indiscretions, has threatened our existence; only the mind has brought fear to motherhood by discarding the ageless lessons of natural law.

11

Diet in Pregnancy

Marcus Aurelius Antoninus wrote in the *Twelfth Book of his Thoughts*: 'Cast away opinion; thou art saved.' This is comforting for during the last thirty-five years I have witnessed many changes in the accepted opinions of authorities about the diet necessary for a pregnant woman.

Today women are no longer passive receptors of routine. I have frequently been astonished at the intelligent questions that have been put to me during antenatal instruction; strangely enough it is not always the so-called educated who are the most enquiring. Expectant mothers are interested in childbirth; they read and learn and are taught to understand how babies are carried and nourished in the womb; they become educated in childbirth and all its phases and implications. Diet is a topic particularly subject to enquiring and searching questions. Doctors are no longer able to say do this and do that for they receive at once the challenge: 'Why?'; and it is my opinion that some explanation should be given if the interest of the mother is to be maintained. I will give, therefore, some justification for those principles of dietetics in pregnancy which experience has proved of benefit both to the mother and the child.

It was believed in many quarters until a very few years ago that a pregnant woman must eat for two people, therefore she ate large quantities of food, quite irrespective of whether it was meat, vegetables, bread, cheese or anything else. The food to which she was accustomed was taken in increasing amounts.

About twenty years ago, the general teaching was that proteins should be cut down considerably because, we were taught, 'they throw too great a strain upon the kidney function'. Today in many countries there is a strong belief that proteins must play a big part in the diet and many diseases of pregnancy have been assigned to the shortage of protein substances in food. With the advent of a knowledge of vitamins, our interpretation of food values rapidly expanded and with the increasing understanding of the chemistry of growth, the importance of certain mineral substances was recognised.

It has become the custom to estimate the adequacy of a diet in terms of the number of calories it contains. A calorie is the amount of heat required to raise the temperature of one kilogramme of water one degree centigrade. The science of dietetics has become so intricate and involved that very few medical men can be called expert dieticians. It is obvious, therefore, that we cannot always teach women exactly why they have to eat a balanced diet during pregnancy, not only because dietetics is a complicated subject, but because no two women are alike even if they are members of the same race and living in the same community.

In the country in which I am writing, South Africa, there is plenty of food of all sorts, although there are complaints that mutton is scarce, but the amounts of fruits and vegetables and the quality of these provisions is excellent and unlimited, and there is usually enough milk.

But in Central Europe, to obtain these luxuries would be impossible for most women because of the price that they would have to pay for them. The Indians live only on fruit; the Chinese staple diet is rice; the African natives in some of the tribes know very little other than mealie meal, an occasional piece of meat, an egg and some milk. There are many vegetarians among the Japanese who have demonstrated that it is possible to be first-class athletes and men of great physical strength without touching meat or estimating the number of calories of which their diet is composed. I can think also of those healthy, happy people, some of the tribes of the Eskimos, who know only flesh, who have lived on it and been born and brought up on nothing other than mother's milk and fish.

It is practically impossible, therefore, to lay down a general rule which is applicable all over the world for the diet of pregnancy. Today it is not that which is best for a mother but that which a mother can obtain, that we have to accept as the basis for her diet during pregnancy. Our responsibility is to see that as far as possible the constituents necessary to health are in balanced proportions and adequate both for the mother and the growing fetus.

The general principle, therefore, is that a woman who is healthy and becomes pregnant and who has acquired a certain regime of feeding, enjoying constituents of diet which may be environmental or necessitated by social conditions, should continue to eat as she has been accustomed. There is very little reason to change the food of a healthy woman leading a normal life because she is pregnant, but there are certain points, however, which should be observed by those who attend to women having children.

EXTRA FLUID is beneficial. Eight or ten glasses of LIQUID a day can be used by the body and assists in the metabolism of other foods. An adequate amount of PROTEIN should be taken – by that I mean lean meat, eggs, milk, peas, beans and nuts. FATS should be eaten as they are fuel for heat and energy in the body and are found in cream, butter, cheese and some of the fat meats. CARBOHYDRATES are energy-making and are found in sweets, flour, sugar, potatoes, also in milk and rice. If there is not enough IRON in the food, there is a possibility of a woman developing anaemia. If the quantities of CALCIUM and PHOSPHORUS in the diet are smaller than the body requires, types of illness might arise which could easily have been avoided or corrected if this deficiency had been recognised. The growth of the teeth and bones and the resistance to disease are largely dependent upon adequate MINERAL supplies. These observations also apply to VITAMINS, which will be referred to lower down.

It is usually suggested that a pregnant woman should take one quart of milk a day. Well, this is very pleasant for those who can both afford it and obtain it, but there are many countries in the world today where it is quite impossible to obtain that amount of fresh milk. This also applies to the sound advice of dieticians who advise that one serving of meat a day, fish or chicken, with liver once a week, an egg at least every day and three or four slices of wholemeal bread should be eaten. In many countries it is quite impossible to obtain such luxuries. This is the advice of idealists and optimists in a hard world.

For my own part, rightly or wrongly, I have become sceptical about the accurate implementation of the principles of dietary to pregnant women and my reasons may be summarised as follows.

I have had the privilege of seeing women of many different races have their babies; not only women of European origin but also Chinese, Indians, Africans and those who have followed various cults such as vegetarians and fruitarians. I have also delivered women who are almost entirely meat eaters, women who have eaten meat and fish up to two, three or four pounds a day and very rarely touch milk and eggs, or even bread.

An interesting observation that one can make is that, on the whole, providing that the woman's diet has suited her for a number of years prior to her marriage and pregnancy, there has been no evidence of higher rate of disease in any one group and no difference in the manner in which their babies have been born. In fact, I have found that the diet of people has tended to make very little difference providing that it is the accepted diet of the mother and that upon which she has been brought up from childhood. I refer only to healthy women, not to those who are ordinarily undernourished and who show signs of deficiency diseases before they become pregnant.

I must advise simplicity, however, and I do not like women to continue to take alcohol because it was their habit before they became pregnant. It is my custom also to restrict table salt. There is quite enough in food prepared in the ordinary way and any excess may precipitate illness especially in the later weeks of pregnancy. The Chinese women are first-class mothers and breast-feeders. They eschew all salt from the beginning of pregnancy until they cease to feed their babies. The custom has been evolved from years of wisdom and experience.

From these comments, which may be accepted as generalisations, we must draw certain deductions.

First and foremost, the question of diet in pregnancy is an environmental matter, which must be solved on the spot. Secondly, in most countries today, women who are going to have babies can get in touch with medical men or members of organisations which care for pregnant women and advise them when there are signs or evidences that their health may be impaired by their mode of living. The health of the expectant mother has, in most countries, become a national responsibility.

In countries with highly organised communities, medical advice is available for pregnant women and it is the doctor who should give the final instructions upon the adequacy or otherwise of a woman's diet or her manner of living. The adviser should give his opinion upon, first of all, the AMOUNTS OF FOOD and the NUMBER OF MEALS to be taken during the day and the constituents of the meals.

During the first twelve or thirteen weeks of pregnancy, possibly 50 per cent of women who are having babies have some feeling of nausea or even vomit. This is very largely a nervous complaint but can be influenced by a correct method of feeding.

There are also women who suffer ACUTELY FROM HEART-BURN, or acid risings as this complaint is sometimes called. Here, again, changes in diet may help to relieve this unpleasant condition and not infrequently it is found to be associated with the wrong quantity of food or the wrong combination of foods that the woman is taking. These are matters that the doctor should decide when he makes his examination during the antenatal phases of early pregnancy.

There are the women also who suddenly DEVELOP AN ENORMOUS APPETITE for some particular type of food, such as half a pound of chocolates a day. Other women may have a strange and unusual liking for beer; in fact many changes of desire for different foods and flavours may occur during pregnancy. It is a recognised condition known as Pica. Apart from the QUANTITIES, the doctor should and will observe if there is any evidence of a MINERAL DEFICIENCY.

Minerals. It is possible that he may find CALCIUM is not being taken in sufficient quantities. This is environmental; there are places where calcium is not found in either the water or in the earth from which the vegetables are grown and in some parts of the world calcium deficiency plays an important part in the health of pregnant women. In Ceylon the soil is so deficient in calcium that domestic animals have to be fed on it to remain healthy and in parts of South Africa the soil is very poor in this mineral. In some of the large coastal town areas there is a marked deficiency in calcium in both water and soil. The incidence of certain diseases of pregnancy is relatively high and the breeding of pedigree horses and cattle in these apparently lush districts has never been a success.

This information emphasises the wisdom of drinking milk during pregnancy, but it should be remembered that the routine administration of relatively vast quantities of calcium in tablets and powders is quite unjustifiable – very little of it being assimilated. Unless especially indicated by disease, calcium taken in MILK or MILK PRODUCTS is best because it is absorbed from these foods in sufficient quantities to provide the 1-2 grammes a day required by pregnant and lactating mothers. Fruit, vegetables and greens also add to the daily quota of this essential mineral.

There are also areas in which there is very little IODINE, places where people develop goitres and show evidence of iodine shortage. Here, again, simple remedies may be advised by the medical attendant. I say simple because in most cases there is no difficulty in overcoming these deficiencies. IODINE can be supplied by eating sea fish once or twice a week; if that is not possible, iodised salt or medicines can be prescribed. PHOSPHORUS is another essential food which acts in collaboration with calcium and is present in protein, so that if an adequate amount of lean meat, liver, eggs and milk is taken very few women will be short of this mineral.

SODIUM and CHLORINE are minerals which also occur in the body, generally in combination as SODIUM CHLORIDE, which is common salt. This is found in most foods and since the total body requirement is not more than 2 grammes a day to maintain good health, we find the majority of people eat far more than is necessary; the excess is eliminated by the kidneys, but its absorption into the body fluids predisposes people who are drinking a lot of water to store up fat.

But IRON is very important and must be absorbed in relatively large quantities during pregnancy. The average pregnant woman will need as much as 15 milligrams of iron a day and even then it may be found that the amount in her blood is only 55–60 per cent of what it should be when she is twenty-five to thirty-five weeks pregnant. This can constitute a serious menace to her well-being and the health of her child. The problem of iron deficiency must be solved by her medical attendant; it is a complicated subject and there is no rule-of-thumb treatment. Each case must be treated on its merits, but one fact will be of interest to mothers – iron is essential to life, it makes the substance of our red blood corpuscles which enables them to carry oxygen from the lungs to the tissue of the body. A cubic centimetre of a newborn baby's liver has five times the amount of iron that is in a cubic centimetre of its mother's liver. Mother's milk, however, contains practically no iron, so iron taken from the placental blood is stored in the fetal liver to enable the newborn to have a sufficient oxygen-carrying substance in its red cells during the period of breast-feeding. The importance of a liberal iron intake will be impressed by these facts upon the mind of a pregnant woman. Foods rich in iron are liver, kidney, lean red meats – eggs are very good, green vegetables, carrots, prunes, apricots and other fresh dried fruits.

We have mentioned the importance of FLUIDS, PROTEINS, FATS, CARBOHYDRATES and MINERALS in the diet of a pregnant woman. Lastly, we must give a short explanation of VITAMINS.

There are innumerable vitamins described these days, but they are present in adequate quantities in all sensible diets – that is to say, the diets of those other than faddists. They appear in fruits, vegetables, cod liver oil, meat and in practically every fresh, unspoiled food that we eat. This, of course, varies in different countries. In countries where there is a lot of sunlight there is a much better supply of vitamins. In countries where there is little sunlight and a limited supply of fresh food, extra vitamins, such as fish oils, should be prescribed. Inadequate vitamin quota in the food affects the growth of the fetus and, indeed, may be responsible for miscarriage in the early months of pregnancy.

In spite of much research into the principles of dietetics, it was only about thirty-five years ago that the intensive study and discovery of many vitamins was made. A tremendous amount of work was done and, for nearly thirty years, on average three thousand original papers were published each year on this subject. It was soon discovered that as the bulk of the people became urbanised by leaving the agricultural areas for town and factory work, the health of a high percentage of the population deteriorated.

My friend Franklin Bicknell states (*Vitamins in Medicine*, Heinemann, London, 1953): 'A survey of the diets of more than a thousand workers in a large aircraft factory revealed that over four-fifths consumed diets which were deficient in vitamins and of those who fed in cafeterias only one-half selected good lunches although they were available on the counter.' He gives the reports of many investigations which demonstrate dramatically how growth, efficiency and good health depend upon an adequate quota of vitamin-containing foods in the diet.

Even so, vitamins are required in only small amounts. They do not furnish energy, but by their presence enable various life functions to be carried out efficiently and without them neither body building nor survival is possible.

Bicknell describes in detail the absorption and uses of Vitamins A, B_1, B_2, B Complex, C, D, E, K and P in the pregnant woman and the fetus, as well as the transfer of some of these substances from the mother through the placenta to the developing child.

Of these, B_1 is important, for a marked deficiency may lead to a number of minor and some major disabilities and discomforts. This substance is found chiefly in cereals, not much in milk or meats, except pork. Wholemeal bread has five times the amount of B_1 that is found in white bread, breakfast oatmeal nearly ten times the quota of white bread and quaker oats even more. Bemax and Marmite (flavoured yeast) have one hundred times and brewer's yeast nearly one thousand times the B_1 quota found in cheddar cheese. Nearly all fresh meats contain this vitamin in good quantity. Peas, butter beans and soya beans are good, having approximately ten to twenty times the value of white bread. This vitamin can be destroyed easily or seriously reduced by overcooking or boiling the foods in which it is found. Whenever possible fruit or vegetables should be eaten raw or lightly cooked.

A deficiency of Vitamin C used to give rise to scurvy in sailors of the olden days, when their diet largely consisted of salted meat, no fresh food or vegetables; its presence not only avoids such diseases but assists in the rapid healing of injured tissue. We also know that Vitamin D, which is largely concerned with the bone formation, is necessary for the development of healthy babies. It is interesting that very little Vitamin D is present in human milk, but more than sufficient is rapidly formed if the infant is exposed to sunlight or ultraviolet rays. Vitamin A not only assists in the growth of the child but has the power of reinforcing the efforts of the body to overcome infection by some of the common organisms.

But the summary of this is that in a well-balanced diet which contains fresh food, milk, calcium- and iron-containing foods, and citrus fruits and vegetables there is no need to be worried about the vitamin intake. I cannot recommend a woman to swallow, as is so frequently advised these days, vitamin and mineral tablets until she is taking six or seven different sorts of pills a day in order to replace the deficiencies which she is told that her diet is likely to exhibit. This is not really true. For my own part, unless there is some diagnosable deficiency I rarely, if ever, prescribe either calcium or iron or vitamins to a patient who is pregnant unless her diet is obviously inadequate or unsuitable. This course, however, requires the personal observation of the antenatal attendant.

I have in front of me now the diets of six different countries for women in pregnancy. The differences in advice are not without interest, but the general principle remains the same. The simpler, the fresher and the nearer to the natural foods that women can take during pregnancy, so much the more effective will their diet be both for themselves and their babies.

There may be some who are more interested in the details of the problem. Let them consider therefore that the average pregnant woman, that is to say the woman of about 130–155lb weight, should have approximately 2,000–2,500 calories daily. This can be made up if she will remember that 1 gramme of protein will liberate 4 calories approximately and she should take 70–85 grammes. One gramme of fat provides a little over 9 calories and a gramme of carbohydrate a fraction over 4 calories also. If the amount of protein, fat and carbohydrate food is weighed, although this cannot be accurate, a very good idea can be obtained as to her total caloric, that is to say, her total heat energy, intake during the day.

It must be generally accepted that women who are on a good, well-balanced diet usually enjoy good health and their babies are born well-nourished. A good or a bad diet does not really seem to influence the birth weights of infants; neither does it appear to interfere with the child's resistance to disease after it is born. There is no obvious change in the manner in which a baby is born because the mother's diet is below standard, unless it has been so poor that deficiency symptoms or disease intervened during pregnancy.

There is, however, reason to believe that premature births are much fewer when the diet is adequate and balanced from the beginning of pregnancy onwards. This was shown in a large experiment carried out by ten hospitals in London at which records of these observations were made. There was, however, one observation which is worthy of particular attention for it was demonstrated both by the People's League of Health Investigation in London and also in what is known as the Toronto Experiment, carried out in 1941 in Toronto General Hospital. However good a diet, there is no reason to believe that because of food alone a woman can avoid the possibility of suffering from some forms of anaemia, although the incidence of other illnesses and diseases was very definitely lowered by a good diet. Therefore I repeat, when a woman is pregnant she should visit a doctor or some institution where the condition of her blood can be ascertained and her haemoglobin quota assessed. Unfortunately, we cannot overlook the fact that the feeding habits of many women today, who should really know better, are extremely lax. This does not only apply to pregnant women, but to practically all so-called civilised countries. We have become 'speed and flavour seekers' – food is overcooked and sauces and flavourings are added to make the meals more acceptable. We have adopted the habit of eating at certain times, rather than eating when the stomach requires food. I think it was Nietzsche who made the comment: 'Through an entire lack of good sense in the kitchen, mankind's development has been retarded more than through anything else.'

The same principles apply both during gestation and lactation. The feeding mother should continue to take milk up to two pints a day and drink more water than before the baby was born. She must not take salt other than that which is used for the cooking of food. There may be articles of diet incompatible with the baby's digestion. For instance, green stools and colic have been observed to occur when vegetables and certain fruits have been taken in large quantities by the breast-feeding mother. There is no rule – some infants will have pain if their mothers have taken strawberries, oranges, rhubarb, or even sauerkraut and coleslaw. The majority of women, however, do not meet with these difficulties when feeding their babies; although attention must be drawn to them, they are rarely of any importance.

In short, the principles of diet in pregnancy may be epitomised as follows: eat sensibly, simply and discreetly, recognising the essential constituents of food, and including in them sufficient, but not excessive, quantities to maintain good health and provide for the development of the baby. Look upon meals as important and pleasant pauses in the daily round. Put aside for an hour all ambitions and anxieties – eat slowly and enjoy the natural flavours of food of which quality not quantity is the quintessence. Be restful and relaxed in comfort and conversation, finish before you feel full and have time for fifteen minutes quiet reading or rumination before returning to the duties of the day. This aids digestion and prevents the signs and symptoms of dyspepsia which are so often avoidable discomforts.

12

The Phenomena of Labour

It is one thing to assess the strength of the enemy, but it is another to conduct a campaign in order to win a battle. So far we have considered the association of pain and fear with labour. Whilst disbelieving in the necessity for pain and deploring the prevalence of fear, both are almost invariably present in what is known as normal labour. Not only the lay public but the medical profession as a whole accept pain and have overlooked fear. It is obviously a very difficult position to uphold and although from a careful scrutiny of the facts that have been collected the theory of natural childbirth appears to be logical, the majority of the civilised world had good reason, from practical experience, to regard the theory with suspicion.

What 98 per cent of childbearing women have felt and 100 per cent of obstetricians have taught and believed since man became civilised is quite likely to stand the test of assault, especially when that assault is made by a lone voice crying in the wilderness. Theories alone are useless; they must have practical application and even then, however successful the results of practice, they will probably be scorned by those in authority who are not prepared to give them fair trial or for whom it is inconvenient to be impressed.

These considerations, however, have in no way influenced me to give up what at first sight appeared to be an impossible task, and the decision was taken some years ago to manage normal pregnancy and conduct uncomplicated labour in the belief that intense pain is unnatural and pathological. Pain was caused by tension and tension by fear. For years an aphorism was imprinted on my mind, 'Tense woman; tense cervix.' All obstetricians know the effect of a tense cervix: pain, resistance at the outlet and the innumerable complications of a prolonged labour with probably an operative finale.

It became obvious that the first place to strike was at the cause of tension. I believed that to be fear; therefore, a closer study of fear in relation to childbirth became necessary before it was possible to try to eliminate it. In the previous chapters there is sufficient evidence to show the fear of childbirth originates from so many sources and from such high places that the whole scheme of society would have to be altered if the attack were made at the source. It was equally obvious to me that those who have suffered were very unlikely to refrain from saying so, and even less likely to preach their suffering was unnecessary. It was also rather difficult to go round saying that the Bible and the Prayer Book do not really mean what they say. And finally I came to the conclusion that it would not be much fun to shake a theory in the faces of my confrères as a means of persuading them that all the greatest obstetricians were wrong and that on no account should anyone believe what they said. It appeared to me to be rather like a flyweight squaring up in the corner of the ring to, not one, but a dozen professional heavyweights.

It will be seen the correct line of procedure was not obvious. On the other hand, I must own to a profound affection for my theory and that, combined with a modicum of quiet pigheadedness which always stimulates a Norfolk man to discount odds, prompted me to get on with it without further 'quavery mavery'. An effort was made, therefore, to educate women in the facts of pregnancy and childbirth; to promise them nothing, but to assure them of relief from their doubts. I soon received encouragement, for many women instinctively felt the truth and disbelieved in the necessity for suffering. That did not appear to be enough, for it was found as soon as labour commenced, the accepted principles upon which it was conducted actually produced a state of tension in the body. Exaggerated receptivity of the mind to all forms of stimulus, both physical and psychical, swept aside their good intentions and defeat had to be acknowledged. Some method had to be found to overcome this main weapon of the enemy, which was tension.

So the practice of physical relaxation was introduced, not just at the time, but during the last four or five months of pregnancy. By applying this to the conduct of labour it was found that the mind remained at rest, muscular control was possible and, what was more gratifying than anything, the interpretation of the sensations experienced during labour was not invariably that of pain.

In a short time I was more astonished than my patients. In the absence of turmoil, anguish and misunderstanding, many of the phenomena of labour appeared in their true light. After not more than two years, the results of the application of these procedures had not only established my own belief but – what was more important – the large majority of the women whose labours had been conducted in accordance with them had an entirely new attitude towards childbirth.

As time went on and experience increased, a closer understanding of the minds of women in labour became possible. Education and explanation dispelled their doubts; a good courage was born of that confidence; they became interested in the performance of their own parturition. To my astonishment they held the apparatus of anaesthesia in their hands with full knowledge of its use, but refused to take it. They were able to criticise their own sensations during labour, and to differentiate between hard work and pain. Those who had learnt relaxation not infrequently lay peacefully at rest throughout the latter part of the first stage, awaking only to control their breathing during contractions but continuing to maintain physical relaxation of the body apart from the respiratory apparatus. Throughout the second stage their receptivity to stimuli was lowered to such an extent that many were unconscious of incidents occurring and words spoken during that time.

It is necessary, therefore, to explain what is meant by 'education'. There is no rule of thumb to such teaching, for no two women will or can accept facts in the same words. It is not a question of social class, for similar varieties of women are represented in all classes of society and judgment must be used in each case. The same applies to the ability to attain relaxation; some are better than others and the results vary accordingly.

When labour starts, each woman must be treated according to her understanding and having outlined the general conduct of labour so that all fear may, as far as possible, be eliminated and physical relaxation attained, I propose to relate what has actually occurred during the labours of different types of women.

Then the observations of the women themselves will be reproduced over a consecutive series of normal labours. These will include remarks upon relaxation, the conduct of labour from the woman's point of view, anaesthesia and their impressions of the birth of a child. These few chapters will constitute a record of the ways, means and results of the practical application of the theory that has been set out in previous chapters.

There will be certain clinical observations to make upon the phenomena of labour and philosophical considerations of motherhood, all of which are in direct relationship to my efforts to change the existing teaching and all of which are to the end that the Fear-Tension-Pain complex as a necessity in childbirth may cease to cast its shadow across the glorious art and science of obstetrics.

The expression 'phenomena of labour' has been used several times in preceding chapters. It does not appear to be generally recognised that parturition is divided into three definite stages by signs and symptoms. The first stage is not just the dilating of the cervix uteri; it is a part of the process of labour which presents certain features, all of which can be shown to be purposeful. If a woman comes into labour with her neuromuscular mechanism deranged by fear-tension influences, she does not experience the phenomena of normal labour. For fear-tension is pathological and the resultant corticothalamic impulses produce abnormal conditions of mind and body which override and inhibit the natural processes. In the presence of fear, elation is impossible, but where education has been satisfactory and the commencement of labour is the joyful prelude to her child's arrival, a woman is conscious of each uterine contraction as a harbinger of her highest ambitions. Elation, rejoicing, and a strong sense of contentment and relief is the natural emotional reaction to the onset of labour.

There is abundant evidence to show that 'pains' under these conditions are painless. A woman may be conscious of uterine contractions for hours, but have no discomfort until she is told that she is in labour. The association of parturition with pain is so firmly implanted in the minds of many women that the only interpretation of these new and mysterious sensations is pain, unless they have been well and truly educated in the art of labour before its onset.

I use the term 'elation' in its strict meaning. It is not a simple happiness, but an exaltation of the mind resulting from the feeling of success and pride in the confident approach of the reward of pregnancy. Many women become conscious of their own importance at this time and the strong instinct of self-assertion may be observed. This state is not often seen by doctors because they are rarely, if ever, present at the beginning of a normal labour. But the good midwives know it well and do their best to preserve it until the doctor arrives. The majority of women who do not fear labour ring up on the telephone in a cheerful spirit when they think they have started. Such phrases as, 'I think I have started. Isn't it heavenly?' or 'Things are happening; I am so thankful.' This emotional state was described to me by a vivacious, intelligent girl in simple yet dramatic words. I have previously quoted them in *Natural Childbirth*. 'I have never known such a sense of joy,' she said. 'I walked out into the garden; I felt an irresistible desire to parade myself. I made a point of going to speak to the gardener; I told the chauffeur to be ready to go out in the car at any moment; I have no idea why, but it seemed as near as I could reasonably go to telling him that my baby was coming. I walked down the drive and up and down the road for five or ten minutes, feeling in the back of my mind a hope that I should meet some of my friends. My time had come; my baby was on its way; after all it was true. I believe now that I actually exaggerated my shape.'

This is only one example of many instances that have been recorded to me. Women do not hesitate to say they are glad when their baby is coming at last, but few will volunteer, without questioning or inquiring, to describe the profoundly stimulating emotions that accompany the onset of labour when complete confidence in its outcome dispels all fear.

The mental state is of the utmost importance. The sequence of events from elation is – determination, calm, relaxation and neuromuscular harmony with sympathetic nervous-system inhibition. Fear, however, promotes a desire to escape, mental turmoil, tension and disturbed neuromuscular harmony with the sympathetic nervous system impulses overriding the pelvic autonomic. *Elation* maintained under these normal psychological sequelae produces an easy, unimpeded first stage and is natural and primitive, but *fear* maintained until the vicious circle of its influence has produced the state of resistant tension, pain and exhaustion is pathological and cultural.

To all nurses, mothers, midwives and husbands, I say: do nothing to destroy the cheerful courage and confidence of the girl who has commenced labour with her mind in that state; bury your own anxiety and fear and share with her the spirit of victory about to be achieved. You will thereby assist in paving the way for her progress to uncomplicated motherhood and ward off the greatest enemy to her neuromuscular perfection. There are few greater obstetric crimes than to become a serious busybody, who demands compliance with illogical and baseless conservative principles, such as those who request silence, speak in whispers, parade a mass of so-called essentials ready to deal with all emergencies. The kindly sympathy and word of warning advice is disturbing to a happy girl; she does not wish to visualise her labour as progressing from one horror to another, culminating in a 'when-the-pains-are-too-bad' time. She sees only the impending joy of her child's arrival, and believes that it will come quickly and easily. Elation is an emotional state, but it has profound physical manifestations; it is not only a part of the reward of childbirth, but it is a phenomenon of which nature takes most subtle advantage to facilitate the safe reproduction of her species.

I was speaking to a midwife in charge of a large area south of the River Thames. She had been assiduously carrying out antenatal education on the phenomena of labour. By explaining what happens when a baby starts to come, an intelligent interest had been awakened in the minds of the women whom she attended. The ignorance amongst such women appalled her at first. 'What do you know about child-birth?' she asked. 'Only what Mum has told me.' 'And what has she told you?' 'To be sure and do as the nurse tells me.' And that has been for generations their only prenatal education. Unfortunately the nurse cannot always remain with primiparae; her busy life demands visits to other women whose babies have arrived during the previous fort-night. So for a time many young girls are left to the tender mercies of friends and neighbours during the early first stage of labour. 'That is where my greatest difficulty lies,' this nurse explained to me. 'Not only mothers and mothers-in-law, but friends and neighbours crowd in and offer with one accord the time-worn advice, "'Ang on yer pains, dearie; 'ang on 'em"!' So from the beginning of labour the poor child is encouraged to push and bear down, pull on arms outstretched to help her and exhaust herself in an effort to help which results only in hindrance. It seems impossible for some women to realise that the first stage of labour demands peaceful relaxation, quiet assurance and disassociation of the mind from the mechanism of the uterus.

Any effort to assist actively or to reinforce normal first stage con-tractions is designed to defeat its own ends. The secret of rapid cervi-cal dilatation is disassociation; the more flaccid the abdominal muscles and the muscles of the pelvic floor remain, so much the more easily can each uterine contraction pull the cervix over the head that is being gen-tly pressed down into the birth canal. General tension of extra-uterine and skeletal muscles brings into play the circular fibres of the cervix and lower uterine segment. Determined and fruitless bearing down diminishes the elasticity of the pelvic tissues and produces exhaustion from the use of power in its wrong place and at the wrong time.

Relaxation must be recognised as a necessary phenomenon of nat-ural labour and it should be accompanied by an alienation of the mind from any active interest in the uterine function. How often have I said, 'You can do nothing to help yet; allow your uterus to get on with its work undisturbed by your inquisitive interest. If you interfere it will resent it and hurt you.' Almost invariably, that advice, when acted upon, results in the relief of pain and discomfort caused unwittingly by efforts to assist.

But even if efficient relaxation and disassociation are practised, there is always the possibility of a few relatively painful contractions at the end of the first stage – the final dilatation of the cervical canal. The pain is referred to the mid-sacral region and can be relieved by firm rubbing, or more often by really hard pressure on the sacrum. It is described as an acute ache and sometimes persists between contractions. It is caused, in the main, by the maximum stretching of the lower uterine segment and cervix. There may be small lacerations of tissue, for not infrequently such contractions are followed by a definite show of blood. I suggest that this is a simple mechanical phenomenon, for when a ring is expanded by a sphere, the mechanical advantage of the downward thrust of the sphere increases as the diameter of the ring enlarges. Similarly, if a series of rings is pulled over a dilating spherical object, the larger the rings become, the greater the expansion caused by a given force.*

Normally, a cervix is dilated much more rapidly from three inches to full than from half an inch to one and a half inches. The last few contractions increase the tension in the already well-stretched tissues of cervix and lower uterine segment and the normal nociceptors record pain stimuli as reaction to stretching and laceration. This is referred to the area of the sacrum and lower end of the spine. If, at this stage of labour, there is pain anywhere else it is probably due to some factor not usually present in normal labour. For instance, acute pain in the twelfth dorsal or upper lumbar region is not uterine in origin, but arises in the structures which take the strain of labour, but which, if healthy, should do so without discomfort. On many occasions I have formed the opinion that the only true pains of normal labour, if present at all, are the last few contractions which completely dilate the cervix. When this discomfort is recognised and its significance appreciated, a woman may confidently be asked to put up with about six or eight such contractions. The reaction to such a request is almost invariably an easy compliance. 'If it is only six or eight, I don't mind, but I thought it might be going on and getting worse all the time now.' And so it proves to be true; this short phase passes into the more definite but completely different second stage. The discomfort of the end of the first stage lifts, either gradually or suddenly, and this appears to depend upon the mode of onset of the bearing-down reflex.

Sometimes a uterus calls for external help immediately the cervix is fully dilated, but, on the other hand, the cervix may be fully dilated for some time without any reflex demand for assistance from the extrinsic muscles of expulsion. Therefore, it is advisable to introduce to the contraction a stimulus to this important reflex. This is done through the respiratory function.

Vide Natural Childbirth (Heinemann, 1933), Chapter VI, pp78–81.

In the first stage, respiration is naturally free and as dilatation progresses, increases in rate and depth. From twenty-four to twenty-eight full breaths in a minute is normal at this time, followed by one or two deep breaths as the uterus relaxes, as occurs after the prolonged use or strain of any muscle in the body. But in the second stage, as a contraction develops to its greatest tension, a deep inspiration is made and it is held during the bearing-down effort. Now, if the cervix is dilated fully, the woman should be made to draw a deep breath and hold it at the height of the contraction. Not infrequently, after doing this once or twice she will begin to bear down and will remark upon the satisfaction the effort affords her. Once the reflex is started in that way it continues and the distinctive phenomena of the second stage become increasingly apparent. With the uterine contractions, somatic relaxation is impossible, but between them it is easier than at any other time during labour; in fact, as the uterus works more violently in its effort to expel the baby, a relaxed sleep in the intervals between contractions is commonly observed. It is not easy to explain, however, why the 'pain period' of labour, when it occurs, may persist until the second stage is relatively advanced. I suggest that a possible explanation of this may be found in the initial changes that occur in the mentality of a woman at this time. As the second stage becomes fully established, acquired social habits and manners are thrown off. She becomes aware of the conscious effort demanded of her to help, so far as possible, in the expulsion of her child. She is engrossed in her task and concentrates upon the all-important occupation of the moment; she demonstrates the relative inactivity of her senses of discretion and discrimination, she becomes oblivious to her surroundings and careless of her appearance, expression and speech. Normally, that is, in the absence of any dominating fear – she is devoid of any consciousness of herself and employs all her energies in the fulfilment of the immediate purpose. When the muscular effort ceases, her mind and her body relax and she passes into a restful, sleepy state, sometimes into a deep, snoring slumber. This condition of complete alienation from other thoughts and associations either causes or passes into a state of amnesia and partial anaesthesia; the perception is dulled and the interpretation of stimuli through the normal channels clouded.

Some years ago I wrote: 'It is possible that the initial stages of the lowering of mental acuity which results in the typical amnesia of the second stage may have a direct result upon the interpretation of sensations that arise at the end of the first stage. As the mind becomes clouded and the awareness of the woman decreased, so the interpretation of pain appreciation must be temporarily intensified with the gradual release of conscious control, just as our mental images as we sink in sleep are more vivid though less accurate than those we see when widely awake.'

This may or may not be the case, but it is an observation made beside the beds of women at that time. So frequently does the drift towards amnesia or dulled consciousness coincide with the phase of pain interpretation of normal sensations, that some association between the two phenomena is possible. As the level of consciousness is lowered still further, so the sensations of labour cease to be painful and only the truth of the inborn subconscious mind remains.

A school of thought has arisen which ascribes the excellent results of the natural childbirth procedures to some form of hypnosis. Experienced midwives have observed that, when arriving at a house late in labour, they have frequently found the patient in the carefree, semi-conscious state that I describe. These women had received no instruction, but they were not afraid although alone in the house or hovel of confinement. The question naturally arises under whose or what hypnotic influence have such women acquired the state alleged to be 'waking hypnosis'. There is, in reality, much evidence to show that the awareness of the second stage of labour has no relation to any previously recognised hypnotic state. The native woman who squats on the polished cow-dung floor in the corner of her hut displays a similar dullness of the mind in the same stage of labour; this I have seen myself. It is a symptom with a physiological purpose and is present in all labours uncomplicated by fear.

I cannot lay too much stress upon the necessity for recognising this *amnesic state*, and the changes in perception, interpretation and reaction that accompany it. It is a phenomenon of first magnitude and importance, for if this state is acquired with the mind in a turmoil of doubt and fear, frontal areas of discretion and discrimination react to the most potent and unimpaired stimuli, which are fear and self-protection. This accounts for the unbalanced behaviour of the woman who is afraid during the second stage. If control is removed from a mind which is undisturbed and confident, a quiet peace remains; but if control is removed from a mind struggling against doubts and fears, the reactions to fear become apparent and the effort to escape at all costs, by any means available, resolves itself into an appeal to the sympathies of those attending her that she may be released from her turmoil.

It is because of the lowered state of consciousness, and therefore impaired control, that fear prompts them to escape. How often has the obstetrician heard, 'Can't you do something, anything, to get me out of this?' The fundamental belief in pain permits only the interpretation of all sensations as agonising in the absence of her discriminating senses. The onset of every contraction is the harbinger of renewed torture; the expectant tension of her mind results in early exhaustion and the excessive drain upon her nervous energy produces symptoms of profound shock. There is no pretence or play-acting in this; the woman suffers; and her pitiable appearance rightly calls for all the encouragement and relief within the power of the physician to give. Her cry for anaesthesia is an escape demand. How infrequently is it realised that the majority of women fly from fear into unconsciousness and not from primary physical pain. This is best demonstrated by the relative absence of discomfort when a woman retains both confidence and courage. 'Hard work, yes; the hardest work I have ever known,' was the criticism of a fearless woman. The physical reactions to the emotional state in the second stage must be more clearly understood if interference is to be avoided in normal labour.

Constant assurance of adequate progress sinks into the dulled mind if quietly and considerately given. Your patient desires the unwavering strength of confidence you share with her in the successful issue of her trial. And trial indeed it is; for in labour a woman shows her true colours – the patient and impatient; the courageous and 'gutless'; the 'I-can-and-I-will' women and the 'Oh-please-I-can't-and-what's-more-I-won't' women are all met and all require different handling, but with one accord they seek encouragement and comfort in the support and strength of their guide and protector in labour. The obstetrician, alas, is in an unenviable position if he has not educated her to understand the experience before it commences and she is indeed in an unhappy dilemma if the significance of the phenomena of normal labour is not understood by her physician.

But let us take another view of this picture. It is absurd to expect a sympathetic man to sit by and watch a woman suffer when he has at hand all the means of preventing it. The suffering is so real, so acute and above all the long-drawn moans sometimes resolving into sobs of desperation and hopelessness, are sure evidence of her agony. This aspect of labour is accepted and taught and in the honest belief that these manifestations are immutable and unavoidable, humanity with its noblest gesture has stepped in to slay the dragon and so free the princess.

This is no satire upon the escapades of modern science and certainly no lampoon upon any erudite contemporary, but a simple justification of the ways and means at present employed for the relief of women in labour.

So long as the phenomena of labour are not observed and the design of nature in the series of events that occur throughout parturition is not recognised in its full importance, no other way lies open to those who would relieve pain. Until the mind and its emotional forces are understood in an elementary manner it is obvious that the physical manifestations of cortico-thalamic impulses are likely to be misunderstood.

Take, for yet another example, the grunts and groans during a second stage contraction. In an uncomplicated labour they vary as the woman's emotional state and not only as the strength of her muscular activity. In a natural labour, these grunts have no association with physical pain. The large majority of undrugged and fully informed women have very little if any discomfort with second stage 'pains', but a deal of hard work. It is the grunt and groan of a man who pulls successfully upon a rope; the physical strain is of the utmost; his determination adds to the violence of his effort; when he relaxes, it is with a groan of satisfaction and relief that he may rest in preparation for the next pull and having rested he is ready for a renewal of his exertion. So he struggles in the sure confidence of victory until at last his objective is attained and, according to his valuation of the prize, so is the joy with which he hails success. His contortions have not been accompanied by physical agony, though his facial expression may well have represented it. His groans have been physiological, for our bodies abhor a sudden change of tension and most of all a sudden drop in intra-abdominal pressure. The diaphragm must be gradually released and the muscles of the chest slowly relaxed from the strain of their rigidity. There is nothing to cause purely physical pain, but the partial closure of the larynx which produces the grunt, groan, or long-drawn moan is a part of the design for safety after effort.

But consider the man whose rope is irresistibly pulling him towards agony and death. As he takes each strain, terror fills his heart; each violent and prolonged effort seems to bring him nearer to inevitable torture and with each relaxation from the tension, his expiration is released with a cry of anguish that is born of exasperation. He will seek to fly from his torment, but cannot break away from his task; he will call long and loud for help which cannot reach him. He knows the certainty of his appalling fate and as he feels the dreaded moment approaching he is filled again with apprehension that saps his strength and drains the courage from his spirit. This is not physical pain, but the anguish of travail. He has heard, he has been told, and he believes that all who have fallen into the clutches of this inquisition have suffered.

How can he escape? He does not escape unless help is available, for he has but one interpretation of his experience and to its influence he succumbs.

These two pictures represent closely the difference between fearless, natural childbirth and the parturition of a terror-stricken woman unaided by sound instruction and unfortified by elementary education in the nature and conduct of her task.

This moan and cry which prompts solicitude and kindly interference is a natural, painless phenomenon and should be encouraged, but controlled. Women have inquired of me many times, 'Why do I make such an awful noise?' It has been explained that it is as it should be and is nothing to be ashamed of; it has a purpose and I like to hear it. 'But,' they have added, 'I don't like to make such a fuss; there is no need for it.' How many obstetricians have heard after the baby has been born, 'I am so sorry I made such a noise. It seems so unnecessary, but I simply couldn't help it.' If unexplained, this crying out may increase the fear which until that time had been well-controlled. The old question arises: 'Do we fly because we fear, or do we fear because we fly?' If for 'fly' we substitute 'cry out,' it is exactly the same problem. Women are often afraid because they hear their own strange, uncontrolled cry. This has so frequently been the opinion of intelligent women with whom I have discussed the question, that the well-known Amand Routh's case (*Obstetric Transactions*, Vol XXXIX, 1897) will help to confirm the view expressed above:

A multipara, aged twenty-two, who had had three deliveries previously, had an accident which caused complete paraplegia below the level of the sixth dorsal vertebra. She had fallen fifteen feet through a trap door, holding a baby in her arms. She was one hundred and ninety-six days' pregnant. The accident resulted in complete anaesthesia and analgesia below the sixth dorsal nerve distribution and motor paralysis. (Absolute paralysis, both motor and sensory.) Sixty-four days later she came into labour and had a child weighing 5lb 12.5oz. During the *first stage* the patient was quite unaware of what was going on, feeling no pain whatever.

At the *end of the first stage*, the contractions were strong and prolonged, with small weak ones in between them; there was no pain or discomfort.

Second Stage. Contractions every two minutes lasting forty-five seconds approximately; strong and useful; head descended well. She then stated she was conscious of a tight feeling, not painful, but which restricted her breathing.

About one and a half hours later contractions were strong, and there were more signs of distress in the patient. She complained of no pain and only experienced a feeling of tightness at the epigastrium. She held her breath involuntarily and cried out on expiration. The crying out was especially evident as the occiput emerged from under the pubic arch.

These reactions to late second-stage contractions occurred in the absence of any pain or discomfort. Can it be correct, therefore, to assume that such reactions must necessarily indicate pain or discomfort?

There is yet one more observation upon the anaesthesia and analgesia of the second stage. The stretching of the vulva is felt as a burning sensation. A woman must be forewarned of this for it may be very frightening. The burning varies in intensity but is rarely of such significance that the patient feels it desirable to resort to the analgesic inhaler. The sensation is intensified by an alarmed woman – she may resist by squeezing up her pelvic muscles. An understanding attendant will overcome the slight and transient discomfort and with full crowning of the head the sensation ceases. The actual passage of the baby through the vulva is often accomplished with so little sensation that the woman is with difficulty persuaded that her baby has arrived; until she sees or hears it she is unwilling to believe it is born. In a natural labour the perineum is practically insensitive. When a tear of the fourchette occurs it is rarely felt to any degree comparable to a similar laceration of surface tissues in other parts of the body. We are not told, 'I have split and it hurts.' But the fieldsman at cricket who does not quite get to a hot one and splits between his fingers knows whether it hurts or not. When this small perineal laceration occurs, I invariably put in one or two stitches required at once and by using a semicircular needle of an inch or an inch and a quarter in its greatest diameter, the operation can be done with little or no discomfort, especially if the point of the needle passes quickly through the skin at right angles to the surface both in and out. I have never had a patient who considered that an anaesthetic should have been given. These stitches are not tied until the placenta has arrived and it is interesting to note that the tying, if not very gently done, is likely to prove much more uncomfortable than the insertion. This is probably due to the sensitivity of the perineum returning after five to ten minutes.

This relative anaesthesia persisting in the early part of the third stage of labour is worthy of note, for it allows of immediate suture of all small lacerations. It is probably true also that lacerated surfaces brought into apposition before coagulation has occurred heal more quickly and more firmly than those which remain open before they are repaired.

There is one phenomenon of labour to which I must refer in considerable detail. It is the arrival of the baby. To women who have been unconscious at that moment this conveys nothing but an extravagant mental picture. To those who have suffered the prolonged agony of anxiety, doubt and pain-producing fear, this only reads as a myth without any foundation of truth. Many such women find it hard to welcome the child who has caused them to suffer so acutely. But to those who have been educated and trained both physically and mentally for the final episode of pregnancy and who have borne their children according to the laws of nature, the truth of these observations will recall the tenderest memories of mother love.

It is my custom to lift up the crying child, even before the cord is cut, so that the mother may see 'with her own eyes' the reality of her dreams. I have been told that no woman should see her baby until it has been bathed and dressed. My patients, however, are the first to grasp the small fingers and touch gingerly the soft skin of the infant's cheek. They are the first to marvel at the miracle of their own performance; to them indeed is due the inspiring reward of full and conscious realisation. That there is anything unsightly in the appearance of a newborn babe is nonsense; that a mother might be shocked at her own baby is fantastic. Its first cry remains an indelible memory on the mind of a mother; it is the song which carried her upon its wings to an ecstasy mere man seems quite unable to comprehend. But like all other natural emotional states, it is part of a great design; its magnitude is significant of its important purpose. No mother and no child should be denied that great mystical association. Its purpose is not only to perfect the restitution of the structures concerned in parturition; it is not only advantageous for the immediate present, but it lays a foundation of unity of both body and spirit upon which the whole edifice of mother love stands.

Many times I have called attention to the wonderful picture of pure ecstasy that we see at a natural birth. Women of all ages and types have testified to this 'greatest happiness in their lives.' It is a moment when, in the full consciousness of their achievement, they experience the most intense emotional joy. 'I have never felt anything so marvellous; it cannot be compared to ordinary pleasure.' If this is intended and is one of the series of physical and emotional states in the natural law of parturition, what reason can we assign to it? Why should the serious hard work of the second stage, with its dulled senses, lowered receptivity to certain stimuli and sleepy relaxation between the contractions, suddenly disappear? It is not just an accident that the brilliant sunlight of motherhood breaks through and dispels for all time the clouds of her labour. No change in human emotions is more dramatic. The quick temper that flashes from calm to rage, with all its disturbing variations of sound and appearance, is dull and crude when compared with this amazing metamorphosis. I have sometimes been constrained to desert my established custom of observing with impersonal interest the phenomena of childbirth. Such an aura of beauty has filled the whole atmosphere of the room and such superhuman loveliness has swept over the features of the girl whose baby is crying in her hands that I wonder if I am right in my stolid abstinence from spiritual participation. 'Strange talk,' my reader may remark, 'from fourteen stone of Norfolk brawn.' But with all sincerity I repeat, I have experienced a sense of happiness myself much more akin to reverence and awe than to the simple satisfaction of just another natural birth.

This phenomenon is so definite and so inevitable if preceded by the uncomplicated events of a relaxed and relatively painless labour that it is not unreasonable to ascribe to it some result. All emotional states have a definite purpose and the more closely we examine the physiological changes consequent upon emotional activity, so much the more clearly the functional advantage of such states becomes apparent. The poise, facies and movements typical of horror, terror, sorrow, pain, anxiety and rage are not for the benefit of those who observe them. They are physical reactions to emotional states and part only of the general reinforcement, fortification or escape necessitated by the stimulus. Digestive, chemical, endocrine and excretory processes are subjected to these emotional states, so that the most advantageous conditions may prevail in the individual to meet the emergency. In comparative degrees, these emotions are less important and the facies are not so easily defined. Mild disgust, slight fear, disappointment, discomfort, doubt and annoyance are minor causes of excitation or irritation of the central nervous system which do not produce major general reactions. The gradual and persistent inroads of these harmful emotions take toll of the nervous energy over a time; the insidious disease not only saps the vitality of the higher centres of control, but the harmony and balance of all bodily functions are disturbed. Both mind and body show signs of illness. The working of the brain, the secretion of the glands, the reactions of nerve centres may be disordered and cause uneasiness and distress.

This state of chronic mental tension is frequently the cause of minor ailments of pregnancy, such as vomiting, heartburn, tiredness, salivation, constipation and anorexia. Although we are concerned here with pregnancy and parturition, how easy it is to see the major causes of illness in modern civilisation. It is indeed rare to meet a disease that has not a background of some irregularity of nervous impulse underlying its physical manifestation.

These things are the negative forces of health; they are the militant and destructive ranks of unsublimated emotional tension; they are of the omnipresent powers of evil from which injurious suggestion flows through all civilised communities.

But fortunately there are positive influences with a fund of pleasure and health-giving happiness about us. Legions ranged along the frontiers of the natural law are both protective and constructive. We see the rejuvenating pregnancy of women who have faith in the mysterious force that guides them safely through the intricacies of the great adventure. They are aware of their own ignorance and live happily in a state of mental and physical relaxation, leaning confidently upon the belief that all will be well. These are the women who pass through labour undisturbed, who assimilate instruction and so assist the mechanism of reproduction. They are free from the negative influences which bring mental and physical tension. Their interpretation of sensation from the birth canal is controlled and truthful; they allow expulsion without resistance and finally reap the reward of consciousness in the reactions of the body and of the mind at the final moment of achievement. The overwhelming delight activates the sympathetic nervous system and all the forces of that great protective mechanism are brought into play. The inhibitory fibres no longer lie relaxed and passive in the birth canal; the circular bands bind firmly the muscles of expulsion and the uterus, as if in answer to the cry of the newborn child, becomes hard and remains contracted. Let every obstetrician and midwife feel once the brisk contraction of the uterus when the mother hears her child; it is the natural stimulus to close the great blood sinuses and render the placental site anaemic, and so hasten the separation of the useless afterbirth. 'No bleeding at all' is frequently recorded, except the ounce or two of placental blood that comes away at the end of the third stage. Thus the physical reaction to this natural emotional state protects the mother from delayed expulsion of the afterbirth, excessive loss of blood and postpartum shock.

But this is not all. When exhilaration and intense joy are experienced, physical changes occur which are readily diagnosable at sight and strangely infectious. The ecstasy of love that floods the whole personality when the earliest call of a new life awakens a woman to the realisation of motherhood is a transport akin to mysticism. It is the spiritual perfection of physical achievement. Many women have written to me of this highest plane of human happiness: 'Something of which no woman should be deprived,' 'A moment no words can describe,' and so on. What does it mean? I do not know what inference should be drawn from such spontaneous and superlative expressions. The thoughts and words of women who watch their babies born are so constant that in spite of the different terms in which they are couched they must be included in the purposeful phenomena of labour. Excitement, emotionalism or sentimentality may be offered as an explanation but it does not account for the uniformity of these manifestations in that most variable and unpredictable field – the mind of woman. Young mothers with no pretensions to piety have unhesitatingly told me that they felt the nearness of God, or the presence of a superhuman being at the birth of their child. 'A heavenly feeling that they have never known before,' and it is difficult for them to believe in the reality of the present. They spoke with awe and respect for the unpremeditated wonder of their experience.

I have heard the same thing said by those about to die. Maybe the psychologists will flaunt a simple explanation for these phenomena, but let us assume, in meditative mood, that beyond the limitations of science there is a force, a power, an entity of thought which activates our motives. Do these profound experiences divest the mind of human limitation and burst asunder for one sublime moment the mundane screen that hides us from the vista of ultimate truth? Many perfectly sane men accept the metaphysical evidence of continuity of some form after this life; to many, death is a translation only. I have never been persuaded, when in the presence of death, that I am watching the end, no part of that experience breathes finality to me. Whether it has been on the battlefield or by bedside I feel a sadness that is only selfish – I know that the vehicle has run its course and stopped – but the spiritual self has gone on to merge into the confluence of an ordered cosmos. Those of us who have shared with our dearest friends the intimate companionship of their last peaceful hours do not think of the disintegrating body. We realise with Goethe that the purpose of living in this world is to provide a physical basis for the growth of the spirit. We become aware of a living intelligence behind nature. We are frustrated by our inability to understand the essence of this great designing and controlling power. We question: are we part of it or is it part of us? Or is it entirely apart from us? Sometimes in the silent hour the revelation of St John has echoed from the distant past: 'I am Alpha and Omega, the Beginning and the Ending.' The accumulating familiarity with birth and death, Alpha and Omega, that comes to us with the passage of the years increases our belief in the profound spiritual significance of the two greatest events in the cycle of human existence.

And so, when a child is born unhampered by the limitations we moderns put upon the natural laws, I am humbled before the miracle of birth and all the host of wonders that awake its mechanisms. It lives, we do not know why, indeed we do not know the source of life itself. But here, from the indestructible forces of the universe, arrives a new human form. It is unlike any other we have ever seen, different in a thousand ways from its most similar brother. It has, however, the great common denominator of all humanity: life, that inestimable gift which from the first moment is our responsibility – life which arrives, is marred or magnified and passes on. Is it surprising that at a moment of such stupendous significance, the woman who has been chosen to be the perfected instrument in the natural law of survival should be rewarded by a sense of exaltation? A new life, which of its very potential power is greater than death, should be logically heralded with pride and joy. In every newborn child there is a new hope – to every mother the people should give thanks.

But is it not here that the obstetrician should realise his privilege and his responsibility? Labour is the final act which brings a fully developed human being into the world; it has for months been influenced by the thoughts and psycho-physical reactions of its mother; already it is predisposed to a familiar pattern, but we see it suddenly possessed of individuality. It has not the ability to speak our tongue; its cries are not the tears of sadness but commands and demands for essential services. It looks at us and sucks its fingers; sneezes and expands its lungs in physiological song; it kicks and waves its arms; it micturates and grunts to expel meconium; within a few hours it learns the reward of importunity; within a few days it exhibits all the wiles of the physically helpless; by the end of a week, mother love has taken a willing child beneath its wing, or flaps pathetically to satisfy the newborn tyrant's whim.

I am inclined to believe there is an important truth in the statement attributed to Freud that subconsciously a child lives again and again the moments of its birth. From such influences the foundation of a mental structure may be built. Can we overlook this possibility?

13

The Relief of Pain in Labour

Anaesthetics and Analgesics

It will already have become clear from what I have written previously in this book that the relief of pain in childbirth depends largely upon the understanding of the Fear-Tension-Pain Syndrome. Fear eliminated from that syndrome unquestionably relieves pain and, in combination with the relief of tension, pain becomes almost negligible in over 95 per cent of normal deliveries. But there are still a large number of women who have not the opportunity for education and prenatal instruction which enables them to break down this syndrome, therefore pain in these cases is present in varying degrees of intensity. It must not be overlooked, however, in reading the methods by which pain can be eliminated from childbirth that, in a rapidly increasing number of maternity institutions and hospitals, it is being demonstrated that the absence of fear means the absence of unbearable discomfort when labour is properly conducted. Women who hold the mouthpiece of a pain-relieving device in their hands refuse to use it and resent the implication they are suffering physical discomfort. This is an observation too frequently recorded today to be waived aside as mythical; it is a fact established beyond the doubts of the most sceptical observer.

Normal Labour

There are thousands of women every year who are given anaesthetics and analgesics against their wishes to whom I will refer later; let me emphasise, however, it is the relief of pain in normal labour that is being discussed.

But what is this normal labour which allows women to escape the necessity for unconsciousness? It appears that obstetricians have differing opinions upon this subject. Some accept pain as being a symptom of normal labour, others consider a labour normal if they have to do an episiotomy and extract the baby with forceps. Many definitions have appeared in medical literature over the ages. Hippocrates, the father of midwifery, whose teaching remained practically unaltered for nearly a thousand years, in 460 BC divided labour into two kinds, namely natural and praeternatural. W. Smellie[1], in 1752, made three divisions: *1.* Natural or unaided vertex ; *2.* Non-natural or aided vertex; *3.* Praeternatural malpresentation. Robert Barnes[2], in 1874, wrote of two kinds of labour: *1.* Propitious, in which he laid stress on the absence of emotional disorder; *2.* Unpropitious, difficult and complicated labours with anxiety and dread as marked symptoms. This conveys the interesting suggestion that Robert Barnes, as far back as 1875, noticed that anxiety and dread interfered with normal parturition.

However, I would like to make three divisions:

1. Normal or natural childbirth.
2. Average or cultural labour.
3. Abnormal or surgical delivery.

Divisions of labour have been recognised by the earliest observers; there is little doubt that the normal or propitious were, in a high percentage of cases, entirely free from true physical pain. Some phenomena of labour may not have been clearly understood and therefore mistaken for pain, as indeed they are today. The old writings give the impression that natural labour was neither distressing nor difficult; but women who are not distressed and those who present no difficulty are of no special interest, therefore such cases have not been recorded. It is the praeternatural, obstetrically exciting that demand attention. Difficult cases are recorded and they have tainted and flavoured the science of obstetrics, just as a bad egg in a cake will make the cake bad; the other eggs, however good, serve no purpose, for they cannot make the cake good.

So the blind teaching has persisted, generation after generation, each respectfully following in father's footsteps since James Simpson in January, 1847, first used chloroform in labour. His first case was a woman with a generally contracted pelvis; she had already had one infant destroyed by a necessary surgical delivery. It was an abnormal labour and called for the humane and courageous experiment that Simpson performed. Since then there has been no division of labour in regard to pain. Obstetricians have been educated to believe that all labours are horribly painful; they have made a routine of using some analgesic or anaesthetic, whether labour is normal or not. This has resulted in anaesthesia for all types of labour by all sorts and conditions of attendants. Professor Andrew Claye[3] writes in *The Evolution of Obstetric Analgesia*, '...in the last few years there has been a definite move towards universal obstetric analgesia in this country, helped financially and otherwise by the National Birthday Trust Fund and encouraged by the investigations of the British College of Obstetricians and Gynaecologists.' So all the eggs are treated like the bad one! Normal, natural childbirth, free from fear or gross discomfort, is treated in the same way as complicated labour demanding skilled surgical intervention.

Physiological function is complicated by the interference essential only in pathological states. The cultural labour is fundamentally a physiological and natural childbirth which has been rendered pathological by the imposition of unnatural emotional states.

Let us consider briefly the three types of labour that I describe.

First of all, THE NATURAL CHILDBIRTH. That is best defined by the childbirth in which no physical, chemical or psychological condition is likely to disturb the normal sequence of events or disrupt the natural phenomena of parturition. A necessary corollary to this perfect condition of a woman is that she should be educated to understand what labour entails and how to assist herself in its varying phases. Also, and this is very important, she should be attended by those who understand the phenomena of labour and are able to help her to overcome the sequence of 'threatenings' that have been described in another place. There are many women who have had their babies naturally without any help from their attendants. This has come to my knowledge in letters to me from women who have read, practised and understood their duty to themselves and their child during labour. They have had natural labours although attended by medical men who had no sympathy whatever with their efforts to produce the child physiologically. They have persevered and demonstrated to their doctors how it should be done. A considerable number of medical men have been so impressed by their patients' behaviour that they have adopted these methods and used them with great success in their own practices.

When women are in labour there should always be an anaesthetic or analgesic apparatus at hand and, if necessary, they should be instructed in its use. Throughout labour, if they appear to have any discomfort from which they desire to escape, their attention should be drawn to the available means of pain relief. It is interesting that these women rarely desire analgesia; what discomfort there is does not justify its use; their ambition is to persevere and be conscious so that they may be aware of the result and reward of their efforts both during pregnancy and labour. This is what constitutes a natural childbirth and it is attended by all those circumstances which I have described in the chapter upon the 'Phenomena of Labour'.

By CULTURAL LABOUR I refer to women who are physiologically and mechanically well-equipped but not prepared for childbirth. They have doubts and fears and they understand very little of what is going on or the sensations they will be called upon to interpret correctly. Fear inhibits the normal sequence of events during labour. The Fear-Tension-Pain Syndrome is present and therefore they have real pain. Their attendants believe in and accept the inevitability of discomfort and are usually absent during the first stage of labour. Their arrival is the harbinger of anaesthetics and 'assistance' so that the women may be relieved of their turmoil and their infants as quickly as possible. This, with a few minor variations, represents modern obstetric care and attention. Fortunately it is a method which is rapidly becoming outmoded by the spread of natural childbirth methods. *But where it still exists women will have pain, and should therefore have access to anaesthesia or analgesia which should never be withheld.* These women have not enjoyed the antenatal preparation that enables them to avoid severe discomfort in labour.

The vast majority of these women are excellent subjects for natural childbirth, but they have no education to combat the evils of misunderstanding. In fact, most of them are encouraged by their doctors to believe in pain and that is the sum total of their prenatal instruction. Like the early Christian martyrs, they are hurled into the arena, naked and defenceless, to be torn and mutilated by the wild beasts; not lions, perhaps, to bring them to a violent end, but agonising fears which prolong the torture, until they, too, escape into unconsciousness. One brave man with a modern machine gun could have made short work of Nero's lions, yet we as a profession deny these tortured women the machine gun of education and faith with which the forces of fear are completely destroyed. Till this supreme provision is made, the horrors must be blotted out by unconsciousness and all the risks and losses it entails. It is not a situation of which a noble profession ought to be proud.

And finally, there is the third group, in which women have some DEFINITE ABNORMALITY, either disproportion or a malpresentation or one of those rare complications which must be diagnosed and treated by an experienced obstetrician. They are suffering from a pathological condition, an illness and not a normal state; they should receive drugs and anaesthetics in order that treatment may be adequately applied as quickly as possible. *That is one of the greatest benefits anaesthesia has brought to humanity and it should never be withheld in childbirth when a woman suffers the pain of abnormality.*

Summarising, therefore:

1. Natural childbirth women very rarely desire anaesthesia and frequently refuse its use.
2. Anaesthesia in cultural labour is almost invariably required because the Fear-Tension-Pain Syndrome has not been broken down by antenatal education, therefore analgesia and anaesthesia should be used. It must be recognised, however, that 95 per cent of these women could have natural labours if properly prepared.
3. In this case it is obvious that analgesia and deep anaesthesia given by an expert anaesthetist is required.

Indications for the Use of Analgesia

We must answer the question here: why not use anaesthetics and analgesics in all cases? Is there any contra-indication? In short, the reply to this is that no woman should be allowed to suffer pain in labour and every method discovered by science should be used to prevent dystocia. If there is true pain, anaesthetics and analgesics should be exhibited at once; but the absence of severe discomfort contra-indicates the use of analgesics. It is as great a crime to leave a woman alone in her agony and deny her relief from her suffering, as it is to insist upon dulling the consciousness of a natural mother who desires above all things to be aware of the final reward of her efforts, whose ambition is to be present, in full possession of her senses, when the infant she already adores greets her with its first loud cry and the soft touch of its restless body upon her limbs. Each of these two unforgiveable errors is constantly committed. The end result of normal labour brings a physiological reward which is happiness and satisfaction too intense for adequate expression. The strain and violence of muscular effort is swept from the mother's memory by the sound and grasp of her newborn child. Women long for this moment. 'I will have another baby as soon as I can; I must live that divine moment again and again.' This was said to me by a girl of twenty-two whose baby was only a few hours old; and similar statements are frequently heard from women whose babies have been born naturally.

The administration of anaesthetics and analgesics should have definite indication in obstetrics as it has in every other branch of medicine or surgery. Pain is the only justification; it does not matter whether the pain is secondary to fear or whether it is primarily physical. As has been pointed out, natural childbirth has no fear and, therefore, little discomfort, and few, if any, women demand relief. Cultural labour demands anaesthetics and analgesics to provide an escape from terror-stricken and tortured minds which not only give rise to physical pain but to the arrest and delay of the normal progress of labour. Emotional tension justifies relief because of the pain it causes, and frequently a mild fear-destroying analgesic hastens the arrival of the infant by releasing resistance within the birth canal.

Misuses of Anaesthesia and Analgesia

I must emphasise once more the unforgiveable custom of anaesthetising a woman as routine, irrespective of her wishes and demands. In the British Isles, the United States of America and many other highly civilised countries this astonishing and deplorable interference is accepted as normal treatment, without any clinical indication for its exhibition.

The opium pill, barbiturates or pethidine are given in some hospitals by labour ward sisters to all women in well-established labour. As the labour advances, epidural, continuous caudal or pudendal nerve block methods are employed in maternity sections of large hospitals particularly in the United States of America. During the second stage, inhalation anaesthesia is administered with the utmost disrespect for the woman's wishes. It may be nitrous oxide and air (Minnitt's apparatus), the chloroform mask, trichlorethylene (Trilene) or open ether, and the advocates of cyclopropane are making headway.

I find it most reprehensible that such a gross misunderstanding of the phenomena of childbirth should be allowed to infiltrate and persist in the procedures of so great a science. It can only indicate a deplorable lack of clinical observation or a domineering and pompous attitude towards parturient women which says: 'We are producing this baby for you, what we do is not your business, and what you want does not concern us.' I have received from far and wide some remarkable reports of this inhumane and unsympathetic treatment of well-informed and intelligent women during their labours. Many women are more afraid of anaesthesia than of labour and only succumb to the mask under the terrifying suggestion of what may happen if they do not 'take it quietly and do as they are told'!

I was lecturing a few years ago to a large country centre. The MoH and other medical people were present; some two to three hundred practising midwives listened appreciatively to my observations. The matron, whose brilliant career at a London maternity hospital justified her appointment to a large county maternity organisation at an early age, rose to speak. She spoke with simplicity and a charm of manner that accentuated the sincerity of her revelation:

'I feel it is the moment to disclose a secret. For a long time after I became matron I failed to understand why so many women asked to be looked after by the nurses and not by the medical men who attend the hospital. I was constantly embarrassed by the situations which arose and finally decided to enquire why the request was so frequently and so urgently made. The reply I had was astonishing. 'Because the doctors all make us have chloroform whether we want it or not, and the nurses don't!'' It was not because of fear of anaesthesia, but because of the absence of fear during labour that the majority of these women felt no need for analgesia. It must be remembered that they knew it was safer for their babies and they actually enjoyed the thrill of producing an infant. Twenty years ago this was not common knowledge – today it is an accepted and established fact.

But this misconception of the use of anaesthetics is found wherever doctors have had their medical education in the most modern and up-to-date schools. It seems that the slogan is: 'Dope them, good, bad or indifferent...' The ubiquity of this teaching is interesting. I have had appeals from all over the world to try and do something about it, but, of course, I can only write and hope that in due course more consideration will be given to the wishes of those who matter most. The product of one healthy mother will have a greater influence upon posterity than the total product of 90 per cent of medical brains. But let us read a few comments of women which demonstrate clearly the point I raise.

Vienna (first baby). 'They got me gas – I didn't want, it disturbed my work. I knew exactly what was happening – the baby's head was crowning. Then they gave me chloroform. I pushed the mask away and said I didn't want it, but – Bang! they put me out. ... I never heard my baby's first cry.'

Canada (second baby). 'I knew what to expect and was not frightened. I was told I was going to be anaesthetised. I told her (the doctor) I wouldn't have it and pleaded with her not to give me any, but they put the mask over my face and that was that. ... I missed hearing her first cry. ...'

Australia (first baby). 'I felt a sensation of hard work rather than anything else. What was painful was (the nurses) holding the baby in whilst the doctor rushed down the mountain side. When she arrived she immediately gave me ether; by then the child was only too eager to leap into the world. As I "came to" my vision cleared on the sight of my son hanging by his heels.'

South Australia (second baby). 'I was given a strong dose of anaesthetic as the staff saw the baby would be born quickly and the doctor could not be contacted, so my wish for consciousness at the birth was not fulfilled.'

(third baby). 'I felt the baby would be born quickly and easily, I was ordered to take gas by the sisters. 'I don't want any,' I said. The nurse tried to force me to take ether, I was resentful and indignant. I was even slapped for not taking gas when I bore down.' (Eventually the woman's remonstrances were overcome and she adds): 'I was again not conscious for the birth. ... I was disappointed.'

Los Angeles, USA 'Immediately I arrived at the hospital I was brought a pill. I asked why, adding that I was very comfortable, but I felt timid about making a fuss.' (She describes her doped condition, then she rang for the nurse because of bearing down.) 'The nurse immediately gave me an injection. That was all I ever knew until I awoke and was told the baby had been born dead ... determined as I had been to take nothing. I learned later that there was no difficulty in labour; in fact, it was very straightforward – the perfect body of the baby never breathed.'

Long Island, USA (second baby). (First was a natural, easy birth – the mother, an excellent subject, was delivered by myself in London.) The lady described her first birth to the doctor who expressed his sympathy with her wishes. ... 'Once arrived at the hospital, however, deception infuriating indeed. Not only was I injected with something I suspect strongly was twilight sleep, but once arriving at the theatre of operations, I was blacked out from the start. I was completely strapped, which prevented me from being able to protest with the vigour with which I afterwards assailed the doctor.' She came round two hours later and saw the baby after twelve hours. Afterwards the doctor apologised (!): 'It's quicker, we can't waste all that time.' 'We don't call them forceps, we call them instruments. It's for the doctor to do the work!' The baby was smaller than her first and presented no difficulty at birth.

Anaesthesia and Natural Childbirth

It is often said that when this obstetric method is used the woman is not given anaesthesia or anything else to relieve pain. The teaching is quite clear and always has been since 1933 when it was first published: *1.* No woman in labour should be allowed to suffer pain. *2.* Analgesia is always available by the bedside for the woman to use herself if and when she desires it. *3.* Analgesia is given as a drug or an inhalant according to the clinical indication and the judgement of the attendant.

The origin of this damaging myth is of long standing, although only recently it was brought to my notice by a doctor whose wife wanted me to attend her. He had read a book in the medical library in which it states that I do not give anaesthetics. I knew at once the book to which he referred. It is popular with medical students as it is short and easy to read. This inaccuracy persists, uncorrected by the author, who has been fully aware that it is untrue for at least ten years!

Andrew Claye, Professor of Obstetrics at Leeds University, in *The Evolution of Obstetric Analgesia* (Oxford Med Publications, 1939) provides a good example of the type of criticism which used to be made. He outlines the general principles of 'Natural Childbirth' but hastily adds: 'With much of what Dick-Read writes I am in agreement' (this refers to Chapter XX in Browne's *Antenatal and Postnatal Care*), 'but I *question* whether the whole procedure is feasible for the average mother.' He adds, 'But the relief of pain by drugs is also a powerful means of conquering fear and drugs are available which in my judgement provide a much simpler method. Incidentally, though the careful administration of drugs demands much sacrifice on the part of the doctor, it is probable that it is less exacting than the instruction in Dick-Read's technique, and that is a consideration to busy men and women.'

Does this really suggest that had I ever been unfortunate enough to be busy I would have learnt that the easiest, safest, and simplest way to cure a poisoned mind is to poison the body as well? If everyone accepted Claye's bald statement: 'No anaesthetic is given', there would be no material for my technique. With laudable control I reply that this is grossly untrue. All women delivered are instructed in the use of an apparatus which is placed within reach; they may use it at any moment if they have pain. In the absence of fear, pain is diagnostic of abnormality and is relieved in this technique as it should be in all others – by suitable measures. Claye should have written: 'No anaesthetic is accepted, when offered, by the majority of women so educated.' That short remark did lots of harm. One lady wrote and told me my name should be struck off the register; such inhumanity was unbelievable in our enlightened age. A society whispered that I sat and watched women writhe in agony. A doctor who had intended to invite me to tend his wife wrote and explained that he did not think it quite good enough! And so on. I feel sure that my learned confrère at Leeds has enjoyed the joke with me twelve years, particularly since I understand he has not given serious trial to my technique but prefers pernoston. He was more than justified in quoting Gauss, having ably criticised a method he had never tried out: 'As with everything else in the world, the technique must be learnt. Time and trouble, and again time and trouble, must be taken to master these methods.' Gauss is right; a certain amount of time and trouble is necessary if a practice is to be proved authoritatively good or not good. Criticism is so easy before trial.

I have referred to Claye's discussion because it is so typical of a drawerful of opinions that I have collected or received. There is not a single example of these critics volunteering the information that they have seriously applied this theory in practice. They believe in drugs and anaesthetics and therefore they continue to use them as a routine in all cases of labour. I do not ask them to wrestle, as I had to, for almost twenty years, with a problem in order to find a solution that was obviously to be found somewhere. It is humbly suggested that the practice of these methods may be made for six months only or upon fifty consecutive uncomplicated labours. Those who have done this are unanimously enthusiastic about their results.

The Medical Profession and the Relief of Pain

Of recent years much has been written upon the relief of pain, and in order to arrive at the present position of anaesthesia and analgesia in labour a considerable amount of reading has been necessary. Several outstanding facts have come to light; the most significant of these is the almost complete absence of authentic works upon the cause of pain in labour. In the introduction to Balme's[4] *Relief of Pain* (1936) Sir E. Farquhar writes: 'He has not failed, however, to emphasise the eternal truth that the first essential in the relief of pain is a knowledge of its cause...' Unfortunately, however, in the chapter upon the pains of labour, Balme did not refer to the cause of pain in labour, but merely repeated the hackneyed observations that modern civilisation, artificial modes of living, and the heightened individual sensitivity to pain are the main reasons why the civilised woman has pain, whereas childbirth among primitive people is accomplished with comparative ease.

An anaesthetist to the Royal Free Hospital, London, wrote a small book on *Anaesthesia and Analgesia in Labour*[5]. She presumed that labour must be painful; she made no reference whatever to the cause of pain; she overlooked, therefore, the first principle of medical science, which is the removal of the cause of the trouble, but she proceeded to give a very able outline of the methods by which inhalation anaesthesia may be given. She enumerated fifteen drugs that may be given by the mouth, four by hypodermic injection, three rectal administration and four intravenous.

Dr A.L. Fleming, in the chapter upon *Anaesthesia in Obstetrics* published in the *Lancet* Extra Numbers No. 1 (Wakley & Son Ltd), commences as an anaesthetist might be expected to commence: 'Obstetrics presents a large and varied field for *practice* and observation for the *student* of anaesthesia.'

At a British Congress of Obstetrics and Gynaecology in Edinburgh, Professor Chasser Moir opened the discussion with an interesting paper upon 'The Nature of Pain in Labour'. Practically the whole discussion, however, was confined to the relief of labour pain and degenerated into expression of opinion upon the relative merits of the different drugs in use. So an excellent opportunity for rooting out the cause of this evil was lost.

C.F. Fluhmann, in the Stuart McGuire Memorial Lecture for 1940 (Virginia, USA), stated: 'The employment of anaesthesia and analgesia is now so universal in this country that it must be accepted as an established procedure. The question is no longer whether they should be used, but what can be done to make them safer. It is often stated that the ideal obstetric anaesthetic must: *1.* Alleviate suffering. *2.* Not interfere with the progress of labour. *3.* Be safe for the baby. There is no such drug available, and some doubt must be entertained as to whether one ever will be found.'

That is still the most generally accepted attitude towards this subject of relief of pain in labour. It is probable that the large majority of practising obstetricians today agree with Fluhmann. But it is deplorable that such an opinion has been accepted by hundreds of the ablest men in our profession, who must have spent in all thousands of hours by the bedsides of women in labour without having applied themselves to answer the most obvious of all questions: 'Why?' All the leaders of our science know childbirth should be a natural function; for some reason or other it has become painful, particularly amongst the civilised races!

Relatively few years back, Simpson applied a method of relieving that pain; unwittingly he also provided an excuse which has appeared to justify the absence of scientific research into one of the most obvious fallacies of culture. The assumption that uncomplicated labour must be painful is the means by which the modern obstetrician hides his own ignorance and the general use of anaesthetics in labour is the method by which he says: 'What I have neither the patience nor the wit to prevent, I can at least avoid, although it is a little dangerous to mother and baby and may, perhaps, rob her of any reward, physical or spiritual, that nature is alleged to provide.' It is, therefore, on the basis that some evil as yet undiscovered has been brought by civilisation into a natural function, that general anaesthesia for normal healthy childbirth has become established.

A Matter of Public Interest

Those who advocate anaesthesia for women in labour do so, I am sure, from the kindest and most humanitarian motives. The pain of child-birth is no longer a medical matter – it has a publicity value, a political value and a social value. There are many reasons why it is desirable for certain people to associate their names with 'a good cause'. The cause also benefits from the length and quality of its list of patrons. It is not necessary to know much about the subject so long as it is sponsored by the correct people and a few meetings are held in the correct drawing rooms. There are usually one or two ambitious leaders with loud and frequent voices. This 'organisation procedure' has its points, and can be of great service in charity and fundraising, but whether it is a sound method of combating the pain of labour is certainly open to question.

Many of the most influential lay women in the 'Anaesthetics for All' movement have experienced painful labours or at least considerable pain in anticipation of the arrival of the obstetrician and anaesthetist. It is possible that upon this subject some of them sympathise with a distinguished parliamentary lady who wrote to me from the House of Commons, expressing her disagreement with my teaching: 'I have one great advantage over you and that is that I have *had* babies.' Rather than face the genius of such intuition, I closed the correspondence! But it is the prevalence of this type of mentality that necessitates a careful survey of the ways and means by which women in labour can receive adequate help. The National Birthday Trust Fund for the Extension of Maternity Services is an organisation the primary object of which is 'to undertake inquiries and experiments under medical advice which might point the way to the permanent solution of the problem of safe motherhood.' I was given to understand that one of the most cherished ideals that its committee held was the provision of adequate anaesthesia for all mothers in labour. At first sight this might have been expected to have been received enthusiastically by hospitals and nursing associations, for Minnitt's gas and air apparatus was made available by this Fund at a relatively small cost for those who wished to give anaesthetics in labour. I was astonished to hear from an official of the Fund that the demand had been disappointing and money was available to supply many more to nursing associations throughout the country. I was asked why I thought such a situation had arisen; fortunately, I was able to reply from facts I have gleaned when lecturing to many nursing associations throughout the country. The large majority of women of the working classes do not want anaesthetics for normal labours; the large majority of experienced midwives know the 'pains of labour' can be mitigated by other methods and they also know that under our present organisation a doctor can be called, in case of abnormality or distress, and he will bring his own anaesthetic. I suggested if nursing associations knew their midwives were anxious to obtain the anaesthetic apparatus on purely humanitarian grounds, the demand might even have been in excess of the ability of this very wealthy Fund to supply.

When I read through the list of the services of the National Birthday Trust Fund, I wished sincerely that one of them might have been an inquiry into the prevention of painful labour. I do not believe for one moment a single member of that very distinguished committee was ever told that if all women were unconscious of the arrival of their babies, a large number of them would be deprived of the greatest, and certainly the most beautiful, spiritual experience of their lives. I do not ask anyone to believe this who has not seen a natural birth; I need not ask those who have.

THE POLITICAL ARENA and its relation to the pain of childbirth is of considerable importance, but we sincerely hope that dramatising of the pains of labour in both *Hansard* and the public press will not prevent some of the leaders of the medical profession from approaching this problem in an academic as well as humanitarian vein.

Sir William Gilliatt[6] in the Blackham Memorial Lecture is reported to have said: 'It is not possible to stem the demand for the relief of pain, which has today become a political pawn which either party is only too happy to use if it is to its advantage.'

The agitation of certain people resulted in a bill being brought before the House of Commons, the main object of which was excellent, inasmuch as it advocated the training of all midwives in the use of analgesics and the provision so far as possible of the necessary apparatus to enable women in childbirth who desire pain relief to receive it. Unfortunately there were those who immediately took advantage of this humanitarian activity in order to misrepresent it for purposes which suited their objectives. It became known as the 'Anaesthesia for All' bill, which rapidly developed the idea that no woman should bear a child in a state of consciousness.

Anyone with a wide obstetric experience knows that inhalant analgesia is not the answer to the relief of pain and distress in childbirth. This bill demonstrated the astonishing ignorance on the part of those who supported it. They overlooked the established truth that the woman who complains most loudly of the horrors of childbirth is almost invariably the woman who was most deeply anaesthetised for the longest period. It seemed a repetition of the fallacy 'cure a poisoned mind by poisoning the body.' To expend vast sums of money and develop, for either personal or collective designs, great benefactions to mothers suffering in labour by training midwives to use a gas apparatus is poor stuff, to which an honest obstetrician would not subscribe because it will not solve the problem.

This type of misrepresentation does great harm so long as women are not adequately informed of the truth of childbirth. If an organisation for the instruction of women was seriously undertaken, as well as the provision of analgesic apparatus, should it be required, the fear of childbirth would almost entirely disappear within one generation.

The relief of pain in childbirth should be the first consideration of all medical men concerned with obstetrics; they have no right to put any other subject in a more important position. That the manipulation of this humane service should be relegated to political vote-catching by those to whom the women of our time should look for leadership in obstetrics is incomprehensible. The subject is really too serious and of too fundamental importance for this sort of treatment; because of the absence of organised effort, the whole question of the relief of pain in labour is in a state of chaos.

There are professors of obstetrics who hold views upon anaesthesia and natural childbirth which demonstrate that they have interests which are placed before the health of the mothers and babies. In a paper on 'A Natural Childbirth Program' by Professor Herbert Thoms and Robert H. Wyatt[7] of Yale University School of Medicine, the sentence is found: '...neither Dr Dick-Read nor other writers on the subject have ever claimed that childbirth should be conducted without anaesthetic aids, or that the natural childbirth regimen renders labour devoid of pain ... analgesics and anaesthetics are used whenever they are indicated, usually whenever the patient desires them.' This statement is correct so far as it goes.

In a critique upon this paper, published in the *Obstetrical and Gynaecological Survey*, Professor Nicholson Eastman[8] of Johns Hopkins University refers to three groups concerned with this concept of natural childbirth, one of which is described as follows:

> 'Some of our *leading professors of obstetrics* charge that natural childbirth threatens to efface all the advantages that have accrued from many years of research in analgesia and anaesthesia. They further allege that it is a backward step to the pre-Simpsonian days when many women suffered the agonies of the damned in childbirth without hope of relief.'

It is almost incredible that such misrepresentation of natural childbirth procedures and such psychopathic prejudice can exist amongst 'our leading professors of obstetrics', but this is only one example of many. If these authorities knew the subject they criticise, they could add something to the discussion, but they don't and they won't – they stamp their little academic feet and shout with all the perspicacity of the petulant Duchess: 'Off with his head.'

When we read the opinions of authorities from all parts of the world, as well as the experimental and clinical reports from those who are never likely to be authorities, we become lost in a tangle of words. I have spent considerable time searching for reason and stability in this branch of our science only to be reminded again and again of Dr Fleming's statement upon anaesthesia in obstetrics: 'Obstetrics presents a large and varied field for *practice* and observation for the *student* of anaesthesia.' Walt Disney could hardly do justice to the silly symphony of obstetric analgesia.

I could only picture a crowd of men in white coats and large horn-rimmed glasses, seeking fame and fortune searching for a weapon with which to protect all women from an enemy which in 95 per cent of cases did not exist, and their chosen method of protection was to risk the life of the woman and her baby by using the weapon upon them, not upon the enemy which they erroneously presumed to be present! It did not seem to matter how a woman was robbed of her consciousness but the more awkward the means of administration, or the longer the name, so much the more likely was it that fame might be achieved. Simple inhalation of gas, ether or chloroform was soon left behind. Drugs were put under the skin, into the stomach, into veins, deep into muscles, into the rectum, into the spinal cord, into the sacral nerves – in fact, anywhere that things can be put into the human body. Those who 'did' a certain number by their own peculiar method wrote up the results, which appeared in big print in scientific papers as the latest improvement; they enlarged upon the absolute perfection of labour under its influence, its safety to both mother and child, and usually gave statistics of forceps deliveries with maternal and fetal death rate. The length of the names of these inflictions increased as the field of operations spread. Pentothal and thioethamyl[9] swept aside our old friend paraldehyde[10], which appears to be equally effective whether introduced from below or from above, but sodium prophy-methyl-carbinyl-allyl barbiturate scopolomine[11] won in a canter.

And after each report the phrase adopted is: 'No harmful effects were noted in the mothers or babies.' Joseph De Lee in the 1939 *Year Book of Obstetrics and Gynaecology* made an editorial note about this phrase: '(The last ten words are getting somewhat monotonous. Why are so many drugs offered? Why do they live so briefly? – Ed.)'

Robert H. Hingson[12, 13] has done magnificent work upon the use of anaesthetic injected either around or within the spinal cord. In many abnormalities and illnesses his methods have been of lifesaving service, but, unfortunately, enthusiasts incarcerated in the overnight cobwebs spun with all the technical brilliance of the great scientific araneida endeavour to simulate his genius before they pass into nothingness. Thousands of normal labours have been mutilated by this dangerous and unjustifiable procedure. Nearly all babies are delivered by forceps extraction – the majority of mothers have deep episiotomies performed. Women rarely know the joy of spontaneous delivery of their child – it is a painless, sensationless birth without emotional rectitude. There is no sense of personal achievement, the satisfaction is of ultimate possession not the pride of accomplishment. An offspring is produced by a magician from a paralysed birth canal. Nine months of happy anticipation of her highest natural ambitions, finished off by unnatural interference. Are there any advantages in this to offset its disadvantages? Professor Nicholson Eastman[7], one of our greatest contemporary authorities, believes spinal anaesthesia is to be blamed for more maternal deaths than any other form of anaesthesia. How long, oh, how long will this nonsense go on? Why do not at least some of these first-class brains settle down to try really harmless methods of preventing pain in labour?

Can the scientific mind see no further than drugs and anaesthetics, or is the incidence of natural amnesia beyond their powers of observation? We know deaths occur from the use of these things; we believe undesirable results are produced by their use; harm to both mother and child is recorded by a large number of competent observers[14]. What is the urge to persist in this search for an elixir to cure all ills which in the vast majority of women are preventable, with the utmost safety?

Let it be clearly understood that I am not criticising anaesthetics and their justifiable uses. There is no greater humanitarian work in the science of medicine than the magnificent advances in the use and knowledge of anaesthesia and relaxants. It gains ground every year and its application in a thousand different fields is made with ever-increasing safety. Doctors and patients alike turn with sincere gratitude to those whose studies have evolved new methods, machines, techniques and new reagents. It is the misuse of anaesthesia to which I call attention. Why should an efficient physiological function be distorted in the eyes of women of the world by constant association with the phantasmagorial futilities of interference? Pain is a pathological emergency in surgery, medicine and obstetrics – its signs and symptoms should direct us to the diagnosis of its cause and origin. If by rational means it cannot be relieved, the use of anaesthesia is indicated and justified, indeed, should not be withheld *as has already been clearly stated in this chapter.*

Anaesthetics are used in place of education; drugs are an antidote for misunderstanding; the phenomena of labour are misinterpreted. A carefully introduced mental process will maintain the normal perception of natural stimuli, enhancing the health and happiness of the mother and the vitality of her child. Surely it is safer to introduce a mental process than a dangerous drug.

Science has been carried away by its enthusiasm; it has left common sense unemployed in the pain-relief problem. This whole picture should be shorn of all excrescences. The indications for anaesthesia are not clearly recognised; when they exist, the choice of anaesthetic should be made by an expert who can assess the danger to mother and child in relation to the unnatural occurrence that justifies deep anaesthesia.

Any discomfort that is overcome by the use of light obstetric inhalants can be avoided or relieved by mental adjustment combined with physical relaxation. This is not theoretical but is the experience of hundreds of obstetricians and midwives throughout the world. The mind is the perceptor and interpreter of stimuli; it is in the mind that pain in normal labour arises. The best and safest anaesthetic is an educated and controlled mind; the next best is the simplest means of rectifying false interpretation by the combined use of suggestion and light inhalation anaesthesia. Of my last two hundred normal cases only two have desired and used the anaesthetic available for them; one hundred and ninety-eight derided the idea of being unconscious when their babies arrived. This was made possible by natural childbirth procedures and not by hypnotism or drugs.

Let the obvious contra-indications to the teaching of 'anaesthesia for all' be summarised:

1. No satisfactory anaesthetic for all cases has been discovered[14].
2. No anaesthetic is free from danger to mother or child[15].
3. All narcotic agents are injurious to babies during birth; they are all more or less severe respiratory depressants[16].
4. In normal labour, properly conducted, a high percentage of women do not wish for anaesthetic.
5. Anaesthesia essentially converts a normal physiological process into a pathological state with its attendant risks.
6. Owing to the ease of the administration of anaesthesia, interference at birth is more common than formerly. 'Thus it appeared that in a considerable proportion of uncomplicated cases in the Maternity Home, resort was had to delivery with forceps.'[17] 'A good deal of the instrumental delivery by doctors under modern conditions of medical practice is unnecessary, and this unnecessary interference has played some part in increasing the maternal mortality rate in Wales.'[18, 19, 20]
7. Anaesthesia prevents the occurrence of some of the natural phenomena of labour upon which the safety of both mother and child may depend.
8. Anaesthesia, contrary to a woman's desire, robs her of the natural reward of a perfected function, and renders surgical an event which many women believe is the physical manifestation of a spiritual experience.
9. Childbirth without anaesthesia enhances the natural mother child relationship to an intensity unknown to the mother unconscious of her baby's arrival.

But in spite of all these contra-indications, and many others quoted by different observers, we must offer the least unsatisfactory method of pain relief, for no woman should be allowed to suffer greater discomfort in labour than she is willing to endure for her child's sake.

In my experience the use of anaesthesia presents no difficulty. If there are clinical indications or if the woman in labour desires it, it should be administered; the signs and symptoms determine the most suitable method of pain relief. There is no rule of thumb, but speaking generally, heroin, pethidine, the trilene inhaler and a local anaesthetic for hypodermic injection is the total analgesic equipment necessary for practically all cases of childbirth, except those which require surgical interference. I do not refer to the mild draught or pill that has a salutary influence upon a labour which is slow to become fully established. A few hours sleep, particularly at night, during the early dilatation of the cervix evades the weariness of mind and body that predisposes to pain interpretation of the sensations of parturition. This therapeutic common sense should not be confused with the use of drugs to relieve pain. It is an adjuvant to avoid pain in a well-conducted labour.

But even with these simple and very effective methods of pain relief, considerable experience is required in order to obtain the desired results. It should not be overlooked that if any reagents are used contrary to clinical indication at the wrong time in labour, serious trouble may ensue. The most important factor, therefore, in the use of anaesthesia and analgesia in childbirth is the skill, experience and judgement of the attendant. Without these nothing is either safe or effective. And it should always be borne in mind that in properly conducted normal labour more than half the women want nothing and of those who have discomfort, over 80 per cent benefit from the relaxing influence of a single small injection of pethidine administered at the right time. Inhalant analgesia is not used today by more than 3 or 4 per cent of women; they prefer to be present and help in the delivery of their child.

THE PRINCIPLES OF THE RELIEF OF PAIN IN LABOUR, quite apart from the discussion of anaesthesia and analgesia and the main principles upon which the diminution or obliteration of pain from childbirth are based, must be mentioned.

If we refer once again to the Fear-Tension-Pain Syndrome, we will realise that the previous pages of this chapter deal almost entirely with the breaking down of this syndrome by the forcible removal of pain. We know, therefore, that if fear and, therefore, to a large extent, tension which causes pain, is removed, the use of anaesthesia, analgesia and drugs becomes either entirely unnecessary or minimised in amount and duration of administration.

The FIRST PRINCIPLE of the relief of pain in childbirth is the progressive education of the young; by this means only can the ignorance and the fear of parturition be forestalled and replaced by confidence and understanding. In order to do this, changes must be brought about in the attitude of men, women and children alike towards childbirth.

This most wonderful and satisfying of all human experiences should be placed in its correct perspective in the upbringing of children and in the education of young girls.

The SECOND PRINCIPLE is the education of the pregnant woman so that throughout the antenatal months she becomes familiar with the changes within and about her and finds confidence in understanding the processes of childbirth.

This prenatal instruction is probably the most invaluable asset in the hands of the obstetrician for the relief of pain in labour. We see, therefore, that the woman herself can take part in the pain-preventing preparation for parturition.

The THIRD PRINCIPLE of pain relief is to have an educated labour-ward staff. Whether this is in the hospital, maternity home or the private house is of no consequence. The nurse, sister or midwife must be a bulwark against the onslaught of fear and a tower of strength in time of doubt, weakness or wavering self-control. In order to occupy this position the attendant must have an accurate knowledge of the psychological as well as the physical phenomena of labour.

The FOURTH PRINCIPLE is that the obstetrician should observe the significance of the Fear-Tension-Pain Syndrome and should protect by his comprehension the minds of women as well as observe their physical activities during labour.

Where these four principles are fully implemented there is rarely reason, in uncomplicated childbirth, for the use of inhalant analgesia. A certain number of women do better with pethidine to assist their relaxation, but as I have repeated, and continue to repeat, over 95 per cent of women so prepared, attended and treated, prefer to remain conscious and witness the birth of their babies and will remark afterwards that they are now ready to have as many babies as they can afford.

The relief of pain in labour, therefore, depends upon the adoption of a new approach to obstetrics and the routine of childbirth. And I go further: it is rapidly becoming clear that within the lifetime of many who are bearing children today, the use of inhalant anaesthesia will be restricted entirely to gross abnormalities and its imposition upon the healthy woman in normal labour will be resented as an aspersion upon her ability to bear a child in the natural and healthy way.

Bibliography

1. W. SMELLIE. *Treatise of the Theory and Practice of Midwifery*, London, 1752.

2. ROBERT BARNES. *Obstetric Operations* (1870) and *Clinical History of the Clinical and Surgical Diseases of Women* (1874).

3. ANDREW CLAYE. *Evolution of Obstetric Analgesia*, Oxford University Press, 1939, p95.

4. ALECK BOURNE. *Synopsis of Obstetrics and Gynaecology*, 1937, pp99–100. H. BALME. *Relief of Pain*, 1936, pp291–2.

5. *Vide* most authorities on this subject.

6. MISS LLOYD-WILLIAMS. *Anaesthesia and Analgesia in Labour* (1934).

7. SIR WILLIAM GILLIATT. The Blackman Memorial Lecture, London, 1951.

8. HERBERT THOMS and ROBERT WYATT. 'A Natural Childbirth Program', *Amer Journ Public Health*, 1950, 40, p787.

9. NICHOLSON EASTMAN. *Obstetrical and Gynaecological Survey*, April, 1951.

10. WESLEY BOURNE and A.J. PAULY. *Canad MAJ*, May, 1939, 40, 437–40.

11. E.D. COLVIN and R.A. BARTHOLOMEW. *Internat Clin*, December, 1938, 4, 191, 201.

12. FRENCH, VOLPETTO and TORPIN. *JMA Georgia*, April, 1939, 28, 147–53.

13. HINGSON and LOVE. *The Control of Pain in Childbirth*, 3rd Edition, Lippincott, 1948.

14. ROBERT HINGSON. 'Continuous Caudal Analgesia in Obstetrical Surgery and Diseases of Women', *British Medical Journal*, p777, October, 1949.

15. WATERS and HARRIS. *Amer Jour of Surgery*, April 1940, pp129–34.

16. JOSEPH DE LEE. *Year Book of Obstetrics and Gynaecology*, 1939, p164.

17. JOSEPH DE LEE. *Year Book of Obstetrics and Gynaecology*, 1939, pp167–8.

18. 'Report on an Investigation into Maternal Mortality', Ministry of Health, London, 1937, p183.

19. 'Report on Maternal Mortality in Wales', Ministry of Health, London, 1937, p118.

20. MONTGOMERY. *Jour Amer Med Assn*, May 15th 1937.

21. BUNDESEN, and others. *Jour Amer Med Assn*, July 25th, 1936.

22. S.R. WILSON. 'Physiological Basis of Hypnosis and Suggestion', *Proc of Royal Soc Med*, Section Anaesth, Vol 20.

14

Hypnosis in Childbirth
as a Means of Pain Relief

Recently, considerable confusion has arisen because of the emphasis I placed on the use of simple suggestion in childbirth. An explanation has been offered by Dr William S. Kroger and Dr Charles Freed in their courageous book *Psychosomatic Gynaecology*. A condition known as 'waking hypnosis,' by which complete relaxation without loss of consciousness can be induced by authoritative personal association between attendant and patient, is described by them. Without posing as a philologist or an expert in semantics, I must say the term is not convincing. Hypnosis means sleep, or a condition simulating sleep; 'waking sleep' is not a state easy to visualise.

However, by waking hypnosis the phenomena of a natural function are explained. This is perfectly all right so far as I am concerned, for it merely allocates to all human function and behaviour a means by which performance can be initiated or controlled. Its application is very wide. A good Christian lives healthily and happily, being subjected to a state of waking hypnosis by reading his Bible. Prayer becomes simply a hypnotic motivator of our thoughts and actions.

The big, bad man who is committed to jail for highway robbery, suffered from waking hypnosis induced by Silas Puttamup Jr in his book *Two-Gun Jake of Rustlers' Rump*. A learner pilot is hypnotised by the instructor who teaches him to fly and not to destroy himself in his efforts. Does a gardener induce 'growing hypnosis' in his chosen flowers by planting them in their natural environment, by destroying the pests that may mar their beauty and by tearing up the weeds that would choke them and rob them of their fragrance? By reading my works upon natural childbirth, it has been suggested, both in America and Germany, women are being hypnotised by, through or because of me, in twelve different languages all over the world. Frankly, when I saw myself in the looking glass this morning I hesitated, for one brief moment, before accepting this distinction.

I do not state that my friends are wrong in their diagnosis of the nature of my teaching because I am not an authority upon somnambulism or waking hypnosis, and I prefer to criticise subjects with which I am familiar. But the results obtained by the teaching of natural childbirth are so constant yet so ubiquitous that neither an individual nor his written work can be held entirely responsible. But we read 'this type of hypnosis is based upon direct prestige suggestion'. Wherever and however the birth of a child conforms to the physiological pattern it is the result of a mysteriously induced state which is not her natural self – in fact, any woman who bears her baby naturally, whether she has an inborn sense of confidence and understanding in childbirth or whether she gleaned her knowledge from the *Reader's Digest*, the local curate or by watching the family cat, achieves her most desirable ambition in a state of waking sleep. If we are to believe that behaviour, accomplishment, the results of education and learning, the simple domestic habits and, indeed, life itself, is lived under this influence, then, and only then, can I agree with my colleagues in America and those who subscribe to their beliefs.

For nothing is more natural or more in keeping with the simple principles of physiological activity than childbirth. Drs Kroger and Freed 'feel justified in asking – what is the Dick-Read Method?' Let me help them to understand what the method is, since they have compared it with hypnosis, made comments upon it and suggested its *modus operandi* – under these circumstances I think they ought to know what it is!

1. The Dick-Read Method is a simple approach to parturition which employs obstetric procedures based upon clinical observation and deduction.
2. It is a method which enables women to have their children by physiological principles and mechanism with which the healthy human female is equipped for that purpose.
3. The method is designed to protect women from the appalling dangers of ignorance. This not only applies to mothers but to those who look after them from conception to the end of the puerperium.
4. The method enables babies to be born with the least possible risk of injury, either physical, chemical or psychological.
5. The method is based upon a complete familiarity with the motivating powers, the mechanism, and the purpose of the natural phenomena of childbirth.
6. The primary objective of this method is to encourage the im-

plementation and maintenance of a highly efficient natural function, which has neither anatomical nor neurological provision for pain or fear in its normal state.

I do not suggest that hypnosis, waking or otherwise, will not remove both pain and fear. We know that some skilled and experienced people can produce amazing phenomena by its use; but severe pain can be eliminated in over 90 per cent of parturient women by substituting understanding for fear. It is a system of elementary education and no one has been able to hypnotise a high percentage of women in labour. Some authorities say that only from 30 to 60 per cent of women are responsive to its influence during parturition. There are thousands of doctors and midwives who practised for years the orthodox methods of pain relief with anaesthetics, analgesics and drugs, but having become familiar with the procedures based on the Fear-Tension-Pain Syndrome, find that women demand to remain conscious and see their babies born. Their discomfort, if any, does not justify the use of pain-relieving reagents. Have these obstetricians suddenly and unconsciously become hypnotists because they learnt and were able to remove the primary cause of pain?

I agree entirely with the advantages of hypnosis over deep analgesia and anaesthesia. Dr Kroger enumerates twenty-one indications for its use, all of which are almost identical with the benefits of natural childbirth procedures. But he also draws attention to seven major disadvantages, none of which arises if the physiological function is preserved.

He states that hypnotic procedure is relatively simple and any physician can be taught. This may be so, and in America where most women are attended by doctors it would undoubtedly be of considerable value in avoiding the very prevalent interference habit. But this teaching is not American; it is all over a world in which the majority of women are still attended by midwives and nurses, who only appeal for medical aid if it is required. Can we instruct hundreds of thousands of assistants in the art of hypnosis and the discretion necessary for its safe usage?

Women are enthusiastic to learn about childbirth; they understand and enjoy the elementary education in facts that so many of them feel are common sense. The majority, however, hesitate to be hypnotised in order to avoid pain that need not be present if they are properly prepared and cared for in labour. Many more people can learn the natural childbirth teaching than can be made competent to exert adequate hypnotic influence over women in labour. It takes much less time and requires human sympathy and understanding rather than scientific ability.

I agree with Dr Kroger and those who hold his views that hypnosis has not a good name with the lay public. There is still an abhorrence of the mysticism with which it has been surrounded since Franz Anton Mesmer (1734–1815) first cured by what he called 'animal magnetism'. It was known and used for many purposes, centuries before he exhibited his prowess. The Persians, Indian fakirs and the Oriental masters were great exponents of the art. But the unscrupulous charlatans who professed to imitate Mesmer brought this important work into disrepute from which it has been slow to recover. Its colourful exhibition in the music halls has helped to mutilate its assets. The association of hypnosis with pain relief in childbirth is by no means generally acceptable. The idea of a young woman being 'under someone's influence' or 'got into somebody's power' still exists, and I have been asked to assure women that natural childbirth procedures are not hypnotism because of their dread of this inscrutable fetish.

Why hypnotise when education and understanding give better results in a higher percentage of women? Surely it is not dissimilar from the practice of anaesthetising women against their wishes, or withholding from mothers-to-be the right to try to have their babies naturally? It is preferable to teach doctors obstetrics if they are going to be obstetricians, rather than to instruct them in the simple procedures of hypnotism, which hides the phenomena of normal labour behind the ephemeral curtain of disassociated consciousness.

The absence of pain and distress in normal labour has caused considerable suspicion and the recent introduction of the notion that it is hypnosis has already proved damaging to a highly beneficial, but essentially harmless, approach to childbirth. Discretion in using this power is so important. The prepsychotic woman, that is one who of her nature is predisposed to major or minor mental derangement, frequently becomes a chronic psychopathic case if this treatment is applied. A maternity unit associated with a large London hospital, after a considerable series of cases conducted under hypnosis, and not without some success, gave up using it because the after-effects were harmful in too high a percentage of women to justify continuing. The disadvantages outweighed the advantages.

It is for these reasons that I have written upon it, in order that the principles and procedures of natural childbirth may be entirely alienated from the conscious employment of hypnotism in the accepted use of the term. The technique is a process of purifying this physiological function by removing pathological inhibitions that have been allowed, by ignorance of facts, to invade and disrupt its supreme efficiency. Our anatomy and physiology have not altered fundamentally in thousands of years. These 'Dick-Read Method' procedures disclose nothing new – they are the activities of an obstetric gardener who plants and tends his most cherished flowers in their natural environment and protects them from the pests that would injure or destroy. He sees, and is humbled by, the beauty and incomprehensible genius of their procreation and strives to foster the happiness they radiate and the infectious laughter in which they flourish:

One is nearer God's heart in a garden,
Than anywhere else on earth.

15

The Conduct of Labour

Many of my friends have asked me to give a detailed account of the conduct of labour which embodies the fundamental principles of what has become known as 'Natural Childbirth.' It will be unnecessary to repeat the teaching of our great masters of obstetrics so far as the ordinary routine of midwifery is concerned. *The general principles of good obstetrics must be recognised and practised by all who undertake the attendance upon women in labour.*

The obstetrician must be fully prepared to meet or provide for all emergencies, and since chapters on the conduct of labour are usually concerned with the imminence of the unforeseen, it would be vain repetition to delve into the abnormal. Let it be presumed, therefore, that all the sound general principles are employed for the safety and care of women so far as the purely physical process of parturition is concerned. Here we will examine the conduct of labour from the point of view of the woman herself, her mental condition and changing emotional states, and endeavour to deduce without elaboration or bias the importance or otherwise of paying more attention to this aspect of childbirth. It is not intended to offer a panacea for all the ills of labour and it has but little influence in rectifying genuinely abnormal conditions or occurrences, but it does raise the question of preventing troubles which appear to be relatively unimportant but which in reality are the roots of many serious evils.

In a previous chapter attention has been drawn to the emotional states and sensory conditions to which women are subjected in what is believed to be normal and natural labour. The necessity for recognising the important purpose of these phenomena has been pointed out. It is not easy, at first sight, to foresee how labour can be conducted along lines so unorthodox. It is even more difficult to assess the value of retaining the natural design when the cultural plan is apparently so efficient. Happily, we have a reply which is incontestable. A large number of women have been willing to give their own opinions, many having had children by the accepted routine and treatment before they became acquainted with the methods about to be described. I am sure that great obstetrician Joseph De Lee of Chicago, had he been alive today, would have modified his opinion (*Principles and Practice of Obstetrics*, de Lee, 7th edition, 1938, pp339 and 340): 'It will take several thousand generations before we can train women back to the state which Grantly Dick-Read speaks of as "Natural Childbirth."' I do not like to consider this a method by which women are trained back to a state, but rather a means of liberating them from the burden of medieval misunderstanding and thereby enabling them to make use of the great gifts of nature which early civilisation has buried beneath the pompous cloak of ignorance. Elation, relaxation, amnesia and exultation are the four pillars of parturition upon which the conduct of labour depends; each, in its proper place, maintaining, supporting and controlling the impulses, both sensory and motor, upon which the neuromuscular harmony of the function survives.

Parturition is the great event in the reproductory cycle of woman. Although in recent years antenatal care has become increasingly important and its value fully recognised, labour is the real excitement for the patient and midwife.

The nature of labour depends basically upon the efficiency of antenatal education, care, and, if need be, treatment, and the act of parturition should be complementary to the conduct of pregnancy. In modern childbirth, the importance of labour is overestimated, and the full significance of antenatal preparation is overlooked. Natural childbirth depends in nearly every case upon the education of the mother; she must be aware of the natural process in order to assist in its design. She must understand and expect the changing phenomena of labour, so that normal actions and reactions occur uninhibited by resistant forces. The four pillars of labour that have been mentioned above must be maintained and fully utilised so that parturition may progress easily and smoothly from one stage to the next. But this is impossible if the woman has not been educated in their significance, does not understand the routine of nature's principles and at the time, when various phenomena arrive, cannot meet them in full confidence, unshaken by the changes in their manifestation. Above all things, confidence must reign supreme; there must be no fear, either for the events of the immediate present or the ultimate result of labour; the earliest sign of anxiety must be challenged, the mind of the parturient woman protected from this great evil – fear.

A sister at a maternity home where elementary education in the physiology of labour is given as part of the antenatal care, was discussing the conduct of a woman whom we had just attended. The whole process had been perfect; a delight to all who had been concerned in it, including the mother herself. 'The more I see of this natural childbirth, the more I am persuaded that education is what really matters. Although, so far, we have neither time nor opportunity to teach our mothers as fully as we would like to, the change in our cases is remarkable. There is a different atmosphere in the wards; those who have their babies have no recent horrors in their minds and those who are about to have their babies are not afraid. Our women are happy and the babies are peaceful. We may have as many as thirty-five to forty babies in the nursery wards, but it has become the exception to hear a crying, restless baby, not the rule as it used to be.' I asked her frankly if there was any obvious difference in the conduct of labour in my cases from those of other obstetricians who also practised the general principles that I teach. Her reply was interesting because she is a woman of wide experience and a midwife of consummate skill. 'Yes, in your technique, but the outstanding difference is in the women. They seem to know their job before they start; they know what first-stage contractions are doing and realise that it may be a long time before the "door is opened". They understand why relaxation helps and why it prevents pain in labour...' She had much more to say, but the point that appealed to me was that although she saw certain differences in my conduct of labour from the methods of my confrères the behaviour of the women themselves impressed her most. That she attributed to prenatal education more than to any other factor. There were still reputable and experienced men attending cases at that home who gave no prenatal instruction, who explained nothing at the time, and who gave relatively deep anaesthesia as a routine.

The usual routine in a case of natural childbirth is as follows.

Women are all asked to go into the maternity home as soon as they are conscious of regular contractions every fifteen to twenty minutes. Multiparas recognise these 'pains' and waste no time, since they know how rapidly labour may develop under the influence of relaxation. Primiparas have more time in which to decide if the contractions are the real thing, but my practice is to ask them to speak to me on the telephone if they have any doubt; there is usually a telephone box nearby if there is not one in the house.

The uninstructed woman frequently asks: 'How do I know when my baby is ready to come and what do I do?' This question should have been answered many weeks before the probable end of her pregnancy.

She will be told that there are three warnings when labour has started or is about to commence:

1. *Water leaks from the uterus* or the *bag of waters may burst* and the liquor come away in a considerable flow. This is probably more likely to happen in women who have had babies previously rather than in those having their first baby, but there is no rule to guide us in that.
2. A slight haemorrhage may occur rather like the beginning of a menstrual period except that there is a good deal of mucus with the discharge. This is known as '*the show*'.
3. A feeling of tightness around the abdomen, possibly even extending to the back, will be recognised as coming and going at intervals. At first not regular, but probably one every quarter of an hour to twenty minutes. These are the *contractions* of the uterus which may continue for some time before full labour is established.

There is still some controversy on what indicates the establishment of true labour. The waters may leak for a number of days before labour starts – in fact on several occasions I have observed that the liquor has stopped, the bag of membranes apparently closing. The 'show' may appear some days before labour is established but this sign is probably the most constant of the three in indicating when labour is imminent.

The recurrence of contractions or tightness of the uterus may be misleading inasmuch as some women who have not been prepared for labour and are still wrapped in anxiety may have contractions of the circular fibres in the lower part of the uterus a fortnight, three weeks or even longer before the longitudinal fibres go into action and true labour starts. I have met women who believed in all seriousness that they were in labour from ten to fourteen days before the arrival of the child but when the signs and symptoms that they had observed were discussed with them, it became clear that true labour lasted for not more than twelve hours.

It is my opinion that the onset of parturition is best diagnosed by the rhythmical contractions at shortening intervals and a sense of generalised tightness of the abdomen without pain so long as the woman remains relaxed. The intervals will decrease from a quarter of an hour to five minutes or even less.

These three major signs usually make it easy for a woman to realise that her baby is on the way. If there is any doubt whatever, she should get in touch with her medical adviser and invite him to direct her whether or not it is time to leave her home and go to the maternity hospital, or whether he should visit her to make sure her labour has commenced.

Having arrived at the maternity home, a hot bath and an enema are given in most cases; this procedure is advantageous from all points of view. If the membranes have been ruptured before labour started, an enema is given but no bath.

As early as possible in the first stage my visit is made to the patient. This is not a hurried rush in and 'Glad you've started; get on with it; I'll be back in time' sort of visit, but a prolonged stay, possibly for an hour or more. The natural anxiety or anticipation at the commencement of the final episode must be overcome by kindly but careful explanation of the sensation she is experiencing. It must not be overlooked that the most cheerful and apparently carefree woman may be very frightened. Beware of an excess of laughter between contractions; it is often a manifestation of tension of the mind and may well turn to tears when real effort and control become necessary in the later stages of labour.

During the visit a calm, reassuring but firm kindliness is desirable. In spite of all teachings to the contrary, I am persuaded that women are best lying down towards the end of the first stage of labour. If relaxation has been practised and acquired as a habit, it will easily be obtained during first-stage contractions. Until a controlled relaxation is obtained, the patient should not be left.

The points to remember are the few deep breaths as the uterus comes into action; eyes open and face relaxed – that is, no frown or puckered brow, no screwed-up eyes, no pursed lips or grinding teeth. There is no need for these exhibitions; they do no good; they are either demands for sympathy or manifestations of fear. Both increase neuro-muscular tension.

With the utmost patience procure a well-relaxed woman early in labour. Such patience is amply rewarded. Speak quietly and with understanding; be honest in your advice and gentle in manner; point out once again the significance of these first stage contractions. They are pulling open the outlet of the womb; step by step it expands and muscle is collected up and shortened, so that it cannot close again until the baby has passed through. 'The uterus must be left alone; it can do all this without any effort to help on your part. Consider it a machine apart from yourself, and in due course the dilatation of the outlet will be complete. There is no hurry; the door will open, but you must not make the work harder for the uterus by tightening the door. If you are rigid and squeeze up your face, then the muscles of the outlet will squeeze up too. But the uterus is astoundingly strong and persistent; the result of your resistance will be pain. The more completely relaxed you become, so much the more elastic will be the mouth of the womb and so much less discomfort will you experience.'

It is frequently observed by women how different labour becomes once relaxation is obtained. They are encouraged to maintain this state because it is common sense that an elastic opening is not only more easily but more quickly expanded.

During this time, reassurance in the normality and straightforwardness of everything may be given. Gentle encouragement to be patient and persevering is helpful. A peaceful, confident atmosphere should be sustained and a close watch kept upon any untoward trend in conversation. At this time a woman is only interested in her own business; she is doing a job of work and wants to concentrate upon it in order to do it well. Most women who understand what is going on are keen observers not only of their own actions, but of the reactions of those about them to every fresh event or incident.

I have laid stress previously upon the sensitiveness of mind of a parturient woman; if you wish to try to deceive them, you will fail. They miss nothing and have a way of turning over in their minds the things they see and the words they hear.

Stand, therefore, in the forefront of the contest, side by side both mentally and physically, with the woman in labour. The attendant is there to prevent trouble and, if he is wise, he will watch and listen, with senses as acute as a lone sentry in the night, for the obvious or insidious intrusion of the arch enemy, which is fear.

I say most definitely that such care in the early first stage lays the foundation of a labour which will stand for all time as a monument of happiness in the mind of a mother. From the midwife and obstetrician it demands patience, peacefulness and personal interest as well as confidence, concentrated observation and cheerfulness. These three P's and three C's may be easily remembered by beginners – and have been referred to in some of my lectures on this subject – as the capital letters of the Perfect Confinement. The percentage of labour which conforms to this high ideal is rapidly increasing. As the importance of treating the mind becomes recognised, this picture of normal labour is more frequently seen.

Let us consider in detail these six cardinal requisites of the obstetrician and midwife.

Patience is the most exacting of virtues, but probably the greatest of all. When a woman is being attended in labour, every other consideration must be of secondary importance. Babies have a habit of arriving out of turn and out of time; they do not respect the ways of adults. On the few occasions upon which I have taken a reasonable risk during the last few years, I have invariably been caught out by the sudden and rapid arrival of a child in my short absence. For three years in succession my summer holiday was planned for three weeks, giving ten days clear at each end from any booked dates for births. Each year from ten to fifteen days of that three weeks had to be sacrificed to infants who insisted upon remaining *in utero*. It is not surprising that my family had a poor opinion of obstetrics as a hobby! To invite friends to dine was to precipitate a labour during dinner, and to fulfil a long-standing promise of a family evening at the theatre was practically impossible. The special days of the school term when the children looked forward to a visit from their 'baby doctor' father were frequently days of disappointment. We still hear of normal cases having the membranes ruptured early so that the physician could get the case over in time to do this or that. We still hear of anaesthesia and forceps being employed to assist in the maintenance of a social programme and even for the purely selfish motive that it is the quickest method of getting the job over. Obstetricians are sometimes busy men, but there is no reason why busy men should not be obstetricians! I am frequently told: 'But, my dear So-and-so, I simply have not time to do all this. There are other things to attend to and other things to be done.'

No specialised calling in our profession demands such dedication to its service or such controlled patience as pure obstetrics. It is a communion with the most noble and the most inexplicable manifestation of the spirit of nature. It has no place for hustle or hurry and should be protected by law from the incursions of the brilliant busybody. It should cease to be the popular playground for practitioners who claim to be specialists in half a dozen branches of surgery and medicine and who in reality are a social and scientific menace. For of all men, the virtue of self-effacing patience is most rarely found in these and to them the art and science of obstetrics is almost unnatural.

At the bedside of a woman in labour we have to await the will of intangible forces. The emotional conflicts and physical reactions of our patients present a constant stream of problems. Initiative, clear thinking and honest exposition must be at hand to control the fearful, encourage the failing and support the tired. No force of mind or body can drive a woman in labour; by patience only can the smooth course of nature be followed.

But patience must be exercised, for without understanding, accurate observation, and clinical experience, it may lead to a peaceful waiting upon avoidable discomfort and trouble that should have been prevented. Natural childbirth is not just sitting by and allowing what comes to take its course. The law of nature has a host of enemies not only in the mind and body of civilised woman but in the good intentions of those who are concerned with her well-being. An obstetrician is a private detective who watches, guards and unostentatiously accompanies a woman during her parturition. He is armed to keep off intruders and trained to recognise those who would disturb the peace. Should unpredictable emergency arise he meets it fully equipped from the various departments of modern science with devices to overcome the misadventure and safely deliver the woman of her baby.

The course and progress of labour must be watched and followed in all its stages, particularly at the end of the first stage, when fear makes its most subtle attacks upon a woman and when a woman makes her most subtle efforts to escape. And so it may be again in the latter half of the second stage of labour, especially if the woman, strong and healthy, is bearing her first baby. The thick perineum must gradually be thinned by successive uterine contractions until it can allow the baby's head to pass. It is so slow – there seems to be no progress, no advance – the weary hours hang heavily upon the attendant's expectation. The woman, amnesic and contented, is not aware of time, she is so noble in her efforts, so courageous in her determination. The doctor hears a voice whispering in his mind, it sounds so gentle, just and humanitarian in the silence of the labour ward: 'Help her; a whiff or two; small straight blades will do it. She is tired, she has been marvellous; she deserves to finish now.' This subtle effort to persuade is fraught with evil; it is the devil standing in the guise of liberator of the oppressed, playing on the kindliness of man's nature, endeavouring to prevail upon him to commit the unforgiveable crime.

Patience – hard put to it – must be heard; it carries safety and health to both mother and child; it is the immutable law of nature, and rarely, if ever, betrays those who have faith in its ultimate beneficence. How many matrons of maternity homes have watched that struggle in the minds of obstetricians; they have judged men on their reactions to those impulses, and they have seen tragedy or joy reward the choice that has been made. One grand old man of obstetrics, whose name is known throughout the schools and universities of England, would frequently turn to the matron of his nursing home when labour had reached the stage described, and say: 'Sister, put my bag outside the door; lock it and keep the key in your pocket. If I ask for my forceps, say "No." Quick, take it away; I am sorely tempted!'

Temper your tranquillity with vigilance lest any harmful thing occur. It is astonishing how often patience will overcome difficulties and solve the host of mythical problems the long, quiet, waiting hours of night will create in fertile minds.

Peacefulness. Nothing is more irritating than noise and restlessness when relaxation is sought. Nothing is more exasperating than inconsequent chatter when the mind is occupied with an all-absorbing interest. Disturbing interludes of tune humming or muffled tap dance rhythm with fingers on the bedside, frequent comings and goings, openings and closings, shufflings and solicitations, are thoughtless actions of those who have no human understanding. Women in labour abhor loud voices and terse commands; they are alarmed by the clumsy incongruity of the bull (or even the cow) in the china shop. I shall never forget the harassed, agonised expression on the face of a nineteen-year-old girl whose doctor had sent for me. The labour had been slow and the mother-in-law – a perfect example of one of the major pests of parturition – rushed dramatically into the drive and flung open the door of my car before the chauffeur could leap from his seat. She tugged my arm, and cried, 'Come, oh, come quickly. They are killing my daughter. Save her! Save her!' I ceased to be popular when I looked down upon her and asked with a smile, 'From whom?' The scene upstairs was one of tribulation and turmoil. The nurse was perspiring and flushed; the doctor had a red apron on and a blue and red striped shirt; his collar was off and his sleeves rolled up. The girl, uncovered from the waist downwards, was biting a towel which had been stuffed into her mouth; the room bore evidence of rapidly disintegrating dignity. When I entered the room, I was greeted with a triple sigh of relief; I think a policeman would have had a similar greeting at that moment. The towel was taken from the 'patient's' mouth; she flung a tired arm across the bed to me, and said, 'For God's sake give me peace.' There was nothing abnormal in her labour, except its conduct. Each contraction had been a signal for loud shouts of, 'Push, shove, pull, hang on!' Pressure on the abdomen alternated with the raising of the left buttock to see if the child was appearing. Nurse, doctor, and even mother-in-law gazed at the inoffensive outlet in an agony of anticipation. But the cervix was not fully dilated. It was suggested that they were all very tired; I advised a large brew of tea – downstairs – away – a cigarette or two, and a cup of tea for the patient and myself upstairs, weak and warm. In one hour a normal second stage had produced a healthy baby. A few whiffs of gas just at crowning time for she was still very alarmed, and peace reigned. The pitiable request of that girl, tortured by the turmoil of her parturition, 'For God's sake give me peace', embedded itself in my mind and left an indelible impression of the power of imperturbability.

Personal Interest. One of the most gratifying features of a normal labour is the personal interest and undivided attention given by the attendant to the parturient woman. This applies particularly to primiparae. However great the confidence and courage, the knowledge that someone competent to understand is nearby affords a comforting sense of security. How many doctors have been told, 'Everything seemed much easier when you arrived.' It is not the doctor himself who brings relief, but the inborn dependence of woman finding satisfaction for its natural demand, which is someone upon whom to depend. This does not only happen to doctors, for the patient and the whole household relax in a feeling of safety when the midwife arrives.

The importance of the obstetrician's presence is not sufficiently realised and one who fills this high office should be sure that no laxity of interest disappoints the woman who relies so implicitly upon his judgment, knowledge and skill.

If mental and physical tension is to be minimised, or even avoided, the first evidence of personal interest is the early arrival of the accoucheur after labour begins. The mind of a woman can only be put at rest by a close personal understanding of her doubts and fears. Fears can only be avoided or destroyed by the maintenance of confidence and confidence is gained most easily by actions which justify its existence. I do not for one moment suggest an aimless fussiness or extravagant show of zeal. The acute sensitiveness of a woman in labour must be constantly borne in mind. Her physical comfort can be attended to without ostentation; her hot drink or her cold drink* – whichever she prefers – may be given without demand for gratitude. Do not desire to make it obvious that you wish to be helpful; very few women have any use for sentimentality and 'sob stuff' in labour. They do want practical, common-sense companionship and that should be dispensed according to the particular woman. No two labours are alike; no two women are alike and there is something new to be learnt from every case of childbirth. No rule of thumb for the conduct of parturition exists and

---

* For years I have used raspberry leaf tea as a drink for women in labour. *Vide* Professor Sir Beckwith Whitehouse on 'Fragarine,' British Medical Journal, September 13th, 1941.

I know no rule that governs the conduct of women. It is at this time you see the true woman. Give her your attention and you will witness the metamorphosis of the female of the human species. Be interested in her elation, encourage it and mildly share it; she will feel that you are in harmony with her and will more readily accomplish relaxation of both mind and body as the contractions become firmer. Then, as the spirit of jocularity wears off, as it does, the reality of her task dawns upon her consciousness with a calm confidence. As the first stage progresses, the word of friendly counsel and authoritative advice is welcomed as a draught of water by a thirsty man. Your interest, your attention, your presence and even your hand are pillars of strength to aid her in the new undertaking. The veneer of womanhood is removed, she concentrates upon essentials and both learns and performs her task with the utmost fortitude.

It cannot be too strongly urged that these changes should be observed, for if they are not expected and received with understanding, the unity of purpose that should exist between woman and obstetrician is likely to be found wanting. The final dilatation of the cervix is the phase that calls for the greatest control. A woman demands that her courage be sustained. There may be real discomfort at this time in the most natural cases, but if her confidence has been maintained by a sympathetic comprehension of her reactions to psychical and physical stress, she will pass quietly into the second stage with its lowered mental appreciation and its modified interpretation of sensory stimuli. Then, with relaxation between the contractions and effort with them – instead of relaxation during contractions as in the first stage – the most profound change of all occurs. She wakes to work and does not stint the violence of expulsive strain. As it passes off, her few deep breaths of recovery precede complete relaxation and even sleep, until, reinforced once more, she calls on you to help and encourage her to get the best possible result. I have been moved to such a height of admiration by the cheerful, courageous determination of good-hearted women in the second stage of their labour, that no service or sacrifice on their behalf has seemed too great – women whose flippancy and foolish behaviour, whose exaggerated cosmetic atrocities and uncontrolled domestic excesses have given them the appearance of decorative but useless butterflies, not infrequently confound criticism by exhibiting a quiet, unbending stoicism during labour, with complete scorn for any word or action that may suggest absence of 'guts'. Give them personal interest, companionship and a good lead and they will follow you cheerfully and what is more, they will find it is not the unpleasant experience of which they may have heard. Do not be mistaken by prejudging a woman; wait until you see her with her baby, for by then you will have had every opportunity of learning her true nature and the environment from which she comes. The quiet, domesticated woman, filled with good intentions and a high estimate of her own ability, may prove deceptive to herself as well as to her doctor. She may have retained her social respectability because of her environment, but she may have feared to venture where more exuberant youth has dared to take a foolish risk. I have been disappointed in many women of this type; the interest that they demand from you is that you should witness a demonstration of perfect behaviour. They accept suggestion coldly and prefer their own methods; they have been adequately informed behind the closed door of the boudoir; the family name, even, may be at stake. I advise a very firm control in such cases, for if you cease to observe and fail to dominate these rigid personalities, you are in for a squall. They have never had the courage of unorthodoxy and crack beneath the first shock that the call for determination and fortitude gives them; they have not given vent to the spirit of adventure which learns to control fear.

For your patient's sake, be interested in her mental and physical well-being during labour; for your own sake observe closely her reactions to its demands. You are dealing with several different women during labour; she who is reacting to her social environment in the early first stage has little physical and mental resemblance to herself reacting to uncontrollable neuromuscular energies of the late second stage.

Varium et mutabile semper femina[*], but never more so than in childbirth.

In general outline, I have drawn attention to some of the advantages of personal interest in a woman in labour, but the evils of its absence are not usually recognised. All sensitive women are hurt by friends who appear disinterested when friendship is most salutary. When, in times of anxiety, the support we expect of those in whom we have implicit faith is withdrawn and when our self-confidence and fortitude are severely tested by the manifestation of a mysterious assailant, we long for the comforting voice of calm; our whole soul cries out for that companionship which compels courage by its very presence. No greater curse can fall upon a young woman whose first labour has commenced, than the crime of enforced loneliness. Why cannot every

* Woman is always a changeable and capricious thing.

obstetrician realise the enormity of this medieval inquisition? Yet, each day and every night, partially or totally uninstructed women are left alone to 'get on with it'. They cannot understand the mechanism of these recurrent contractions from which there is no escape and each contraction, more hateful than the one before, slowly drags the great crescendo of its irresistible might to the very edge of unendurable agony. The agony may not come, but it is so imminent, so terrifying and so real in its proximity that the groan of apprehension is raised to an exasperated wail. Loneliness increases our terrors; under its hideous emptiness we wilt beneath the chastisement of our wild imaginations; we visualise, in its silence, the ultimate horrors of possibility and draw tight the protective cloak of mental and physical tension in readiness for either fight or flight. To be afraid at any time is bad enough, but to be conscious of the presence of a real and justifiable cause for fear, ever advancing to destroy or torture its victim, is an experience that can freeze the bravest heart and scar for all time the strongest mind.

I do not lightly recall my most hideous hour; it was in August, 1915, shortly after we had landed at Suvla Bay. My watch upon the beach commenced at 2am. On the edge of the mud of Salt Lake, crystal-coated and faintly glistening in the brilliant starlight of a moonless sky, was my dressing station. Some three hundred badly wounded men were lying shivering in the cold night air; the fierce heat of day had fled with the fading light and in a few hours men's breath was frozen on their beards. To those who were in pain I gave the maximum dose of morphia; rifles and bayonets used as splints required adjusting; tourniquets had to be released and reapplied. Water was scarce, but some could ill afford to be left without their share of our meagre supply. The monotony of this round was depressing for there were no ships' boats to take them off the beach. From time to time, Death seemed to reach down from the empty spaces and seize this man or that, and on each round I made, a carcass lay where but a short time past I had heard courageous words of patience and gratitude.

I sat to rest upon a mound of sand from which I could hear any call from my stricken flock and wondered if the living knew that their silent neighbours had passed on. It became so still that only the breathing of the sleepers could be heard and suddenly I became aware of utter loneliness. I thought afterwards that some instinctive warning brought that strange desire to fly. In fact, such an impulse was unthinkable, but in theory at least I was reacting to an undefined fear. I had not many moments to wait for the explanation – from only a mile across the bare lake, on Chocolate Hill, a rifle was fired, rending the

stillness so unexpectedly that I started and became alert. But it was followed by a sound of war that still rings in my memory, more terrifying
than the bombs that were bursting within my grounds as I wrote these
words, near enough to shake the lamp upon my table. It was the sound
of a bayonet charge; the Very lights leapt from beyond the hill; the
shrill yells of madness and bloodlust mingled with the wild whoops
and screams of victor and vanquished. A few revolver shots and soon
the lights died down. The stillness was a thousand times more intense
after that mad quarter of an hour. I knew our line was feebly held by
tired and battlestained troops. I peered into the distant blackness wondering who had won. Had the Turks broken through and should I see
the gleam of steel and the fire of mad eyes looming up from the darkness? I would have given anything within my power to have had a
trusted companion with me, even if only to ask him who he thought
had won. But I was alone and that sickening doubt wore down my vitality. I stumbled, tired and frozen, round my patients; my hand shook
as I held the water bottle to their lips; my eyes turned unwillingly, but
half expectantly, to the black mile that stretched to Chocolate Hill. My
mind ran riot and I suffered agonies of apprehension and fear. Not
long after, dawn broke in grey and purple lines across the hills. My
relief came with the first rays of sun and he asked me of the night. I
gave him my report and he looked at me and said, 'You look worn out.
What's wrong?' He was an old Cambridge friend of mine and my answer was, 'I have never known before how frightful loneliness can be.'

The landing of August 6th, the hail of fire over Lala Baba, had been
the reality of slaughter. But that night I had died a hundred deaths.
Later on I was on the Somme, at Ypres, Arras, Amiens and Cambrai; Bourlon Wood, Farbus, Flecquiere Wood, Fampoux, and a dozen
other battles where there was ample food for fear, but never suffered so
acutely as when I learnt what loneliness could mean.

Perhaps that is the reason why I shudder when I pass the door of
those wards where women lie alone, enduring the first stage of labour.
They are not educated to their job; they are told to 'get on with it'. From
time to time, a nurse looks in and speaks some word of hope, but goes
again because she, like other nurses, is so busy. I wonder what goes
through those tortured minds, torn with ignorance and doubt, and
rigidly resistant. Their uterine contractions make pain for themselves
and prolonged labour for their child.

Hospital organisation, we know, makes constant attendance upon
all women in labour extremely difficult, but within the last five years
some few understanding professors have instituted labour sisters who

never leave the patients alone. We sympathise with all who work in hospitals where such service is hampered by inadequate provision of staff and space for individual attention during all phases of labour, but in private practice it is one of the main sources from which troubles in labour arise. Therefore, I repeat, take personal interest in your patient and remember that no woman should ever suffer the mental (and therefore physical) agony of loneliness whilst she is in labour. Stay with her until she understands; demonstrate to her by patient instruction the advantages of relaxation; by simple examination satisfy her that you have reason to encourage her in performing a simple natural function. Remind her of the necessity for patience; hold out no false hopes of rapid delivery. It means hard work and self-control; it is nature's first lesson in the two greatest assets of good motherhood. Children will always mean hard work and will always demand self-control; this is a small cost price to a right-minded woman. If it is desired to do it well for the children's sake, then the initiation into a noble life's work should be seriously undertaken and the significance of the greatness of motherhood in human society should not be obscured by the casual, disinterested attitude of the obstetrician. It is a privilege for any man or woman to guide a beginner; it is a post of grave responsibility and those who care to take it lightly and who, for selfish motives, take advantage of their status to gain all and give nothing, should be forbidden to practise an art and craft of such far-reaching importance.

A large number of written testimonies to the suffering of women is in my possession. It is unhappy reading because we know it need not and should not have happened. Those who have experienced the tortures of the damned have wounds upon their minds that time will hardly heal. They are not to blame; they are to be pitied. The function of parturition bears the brunt of accusation; this is grossly unjust. There is no more beautiful event in the life of a human being than the natural birth of a child. Subtract from modern childbirth the inflictions of ignorance and it becomes a joy to the mother; protect a healthy woman from the influences of cultural contaminations and parturition may be witnessed as a physiological masterpiece. Look with quiet comprehending eyes at the miracle of nativity; each reflex is a reasoned part without which the intricate machinery would break down. No sound or movement of the newborn babe is without significance to its survival; no science knows the origin or the nature of those forces which unite in harmony to vitalise and perfect a new life cast off from the uterus of a woman whose facultative genius has developed, nurtured and ripened the physiological facsimile of herself.

The cultural acquisitions of the human race are not yet comparable to the works of God. Some obstetric scientists may require an apology from me for that assumption, but I suggest that if a closer and more personal interest were taken in the mental as well as the physical influences upon childbirth, the cause of nearly all its evils will be found in ignorance and misunderstanding, for the persistence of which my profession must be held responsible. The first principle for the relief of suffering is the removal of the cause, but in obstetrics there are those who still accept unbearable discomfort as inevitable, and turn the heads of the rising generation towards surgical procedures, drugs and analgesics, when they should be investigating the root of this evil. This could be done in the antenatal clinic, by the bedside or in the nursery. Personal interest and patience will soon direct their thoughts to the source of suffering and their abilities to its eradication. Future generations will recognise in dystocia a pathological state and will employ the science of medicine or surgery for the sufferer's relief, as indeed we do today in abnormal and complicated cases. A great and pleasing surprise awaits the obstetrician who will patiently conduct only a dozen normal labours from start to finish and who will apply himself to understand the mind as well as the body of his patient. It will require concentrated personal interest in every phase, patience to await the issue, and peacefulness of mind from which radiates confidence, courage and self-control.

It may be asked at once: what is this *confidence*, this faith which can remove mountains that have stood since the records of civilised woman have been known? It is a belief in the fundamental perfection of reproduction as the greatest and most complete of all natural functions. It is based upon the experience of those who have seen its possibilities; it is inherent in primitive woman. Accidents and wastage occur in all forms of reproduction, vegetable as well as animal; in the human race there are fewer accidents and the wastage is incomparably smaller than in any other form of life.

Obstetricians must believe, and such faith must be based upon observation and truth. There is ample justification for absolute confidence in the outcome of labour if the antenatal care has been correctly and accurately conducted. Without applied science and with clear understanding the large majority of women, well prepared in both body and mind, produce their babies according to the accepted rule. Confidence rests upon the knowledge of perfect preparation. It is well known that abnormal conditions, which are unforeseen, do arise, but this very rarely happens and it is for such misfortunes that skilled obstetricians exist, for if such things did not occur, then priests, shepherds and old women would be competent to attend at childbirth as they were considered to be but a few hundred years ago. But even in the presence of such dangers, the large majority of women and babies are safely treated and the fact of unforeseen possibilities should not mar the general expectancy of a successful issue. A much smaller percentage of medical men who attend confinements have confidence either in themselves or in their case than is generally recognised. The teaching of abnormal midwifery is so stressed in our student days that as beginners we lose sight of the normal and natural, and unless we observe for ourselves, we may easily fall into the trap of searching only for the abnormalities in antenatal care and suspecting some subtle ambush in every labour from which the devil himself may leap at any moment.

This attitude, which is too prevalent, makes calm confidence impossible; the anxiety of the attendant is to get the case over quickly; he is prompted by his own unfounded fears to do something – anything. It becomes intolerable to sit and wait; he prefers to be called as late as possible and leave the waiting to the midwife who is assisting him. In the early second stage he argues that, the cervix being fully dilated, he is allowed by obstetric law to put on forceps and mentally fingers these adjuvants to his own peace of mind.

An old friend and colleague of mine was discussing with me the midwifery of our time. We were enjoying a pipe and a grouse together when he remarked, 'More than half my obstetric consultations are calls by windy incompetents.' It was not the condition of the patient which required his very expert advice, but the condition of the doctor. In no branch of medicine is there a greater strain upon the nervous system of a medical man. We have all desired the presence of a colleague in a trying case, even if only to corroborate our own opinion. At three in the morning we may be harassed by ruminations and imaginations that raise doubts in our minds and even warp our judgment. It takes a strong moral courage to be able to set out all the facts and review the situation with a calm, logical precision, particularly if the patient has detected a weakening in the support you have given her. During labour, women spot a doubt in a doctor's mind as quickly as a kestrel sees a rat in the stubble. Faith in midwifery is not metaphysical, it is founded on facts and is a bond between patient and attendant upon which rests the integrity of parturition and the natural sequence of its events. However good an actor or however suave a humbug, confidence has no counterfeit. It is neither looks, words nor works, but a special sense born on the atmosphere of truth and inflexible honesty of purpose. To have or to give confidence in labour is the hallmark of one whose calling is obstetrics. Many women cannot share such confidence, but this depends on the success of their antenatal education. Some are so afraid that nothing can induce them to have faith in a function that they insist upon believing is an agony beyond endurance; their minds are irrational; they become abnormal. If a woman's mind is so constituted that it cannot admit a fact, her labour is as pathological as that of a woman whose pelvis is so constructed that it cannot admit a fetus. If it is remembered that natural childbirth is largely of the mind, care will be taken to promote justifiable confidence in all concerned in the case from the earliest weeks of pregnancy onwards. Thus, fear may be attacked and subdued; happy, carefree pregnancy is a grand preparation for an easy confinement.

But always be on the watch. *Concentrated observation* need not be obtrusive, but it must be accurate and keen. You are more likely to find abnormalities by delineating the boundaries of good health than you are to find good health by concentrating upon real or phantom abnormalities. On the day I first wrote these words, a student remarked to me, 'We have only had normal cases lately, but Mr X is coming in later on this afternoon to put on forceps; the woman has been in labour two and a half days; we think she is an occipital posterior; it should be quite interesting.' 'Ah, splendid,' I replied to this lady who, though a student, was a potential mother of the morrow. 'Very interesting. I expect the woman is getting interested by now.' Of course it is exciting to see the abnormal, and necessary for training, but must the normal and natural be considered dull? It is only in these cases that any beauty can be found in midwifery. These simple, straightforward performances are the perfect initiation into motherhood; surely here is the field for observation. Each constituent of the ordinary is so extraordinary when understood. It is so in nature, in every sphere, it is one of its great fascinations. It is more thrilling to watch an avalanche crash in a cloud of snow to the bottom of a ravine, to hear the roar of its thunderous progress and witness the devastation in its path, than to lie on the rand of a Norfolk marsh. Yes, more thrilling until you have looked quietly and closely into the reeds. As the peaceful beauty of nature is observed, its constituents gradually appear; silver fish light up the shallow water, great swallow-tail butterflies flit decoratively from ragged robin to wild angelica; small cotton tufts reveal the newly hatched cocoon of *Epeira Cornuta*; each wee spider is a thrill as it sets out on its great adventure; a moorhen calls and hurries her fluffy offspring past your observation post; a bittern booms in the distance. At every turn of the eye the simplest form of nature is found to be full of excitement and fresh beauty. The more closely we look, so the treasure house opens fresh doors of wonder until we become absorbed in the perfection of simplicity and the magnificence of the ordinary. I have done this so often during the last forty years that the intrusion of foreign bodies in smelly motor boats and multicoloured vulgarities of clothing is equivalent to disease attacking the normal peacefulness of natural beauty. The thought of these disturbers brings resentment; they are not interesting. And so in all observation of a natural state; the more concentrated and penetrating it becomes, so much the more is found to observe, to understand and to marvel at. Normal labour is no exception to this rule. Many people think the Norfolk marshes dull; they abhor the silence, so they bring gramophones and regale the voice of God with ragtime. These are they who love to be with me on the Jungfraujoch and count the roars of avalanches and say, 'Stupendous', while I say, 'Dead ends falling off dead beginnings.' These are also the people who find normal labour dull, but who are thrilled by a forceps operation, a post-partum haemorrhage or a face presentation. If only they would look closely into uncomplicated labour, observing every change in the mind and body of their patient, how much they would find that is of absorbing interest, and how all-important nature would become.

The conduct of labour must be dull to the attendant who sees nothing in it; it is a waste of time to be with a woman if there is nothing to do; why sit there while she groans her way through the long hours of unavoidable pain? If these hours are used sensibly, every word spoken, every smile, every facial expression and every uterine contraction will be found to contain an indication for comfort, help or support. You will notice the change in tone and expression of the spoken word – the flippant courage of the early stage, or the anxious pleading; the laughter of the first stage fades to a tired appreciative smile as the cervix dilates and in the second stage you see the real nature of your patient. Her face tells you the variations of her emotional state; from it you estimate her control, her fear and her ability to relax; and from her uterine contractions you learn of progress and the correctness of the mechanics of her labour. No two are alike and there are a hundred other things to know; every minute has a fund of fascinating information waiting for the keen and concentrated observation of the physician who can piece together the varying phenomena, both mental and physical, and so find the means of help and encouragement his patient requires. Such observation enables an accurate estimate of the personality of the patient to be made. Does she need kindness or enthusiasm, firmness or control? Where her walls appear to be giving way they can be reinforced.

Hear from women who have experienced this truly human attention what aid it gave to them; I suspect you will visualise their labours as something almost unbelievable. But do observe whether your patient wants you there or not; some women dislike intensely the presence of anyone at all; a good many do not want the doctor until they feel they must have him. Tactfully find out why, if you can. It may teach you a lot about your patient that you had not previously suspected.

Cheerfulness if discreetly modulated is quite compatible with shrewd observation. Good cheer is a blessing without disguise; not hilarity and not a giggling futility, and not as I once heard a medical man greet his patient: 'Ha-ha! Cheer up, old girl. You've got to go through hell, but I'll go anywhere with you, so keep smiling. Ha-ha!' I said that we would hate to detain him if he would like to go on ahead.

There is, however, as in all practical work, a margin for common sense and reasonable tact. Such an exhibition of mental inaptitude is worse even than the long face and silent insinuation of tragedy. It is so easy to misunderstand the state of a woman's mind and the nature of her thoughts. A violent physical effort is not infrequently attended by demonstrations of determination or exasperation and its aftermath may well be exhaustion or a transient expression of despair. These are not always true indications of the condition of a woman in the second stage of labour. Between contractions we often hear, 'I am sorry to be making such a fuss, but I really cannot help it.' A kindly word of cheerful encouragement goes a long way at this time; I should be careful, however, not to be too sympathetic. Profound sympathy presupposes suffering, and may therefore act as strong suggestion that suffering is necessary.

Many years ago I was brought to my senses by a woman of twenty-two years of age who had appeared to be in such a state of anguish that I felt genuinely sorry for her and contemplated the means of relieving her from her pathetic state. She caught an expression on my face as she half-opened her eyes and to my astonishment and shame she patted my hand and reproved me, saying, 'Cheer up, doctor; it's nothing like so bad as that!'

During the second-stage contractions, explain carefully to your patient how she can help her contracting uterus. This requires considerable experience. Do not allow her to be violent in the early part of the expulsive phase. There is no need for such exertion. She must hold her breath in full inspiration and bear down when and as the uterus demands. With a first baby this is important for unnecessary tiredness or fatigue which should not occur may create difficulty in the final dilatation of the outlet. When the head is in the mid-pelvic cavity, possibly the bag of waters or the caput is just showing, extra effort may be called for, providing that amnesic rest and relaxation is obtained between the contractions. Wake her up to the conscious reality of her surroundings and be alert to advise her how to get a relaxed outlet and the best method of mechanical advantage for her efforts. But do not presume that she is unaware of what is going on. She may appear to be asleep and behave in a dull and amnesic state, but she is not asleep and will hear and understand everything as her contractions recommence.

Offset the tendency to grim despondency with an element of confident cheerfulness. It may not always be congruous, but in the majority, the large majority, of normal labours, it will be a source of strength to the woman in labour and an indication of the confidence you have in the successful result of her efforts. There is no limit to a woman's courage if you give her faith. A few notes upon labours conducted after the manner described in the preceding chapter will serve as a practical demonstration of its application. It has been my custom upon returning from a midwifery case to record it in considerable detail on the dictaphone. The facts are fresh in my mind, and minor incidents as well as important events to do with the labour are retained accurately without bias or wishful thinking that might result from the happiness of the next visit. It takes only a few minutes and I recommend it to all who wish to examine parturition and its conduct. Such records are enlightening and – although sometimes humiliating if they are kept with fearless honesty – much may be learnt from them. It is undoubtedly true that for some years I met many puzzling phenomena and only time and a long series of records threw any light upon these mysteries. I read, with considerable misgivings, some of my earlier cases, realising how much easier the confinement might have been if certain things had been done differently and certain signs had been recognised in their true significance, as they would be today in the light of more mature experience. The results have more than justified the investigation and the criticism of experimenting upon my patients is not valid, for none has suffered any more because of it and an increasing proportion of all cases have unquestionably benefited from it.

When Isaac Newton presented his 'Theory of Gravitation' to the Royal Society he did so with a simple preamble, 'I beg leave to present to you the results of certain experiments for your contemplation.' It is for those who read these things of which I write to contemplate, not to accept or to discard, for if there is anything of value in them, they become worthy of contemplation and even exhaustive trial, if by such attention they may remove the stigma that civilisation has cast upon childbirth.

And now, some twenty-one years since this chapter was first written, there is a different story to be told. Obstetricians in many countries have turned their minds to, and applied the principles of management of, pregnancy and parturition which have become widely known as 'Natural Childbirth.'

No record has been published, or sent to me in private communication, suggesting that anyone has discarded this approach to childbirth after having given it fair trial. Without exception, they have acknowledged the benefits of these procedures, both to mother and child. From their own point of view, as obstetricians, a number have pointed out that midwifery is no longer the anxiety it used to be; the atmosphere of the labour ward has changed; women demand the satisfaction of personal achievement and their discomforts are so small that they neither need nor use the analgesia at their disposal. The babies, born slightly blue, cry loudly immediately they arrive and rapidly turn pink from unimpaired oxygenation. The need for instrumental interference is greatly reduced and episiotomies are rarely necessary.

Many refer to the supreme happiness of the mothers and their wish to have more children as soon as reasonably possible; others write of the complacent progressive infants, whose unity with the mother is complete in its security for food and warmth and safety. Not only obstetricians and pediatricians have made these salutary observations; the psychiatrists emphasise the absence of signs of frustration in the early infancy of these natural children. It is indeed rare, they state, after the experience of conscious childbirth without distress that post-partum psychopathies develop. The sociologists lay stress upon the enhanced mother-child relationship and the welding, through the father's interest, of the family unit.

The great safeguards of medical science are criticism and opposition. All innovations in the cause of mental and physical wellbeing of the people are purified in the fires of controversy. He who dares to challenge orthodoxy welcomes both the commendations and censures of his colleagues who have applied and contemplated that which he upholds. The critics who are not familiar with the tenets they impugn are ever-vehement and voluble. It is a common manifestation of human frailty – the flotsam of our profession drifts from flower to flower, but rarely carries pollen of creation.

But fear, the noisy poltergeist of pregnancy, that for so long has tapped and moaned its terrifying mysteries, can be laid for all time. Its presumptuous presence in the minds of uninstructed women can be cast out by faith and understanding of the truth.

16

Childbirth in Emergency

There are times when we all have to face unexpected emergency and it is our reaction to such emergencies that is often more important than the sudden, and maybe totally unexpected, occurrence or situation with which we are confronted.

In a country which has within less than fifty years been through two wars, the reaction to emergency has been demonstrated by cruel experience, and valuable observations have been made upon the behaviour of its people when under stress of danger from a variety of assaults upon both mind and body.

Frequently the anticipation of death intensifies the horror of its possibility, but many persons after repeated exposure to danger developed an attitude of submission to the inevitable, and a faith in divine will, which produced an amazingly calm and controlled acceptance of the most violent and cataclysmic bombing.

This we hoped and most of us believed was the last big scale effort of man to mutilate and ultimately destroy life upon this earth. But evidences of insatiable greed for power and riches remain. There are those who would rule the world and we must not turn our backs on these possibilities, however remote. The organisation and education in Civil Defence is carefully and enthusiastically attended to in many towns and communities today, but there is one situation which may apply to the four and a half million women in America to whom babies are born each year. But quite apart from this thought which not unnaturally is more evident in Europe than in the USA, this precaution must not be accepted as an alarmist view, for fires and floods, accident on sea and land and in the air do occur and women all over the world are, and may continue to be, caught in the emergency of unexpected labour – if only because they are alone at home or in the fields or, as I have seen several times, in a public place or vehicle. Labour is not a frightening incident in the life of a woman if she has learnt what goes on and how her body produces the child when it is ready to leave its mother's womb. If a woman has no knowledge of her own natural processes and how to assist and not hinder their performance, she makes many difficulties and much discomfort for herself and maybe for her child.

What can a woman do when and if in circumstances of unexpected emergency she comes into labour – with no competent person to help her and maybe only herself to help her child safely into the world?

Nothing disturbs the course of natural labour more than fear. That is a known and well-proved scientific fact. Fear is caused and intensified by ignorance. It has been demonstrated by hundreds of thousands of women in all countries of the world that knowledge of the facts of childbirth reduces the risk of trouble in 90–97 per cent of all labours – a baby is born to a mother with understanding, without unbearable discomfort and with little if any risk of injury or danger to either mother or baby.

A simple aid to women in this emergency is desirable not as a routine under prepared and equipped conditions, but when, unprepared and ill-equipped, her child decides to arrive.

It is a strange society that teaches women innumerable subjects that concern her mental and physical ability to earn a living and find a home and husband, but no education is made available, as a routine, to teach mature girls, young women, and even pregnant women to understand the most important physiological function for which Nature has magnificently designed them. In a civilised community much requires explanation and instruction that in a primitive tribe might come naturally, but strangely enough, it is the least civilised people and the higher animals who take most trouble to prepare and protect their young females, directly or indirectly, for the reproduction of their kind, so that the best stock may be maintained to ensure that as a tribe or community they will survive.

Let us, therefore, accept this advice as generally applicable to a young woman's education – whether under stress or not – but essential in times of emergency.

Although many mothers of today have an elementary idea of the anatomy of their pelvis and its contents, it is astonishing how many are completely ignorant. We will discuss the question of what to do in an emergency labour, presuming our pupil knows little or nothing about it. When the baby is ready to be born it lies comfortably in the uterus or womb, with its head downwards. It is usual and best for babies to dive, not to step, into the world. It heralds its arrival in three ways – by a *show* of mucous or blood from the outlet of the birth canal, a *leaking* or gushing of water from the uterus, or by *rhythmical contractions* getting increasingly more frequent and stronger. The first two of these warnings, in the absence of the strong contractions of the womb, usually give plenty of time to prepare for the baby's arrival, but under the stress of accident or the threat of death-dealing danger, the intense defensive reaction to paralysing fear is almost complete relaxation and inactivity of the muscles that control the passage of the baby from the womb. Under these circumstances labour is often what we term precipitate and the baby arrives with very little discomfort or difficulty to the mother. This terror paralysis of the muscles of the pelvic floor, allowing spontaneous evacuation of the bowel and urinary bladder, is well known and at the end of pregnancy the same reaction to terror may occur.

When the intensity of fear diminishes and brings conscious realisation of the prevailing circumstances, women resist the effort of expulsion and thereby create a state of tension by opposing the muscles that are contracting to push the baby out and those which are resisting its progress. This is the reaction of emotional stress. There is a very real difference between the emergency or precipitated labour with the primitive defence reaction to violent and imminent destruction, and the labour of a woman in fear of labour itself, for a defensive reaction of the former is emotional and physical paralysis and of the latter emotional and physical resistance. The writer has seen and been able to observe the differences in the trenches, on the shell swept plains and in the rubble of bombed cities, of women in emotional terror who have lost the power of voluntary control and those who are frightened by the visualisation of false childbirth teaching, who lie in the arms of well-meaning attendants whose tender care and hysterical anticipation of pain and trouble bring to women the needless tensions and discomforts they suffer.

May I emphasise, therefore, the importance of elementary understanding of the simple processes of childbirth before a woman is of marriageable age. That is the easiest way in which the fear of childbirth may be removed and remember it is *Fear* that produces all the severe and unbearable pains. A *calm* and controlled woman has little, if any, discomfort, and an *understanding* woman remains calm, awaiting the progression of natural events that she expects because of her learning.

Wherever she is, in a wayside ditch, or a ruin-covered cellar, in a stranger's house, a caravan, or tent, she should *sit down* and lean back against the wall, the bank, or a centre pole. She pulls up her knees and puts her buttocks on a folded coat, a bunch of leaves, or mound of sand or stones washed clean by a nearby stream. If she is alone she must remember some of the cardinal points of this teaching. She does not lie down on her side or her back, but sits as near as possible in a squatting position, taking the weight of her body upon her buttocks. If left alone in labour the body of a woman produces most easily the baby that is not interfered with by its mother's mind or the assistant's hand. If left alone, just courage and patience are required. Faith, if she is a believer, is the secret of having a healthy baby and being a happy mother. If left alone she may escape one of the greatest causes of trouble, which is interference by those who, being kindly but misinformed, feel they must *do* something for her. The safest medical attendant is nature, by whom woman has been marvellously equipped for this purpose. Troubles are rare, even more rare in emergency full-term labours than in the general run of births conducted in modern hospitals.

So a woman should sit and wait for the baby that may arrive inconveniently. She will soon feel a desire to push down, similar to the desire to help the ready bowel to empty. At first the effort to expel is gentle. 'A deep breath and hold it. If the uterus does not ask for assistance wait for the next contraction.' There may be some backache, but it soon goes and if there is no one to rub it, she must not allow it to become too important in her mind; she must relax and not tense against it – it will go. When the expulsive contractions are well and truly established she will bear down with them, not violently at first but firmly, not expecting immediate results. If it is her first baby, it may be one and a half to two hours of repetition of expulsive effort becoming increasingly stronger. Breathing with these contractions must not be forgotten, sometimes two or three deep breaths, in and out, may be taken during one contraction. As the contraction fades she relaxes sleepily, takes two deep breaths and lies quietly resting until the next effort commences. Her drowsiness may be so deep that she concentrates only on the task of producing her child. So much so that I have seen women during air raids, by nature nervous people, who were not disturbed by the noise or the flashes of bombs that rocked the walls about us. On one occasion, being myself disconcerted by the volume and proximity of missiles, I was slow to notice the onset of yet another contraction. My patient of twenty-two years said testily 'Another push, Doctor. Come on, don't worry about the noise.'

Just before the head can be seen some women have a strong wave of escapism. It is not pain but a state of mind, and all should recognise this and remember that two or at the most three determined and concentrated expulsive efforts to help the contraction will get rid of this disconcerting desire to escape. Shortly after that the hair on the baby's head will show at the outlet and if there is a looking-glass from a handbag or other source, it enables a woman to take an active interest in helping her child on its journey; she concentrates upon the baby and its arrival and forgets the fears for her own well-being. The second or expulsive stage of labour is not painful. It may be hard work for first babies' births, but more usually it is a conscious, controlled and painless repetition of pushes to urge the baby to take the normal course and go through the natural twists and turns, flexions and extensions of the head so that damage to the mother and baby is prevented.

As the head starts to distend the vulva a feeling of burning of the labia or lips of the outlet may alarm a woman who has not experienced a conscious labour. Simple remedies overcome this frightening sensation. She must realise it soon passes off if she does not squeeze up against it; the outlet must be relaxed and allowed to bulge as it will. She must not continue to bear down but to breathe in short breaths letting her stomach muscles remain loose and the uterus does all the pushing necessary for a slow and relatively painless birth of the head.

In the meantime she will lose much of the drowsiness and lean upon her back support at an angle of 45 degrees, that is, halfway between flat and upright. She pulls her knees up with contractions and holds them up with her hands, wide open and at right angles to her body. With her feet resting on the bed as the baby is born, with its face looking downwards, she can lean over and put her hand on the perineum to support the head as it arrives so that the baby's forehead and face pass into the palm of her hand, as she directs it upwards towards her abdomen. She should help the baby to be directed upward and over the bone of the front of her pelvis. She must not pull it out straight or she may tear the outlet of the birth canal.

If she is alone or with only inexperienced people she must not become excited and hurried. Slowly, quietly, and gently are the qualities of a good delivery. The crying baby will lie in her hand or on her abdomen, until the cord, joining her to the infant, ceases to pulsate or throb. It will shrink and become pale and flaccid. By this time the placenta or afterbirth may have separated from the womb and be in the vaginal cavity. Soon more contractions start for a few short minutes, the second stage labour is repeated in a diminutive form for the birth of the placenta, or the third stage. The mother should hold her baby, if some bleeding from below continues, and she should put the child to her breast and allow it to nose the nipple, if it does not, as most do, grasp it in its mouth. If the afterbirth does not come of its own accord, put a hand on the uterus, which will be felt as a coconut-size lump above the navel, and give one or two sharp coughs and it may come out easily. In emergency labour the cord should not be cut until after the afterbirth comes away. Till then the baby is kept warm in its mother's clothing, either on the ground beside her or in her arms, preferably held to the breast. When the afterbirth is born it may be wrapped up with the baby until experienced help is available. Amongst cultured races, other than the white or European, this is still the customary procedure.

During labour a woman should pass urine from time to time so as to keep her bladder empty. This is done in a squatting position at any reasonable place, according to the dilemma in which she may find herself.

The dignity and control of childbirth can be advantageously maintained in circumstances incredibly divergent from our accepted civilised standards. Fortunately the writer has seen and attended women in many strange places and does not write without experience. Whatever clothing is available may be used for the baby and for the mother. As little as possible should be put over the birth canal outlet. Do not touch the vulva with the unwashed hand if it can be avoided, but emergency labour seldom becomes infected. Most women after the labour is completed are fit and able to walk with their babies to a place where clothing and cleanliness may be obtained. It may be that medical aid and advice is within reach. There is no rule that can meet all emergencies, but understanding, self-control, and patience are the assets of success and a woman must not forget that faith is not only an ethical emotional acquisition but a state of mind which creates within the body physical harmony of the activities of living, which maintain the highest standard of health and resistance to disease.

17

Breast-feeding and Rooming-in

There have been many changes during the last ten or fifteen years in obstetrics and the approach to motherhood, but there is one which I entirely fail to understand.

It is equivalent in some respects to reversion to the use of wet nurses, but with the knowledge and experience obtained over the last forty years about breast-feeding and its advantages, it is astonishing to find that a number of responsible members of the medical profession appear to be antagonistic to this method of nurturing infants. Naturally those who believe that all babies should be bottlefed from birth have arguments which they use to support their contention. It is necessary for them to defend such tenets, particularly when they are opposed to the natural process and the maternal physiological demand.

It is probably true that over 95 per cent of all healthy women are physically competent to feed their babies at the breast.

The women who do not suckle their babies may be represented in the main by two groups:

1. Those who wish to breast-feed their babies and cannot.
2. Those who do not wish to breast-feed their babies and do not.

Group 1

Those in group one fall under different headings:

a. SEVERE ILLNESS. Women suffering from severe illness, including forms of active disease of the lungs, the kidneys or the heart. Those who suffer from acute anaemias, infectious diseases, prolonged fevers such as influenza, etc.

b. MALFORMED BREASTS. Women whose breasts are malformed to such a degree that the baby cannot suck.

c. THE BABY. Women whose babies are unable to suck. Some premature infants are not strong enough and others suffer from rare nervous or anatomical abnormalities and developments which make sucking impossible.

d. THE ECONOMIC FACTOR. In these days of altered social habits, many mothers have to work to earn their living or supplement the husband's income, which is insufficient to maintain the home at the present cost of living. They continue in their employment until the latest possible week in pregnancy and start work again when the baby is two or three weeks old. It is their means of survival and they must therefore sacrifice the close relationship with their babies in the cause of necessity. These infants see their parents only at night, they are fed by strangers during the day on prescriptions, from a bottle. Some mothers try to suckle their babies in the early morning and late at night, a bottle being used whilst they are away, but the discomforts of full breasts during the day or expressing surplus milk, are difficult to sustain for many weeks.

e. WOMEN WHO HAVE NO MILK, or so little that the baby must have a bottle to supplement the paucity of the mother's supplies. If lactation and the influences that make or mar its efficiency were more generally indoctrinated, there would be fewer women suffering from this disability.

Sub-section *e* is really intermediate between Groups *1* and *2*, for some wish to feed their babies and cannot and others have no milk because of the absence of the desire to suckle the infant. Women feed their babies with their minds through their breasts. The majority of this group suffer from psychopathic inhibition, not physical or hormonal dysfunction.

Before we discuss Group *2* some more general observations on Group *1* should be made.

I reiterate not once but many times – there is no rule of thumb in obstetrics and baby care. Common sense, discretion and experience of the doctor must ultimately be deciding factors in all cases. To preach that all babies must be breast-fed is as ridiculous as saying that they must all be bottle-fed. The fact that there are women and babies who cannot do it must be accepted, but in spite of all contra-indications only 4 or 5 per cent of healthy women are physically unable to feed their babies at the breast.

One English authority records the statement that 500,000,000 gallons of breast milk are wasted each year because mothers do not realise its value and their advisers do not understand the simple technique of natural feeding.

Group 2

a. SELFISHNESS. Unhappily we must recognise that there are a number of women who live entirely for themselves and their personal occupations and enjoyment. Selfishness is the urge that prompts them to wean their babies from birth. They cannot have the normal routine of their lives disturbed by the intervention of a baby which will, they persuade themselves, thrive upon the doctor's prescription or patent food. Many of these people would undoubtedly change their minds if they could be made to understand the importance of mothering their baby – not only to themselves but to the child and the family circle. We can only hope that they will be brought, by conscientious advisers, to realise the error of their ways.

b. VANITY. Many women refrain from feeding their children because they believe that their figure, carriage or appearance will suffer by so doing. Vanity describes this outlook. It is possible to sympathise with those who are rightly proud of their physical assets and who have seen the results of ill-conducted pregnancies of their friends. A woman can lose her good figure and much of her pristine charm, but there is no real necessity for this or for any deterioration in her appearance. With modern instruction and training in antenatal classes, organised by efficient teachers, the appearance of women is enhanced by childbirth and their physical attraction is, in every way, more appreciated by their husbands after, than before, pregnancy. The only excuse for those who will not feed their baby because of these erroneous persuasions is that they have not had the truth brought home to them or have been unable to act upon the good advice they have received.

c. PSYCHOPATHIES. I have drawn attention to the influence of the mind of woman upon lactation and although it is unnecessary to delve deeply into the psychological conditions that inhibit the milk supply, it must be accepted that they constitute a factor of major importance. These illnesses of the mind may either exist beneath the consciousness or within the consciousness; although we are not fully familiar with the exact relationship between the mental processes and the milk supply, we have no doubt of its existence. Under the influence of hypnosis, lactation has been established in a few hours, showing that the breast is able to secrete milk if the inhibitions of the mind are removed.

In practice, we see this in a simple form – the woman who worries about her baby, her husband, finances or any of the other apparently serious troubles, will find her milk supply diminishing. This in itself is an added worry since she is really anxious to feed her baby, but because of her mental turmoil she loses her milk. If her anxieties can be removed, the milk will return in full flow, demonstrating that the breast is not at fault but the mind.

There are certain psychopathic states which make the act of breast-feeding disagreeable and even revolting to a woman. A young girl of twenty-one whom I knew, was unable to stay in a room with a new-born babe – she was known to have been physically sick on one occasion when she unwittingly found a close friend feeding her baby at the breast. Such deeply imprinted states can be removed from the mind by adequate psychiatric treatment – they are recorded only as evidence of the influence of the mind upon lactation.

d. MEDICAL ATTENDANTS. The establishment of lactation can be prevented for social reasons at the birth of the child. For this purpose, whilst mothers are still anaesthetised for the delivery of their infants, they are given an injection which prevents lactation and the breasts do not become active. The school of thought that teaches women to bottle-feed their babies usually subscribes to the belief that they should not be conscious of the birth sensations when the baby arrives.

Unfortunately we hear of women who are very anxious to suckle their offspring being given these injections and to their disappointment and even shame, they have to wean their babies under the instructions of the attendant pediatrician without knowing why their breasts were inactive.

Let us rather consider the advantages of breast-feeding than these unhappy states that we have discussed.

The benefits of breast-feeding can be set in the main under five headings:

THE BABY.	*1.* Physical.	
	2. Mental.	
THE MOTHER.	*1.* Physical.	
	2. Mental, Emotional and Psychological.	
THE HOME.		

The Baby – Physical

When a baby is born it should be put to the breast at the earliest possible opportunity – many of my mothers who watch their babies born and take them in their arms wrapped in warm towels immediately the umbilical cord is cut, notice the child is either sucking its fingers after it has quietened down from its first few lusty yells, or is mouthing when they stroke its cheek. A certain number of them have an immediate desire to put the child to the breast. The effect of this will be discussed later, for there is no milk at this time but a substance known as colostrum, which has been present for some days, possibly weeks, before the birth of the child, and exudes from the well-prepared nipple.

There is still considerable discussion about this thick fluid. We know that it contains a certain amount of milk globules and cells containing fat which we call colostrum corpuscles, but its actual use to the baby is not quite clear. It was once believed that it acted upon the baby's bowels to make it expel the meconium which is contained in the intestines of the unborn babe. Another theory was expounded later that it contained substances which produced within the infant an immunity to certain bacteria that might cause disease. For my own part, I prefer to think that colostrum is of greater use to the breast and nipple than it is to the baby. For nature provides the baby with a considerable amount of fat which, during the day or two before the milk is secreted in the breast, is absorbed by the newborn infant as its own natural nutrition and it is very largely this provision of food within itself that accounts for the loss of weight until the mother's milk supply is established.

About the third day after the baby has been put to the breast, in order to stimulate the activity of the glands, milk is secreted, the alveoli become enlarged and congested and fill the ducts leading from the breast to the nipple, of which there are usually about twenty.

Although it is not strictly accurate to say that the infant sucks the milk from the breast, we will use that term for the sake of simplicity. In reality, it presses the milk out by closing its mouth with a squeezing action. The only real sucking is the action of the baby's tongue in lifting the nipple up to its palate.

Mother's milk has certain qualities; it is fresh and clean and easily available. It is at the correct temperature and contains all the essential elements of food for the baby. It has the highest nutritional value of any known food for the human young. The supply is commensurate with the demand of a healthy baby as it grows and requires more. It is economical and labour saving for there is no necessity to waste considerable time upon sterilising the bottles, teats and preparing the food. It develops within the child an immunity against certain diseases, particularly those seasonal waves of infantile enteritis or diarrhoea which sweep through the land. The mortality rate amongst babies which become infected with this dire affliction is invariably quoted by authorities as being only one-third to one-fifth of the mortality of bottle-fed babies. It has been found that in families which suffer from allergic diseases such as asthma, eczema, epilepsy and urticaria, infants which are entirely breast-fed for the earlier months of their lives are less prone to develop these conditions.

Emotional

Recent investigations upon the mental and emotional development of babies which have been breast-fed up to three months or more and the babies which have been bottle-fed from birth, have brought to light an interesting fact. The newborn infant which is breast-fed exhibits a placidity and absence of the signs of frustration, which enables it to progress in a state of uninterrupted good health – colic or excessive wind, constipation or irritability occurs in only a small percentage of these children as compared with bottle-fed infants. This strongly suggests that however adequate the prescription of the pediatrician, many babies cannot assimilate or digest cow's milk, however accurately the proportions may represent the milk of the human mother. One thing we cannot alter, and that is the solubility of the fat in cow's milk. It requires a medium within the child that is not invariably present and the undissolved portion of the fat gives rise to digestive disturbance.

The breast-fed baby remains in physiological contact with its mother and therefore takes its normal place in the sequence of events that constitute the cycle of human reproduction. The newborn baby has only three demands. They are: warmth in the arms of its mother, food from her breast, and security in the knowledge of her presence. Breast-feeding satisfies all three. The child, therefore, develops upon natural food and becomes familiar with the comfort of being cuddled in soft warmth whilst it feeds, as well as the strong, possessive and protective arms of its mother. In this way the earliest foundation of the mental stability of the child is laid, which is discernible in the ease with which it adapts itself to the new environment of extra-uterine life. An absence of frustration and fear of insecurity are seen in the placid, cooing child who lies awake in his crib and gurgles at the discovery that his fingers belong to him and he can make them do things.

Many psychiatrists have stated from time to time not only that man relives the moment of his birth, but also that his mental development will arise from his earliest association with life. If this is true, the happiness radiated by the nursing mother breast-feeding her child must envelop the infant in an aura of blissful associations with its earliest beginnings.

No hot blanket, guardian nurse or weaning bottle can replace the physiological character formation of the breast-fed baby. There is no substitute for mother love. The relationship between those who love and those who are loved is not a sentimental association but reality. There is a mutual transference of a force which elevates both the mind and body to a higher plane of human development than the implementation of impersonal scientific procedures and synthetic devices.

Man cannot feed the baby within the uterus. What justifies his presumption that he is able to improve upon the physiological provision because the child has recently left the uterus? We can fortify and reinforce with certain substances the adequacy of both the placental and the breast nutrition, but the basic natural nourishment supplies something which no concoction can contain.

Although a skilled physician can write prescriptions for mixtures upon which children will thrive, they cannot include the personality factor of successful mothering. They can build bonnie and beautiful babies whose bodies are the pride of their nurses and a profit to the advertisers of patent foods. Without mothering, a nation of gladiators can arise, as we have seen in the last two generations; but if the seeds of mother love had been implanted in early infancy and fostered in youth, should we have seen the tragedies and the indescribable horrors of the last fifteen to twenty years? Breast-feeding has a sociological value far greater than is generally recognised.

The Mother – Physical

The ability of a mother to feed her baby at the breast is commensurate with her ability to give birth to the child without assistance or interference. The mothers who witness the arrival of their baby and experience the sensations of relief, joy, achievement and pride that are the natural accompaniment to the birth of a child, invariably desire to feed their babies and not infrequently, are able to do so efficiently. We cannot disassociate breast-feeding from the manner of birth.

In my own practice, where not more than 3 per cent of the women who have normal labours accept the analgesia that is offered, 98 per cent desire to be and become good breast-feeding mothers. We learn that where women are subjected to interference either with local or general anaesthesia, the wish to feed their babies is less general. This could be put in another way: that the nearer the birth of a child is to the normal physiological function, so much the more likely is the continuity of the natural sequence of events of human reproduction maintained. When a mother takes her child to her breast immediately after she has witnessed its arrival, not only does the sound of its cry, or the touch of its hands, give rise to an emotional reaction, but a beneficial physical influence is established within the woman herself. It seems desirable and natural for some of them to put the infant to the breast and its contact stimulates, by direct reflex, strong contractions and retractions of the uterus. This activity hastens separation of the placenta and closing of the blood vessels in the part of the uterus to which it was attached.

These observations may be confirmed if a hand is placed lightly upon the abdomen as the baby is put to the mother's breast. One benefit, therefore, and it is indeed an important one, of the physical contact of the newborn babe with its mother, is the rapid separation of the afterbirth and the absence of any excessive haemorrhage. Those of us who are aware of the results of the mismanagement of the third stage of labour can assess adequately the importance of this phenomenon.

The reflex action of the uterus and other structures within the pelvis continues after the placenta has been extruded, for each time the baby goes to the breast it stimulates retraction or shortening of the muscle fibres and diminution in size of the vast blood vessels that have been formed around and within the uterus during pregnancy. This process, known as involution, or restitution, of the uterus to its non-pregnant state, is most satisfactorily completed under the urge of breast-feeding. In the first week or ten days of the puerperium, the activity of the baby may establish within the maternal pelvis a healthy condition which will be a blessing to the mother for all time.

If, as we are led to believe, lactation and the flow of milk are associated with an outpouring of secretion from the pituitary gland, the stimulating influence of that secretion upon the pelvic organs is evident in a breast-feeding mother.

Mental, Emotional and Psychological

The feeding of the child induces certain conditions in the mind of the mother. There is a complacent, peaceful sense of achievement associated with the knowledge that she is giving herself to her beloved possession. Her pleasant physical sensations when the baby feeds not only give rise to uterine contractions, but to a reaction closely akin to eroticism, which in many women stimulates contractions of the muscles of the pelvic floor and activates the glands of the vagina and vulva. I have heard it said that this intrusion of sexual feelings upon the purity of peaceful motherliness has so revolted some women that the conflict has inhibited the milk supply. In my considerable experience I have never met this psychopathic phenomenon. If a woman has accepted, for a variety of reasons, sexual gratification without love, I can understand the basis of conflict when, maybe at long last, she has learnt the power of spiritual love for her baby. Love and sex can be two strongly opposing emotions.

It has been observed that a woman who has breast-fed her baby may require a smaller contraceptive diaphragm than was used eighteen months before pregnancy. I have no recorded case of this in a mother whose baby was weaned from birth. The significance of this is clear to married people.

Apart from these physical benefits and the pleasure that they give to women, there are other aspects which must be considered.

No human being is more sensitive or more receptive than a pregnant woman unless it is a woman during the four or five weeks following the birth of her first child. She lives in the harassing confusion of her anxieties.

It appears that some mothers, through the desire for uninterrupted unity with their baby, unconsciously identify themselves with it and demand for themselves those attentions and considerations that they desire for their child. They become highly emotional, and, apparently without the reasoning discretion and discrimination that we would expect of rational adults, they are carried away by storms of exaggerated reaction to and faulty interpretation of the most inoffensive incidents and remarks. They are babies with their babies. They fear for their infant's well-being and are readily subjected to premonitions of inadequacy, failure and frustration. They suffer from acute depression for no logical cause and not infrequently between the fifth and eighth day of the puerperium will be found weeping appealing womanly tears, but unable to explain why they are disturbed. This may be the simple swing back of the emotional pendulum after the tremendous excitement of the experience of childbirth, but it is usually more than that. I have found that when the baby arrives, mothers often indulge in infantile behaviour devoid of the self-control which was well developed before they became pregnant. They will ascribe the cry of any infant that they hear to their own baby – which *must* therefore be suffering some discomfort or even ill-treatment. I have known women leap from their beds and hastily rush to the baby's cot to make sure that it is still alive, and finding it peacefully sleeping, become lacrimose with relief. One woman, between her baby's feeds, habitually tested her breasts to see if there was any milk for fear lest she should not be able to provide the next meal for her child. Had she had her own way it would have been put to the breast every ten minutes.

This excitable and illogical mental condition so many women experience after their babies are born must be carefully understood and guarded against, for they not infrequently focus their fears and anxieties upon lactation and persuade themselves that they will not and cannot become efficient feeding mothers. Unfortunately this line of thought can actually inhibit the milk supply, which appears to justify their fears, and so a vicious circle is established which is difficult to break down.

Frances Charlotte Naish, who is a general practitioner in the city of York, England, in 1947 was awarded the Sir Charles Hastings Clinical Essay Prize of the British Medical Association on Breast-Feeding. I emphasise 'general practitioner' because they are the only people who have the opportunity of prolonged and close personal study of the women they attend, both in maternity hospitals and later in their own homes. Women and babies owe her a deep debt of gratitude. The book is dedicated to her five children 'who have taught me so much'. From her own practical experience and accurate observations, and from the wide field of domiciliary work she has gleaned truths of superlative value. One sentence she writes should be displayed in every home or hospital where babies are born. I prefer to assume that it refers to childbirth as well as to successful breast-feeding: 'We must try to study our mothers' minds individually.' (What a tremendous advantage these medical mothers have over me, a mere male midwife! I raise my hands to the heavens in gratitude for all that they have told and taught me during their own pregnancies and labours, as well as in discussions upon the woman's point of view.)

If this is done, we shall soon discover ways and means of making breast-feeding a success. With a little teaching it will become a pleasure and a pride to mothers. They will be aware of a satisfactory sense of achievement which has far-reaching results. If their babies have been born naturally, they will recognise again the same joy of success that moved them to tears and laughter when they see their dreams come true as a blue-pink apparition emerged from themselves. If a mother is highly strung or over-anxious, there is no sedation more efficient than successful breast-feeding – each day those five or six phases of pleasing relaxation and calm will bring peace to her troubled mind. Soon she will wait impatiently for her baby's demand for food. She desires the physical pleasure and the comforting relaxation of her mind and body that this hour of unity with her child brings with ever-increasing intensity.

The Home

Breast-feeding does not extend its benefits only to the mother and child. Many fathers are distraught with the troubles of their wives and the cries of a restless baby who does not thrive. It is by no means infrequently the cause of one-child families, the fathers and mothers agreeing that quite apart from the trials that the labour brought to them both, they could never again go through the six or eight weeks of nerve-wracking experience, physical weariness and sleepless anguish that fell to their lot when the baby struggled to attain a standard of health and behaviour in which the parents had lost all confidence.

When successfully breast-feeding his child, a wife is supremely attractive to an affectionate husband. Sometimes when we are writing upon obstetric subjects we forget to call attention to the profound love for the baby that possesses many fathers. We do not remember how deeply they feel the emotional changes of their wives, nor the exaltation and personal satisfaction that they enjoy when all goes well. Husbands fail to realise what indignity their homes may suffer from the alienation of the mother and the baby when it is given at an early age to the care of a nursemaid, to be seen only for a few hurried moments in the evening before its parents change for dinner.

In South Africa, the majority of mothers employ African women to take care of, feed, bath and dress, and embrace their babies and young children. These women are segregated from the Europeans (the appellation the pale-skinned people assume). They enter railway stations and post offices by separate doors and are given no place in society, denied education and even adequate homes to live in, but in order that the social round may be continued and the daily routine of the mother's life shall not be interrupted, the babies and the rising generation of children have the foundations of their future development laid by those whom, in later years, they are brought up to ostracise.

It is possible, of course, that this upbringing has certain advantages, for Mzanyana is often a proud, dignified and loyal woman with a high sense of duty, but even her attentions cannot take the place of a mother's preoccupation in the physical and mental well-being of her child. As we sow, so shall we reap. A little love in the heart today may preclude a weight of grief in a life of many morrows.

Let me offer this solace to the woman who would, but cannot, feed her baby at the breast. She will find in mother love rebuffed a deep and cherished bond which turns the water of weaning into the wine of spiritual communion. The mother-child relationship will be welded by the fire of her frustration and the tenderness of her constant care and companionship will protect the child from any harm it might have suffered from their mutual misfortune.

A gipsy mother, whose breasts had been incurably mutilated by the flames of an exploded stove, was feeding her fifth baby from a bottle. She had breast-fed the four beautiful children who ran to greet me. They were clean, friendly and lovable in their picturesque, highly-coloured clothes and gilded earrings. I sat in the spotless caravan and told her how grieved I was to have to suppress her milk flow, or draught, as she called it. 'Don't worry, doctor, it's all the same if you put your heart into the bottle.' If a mother must bottle-feed her baby, let her give it food herself; with warmth, love and security, snuggled to her heart in the silent serenity of mutual satisfaction. Then little will be lost and much will be recovered. There is no more sentimentality in a mother's love for her child than in the craving of the lungs for oxygen. They are both vital physiological demands upon which the survival of the race depends. There is no logical argument against breast-feeding, but there are incontrovertible evidences of its benefits. Women must beware of false prophets and faddists, lest they be detracted from the truth.

Care of the Breasts

The care of the breasts is of far-reaching importance to a woman both as a mother and a wife. If she loses her figure and adopts an unbecoming posture, it may affect her personality. Some women become self-conscious, develop a sense of inferiority amongst others and an apologetic retiring manner, sometimes akin to shame, before their husbands. They blame lactation and even the infants whom they have breast-fed, although these troubles arise after weaning from birth more frequently than from breast-feeding.

Many women wear false breasts to give the appearance of having the attractive figures they could have retained with proper care and instruction. It is too frequently overlooked by those who attend childbearing women that the breasts are reproductive organs. They have a sexual as well as a personality value, which subjects them to the buffetings of a variety of psychological assaults. Not only have they the supreme function of lactation, but they are the ultimate manifestation of the mother-child relationship.

As surely as the umbilical cord sustains the vital unity of the mother with her intra-uterine fetus the nipple retains that mystic union with the child that is no longer within her. A mother feeding her baby at the breast attains a knowledge of the incomprehensible – the infinite genius of creation. In that blissful hour the infant floods its mother's mind in meditation which brings reality to her most cherished dreams, whilst she radiates the earliest creation of its consciousness with happiness and comforting security. This interchange of mutual possession and dependence enhances the physical and spiritual perfection of both mother and child. Through her breast they are unified in extra-uterine life as closely as in the months of gestation.

A man must be admitted to the masonry of motherhood to be acquainted with the deep emotions and physical pleasures that only women understand. Can we disbelieve the confidential stories given us by tens and hundreds of these healthy, happy people? We cannot write verbatim, words and phrases used in efforts to convey the intensity of their rapture, for it might indeed sound gross exaggeration. Who has the right to deny one woman this gratifying experience if she is fit and able to accept it? What fads and fashions raise their ugly heads to cast a social slur on breast-feeding. Who are the pseudo-scientists who dare to present alleged improvements to a healthy normal physiological process? And what is the object of their presumptuous intrusion upon human intelligence?

Medical science enables us to find successful substitutes when lactation fails – its province is to cure diseases and to forestall or rectify the faults that disturb natural function. But its supreme accomplishment is to comprehend the significance of our structure. The true scientist admits the limitations of his understanding and bows to a creative genius greater than his own. The highest ideal of such a man is to protect and maintain the integrity of phenomena which manifest the harmony of function and design. Nineteen women out of twenty, whose minds and breasts are properly prepared and cared for, can feed their babies faultlessly and experience the inner meaning of the observations I have made above.

Surely it is near to sacrilege to inhibit or destroy by persuasive words or actions, a woman's ability to suckle her child. Obstetricians have a duty – indeed a moral obligation – to direct the desires of women to their own and their babies' benefits. We must be teachers in an ignorant society, with time to justify our tenets, not vendors of scientific candy to please the palates of those who pay fees for our wares.

These thoughts apply to every incident in human reproduction, but to none more solemnly than the education and preparation of women to feed their babies at the breast.

The Breasts

A few weeks after conception the breasts will become sensitive to the touch. With the first baby the areola, that is the pink or pink-brown skin around the nipple, takes on a darker tinge, and small raised spots appear on it known as Montgomery's tubercles, which are early signs of pregnancy. The activity of the breasts is heralded by the appearance of enlarging veins, often showing a bluish tint under the skin around the centre of the breast. These signs are usually accompanied by a sense of fullness and frequently an actual increase in the size of the organs. It is necessary at this stage to wear efficient brassieres, for the shape of the breast may be permanently impaired if the increasing size and weight stretches the skin above the nipple. The distance between the nipples and the top of the breast bone between the ends of the collarbones, will alter very little during pregnancy if adequate supports are worn.

The human body is constructed in such a way that many of the changes due to pregnancy, both in the reproductive organs and the manner in which they carry out their function, conform with the quadruped or all-fours position. There would probably be less trouble with the human breasts if they hung away from the chest and not downwards upon the ribs. The object, therefore, is to retain their shape by supporting them in rounded caps fitting firmly underneath but loosely over the nipple and suspended in such a way that the lift is upwards and inwards towards the manubrium, that is, the top of the breast bone. This takes a strain from the shoulders if the organs are large and well-developed and prevents the drag forwards and in- wards which frequently makes women stoop slightly with rounded shoulders. Further, such support assists in the adoption and retention of good posture and carriage when walking, and facilitates free and full respiration by using the upper lobes of the lungs as well as the lower. It has also been observed that much of the backache that afflicts pregnant women is avoided by this simple measure. The necessity for correct supports for the breasts as they increase in fullness and weight must be recognised.

Assuming that the breast is healthy and well-supported there is very little further preparation, but what has to be done should be done thoroughly, for it has a great advantage in making the milk flow freely when it is first secreted. General, light massage of the breast after the twentieth week of pregnancy is advisable; it appears to stimulate the formation of the milk-producing glands and possibly prevents excessive deposits of fat that sometimes occur when a woman is eating well and taking too much salt during her pregnancy. This massage should be gently done and it is best to use powder so that the hand slips smoothly over the skin. It may be noticed even as early as the sixteenth week that small flecks of secretion dry upon the nipple, which should therefore be cleansed each day with pure soap and warm water. I do not advise any application to make the nipple hard for this predisposes to cracking of the skin. I have heard of midwives who strongly advocate using a nailbrush or a piece of loofah sponge for scrubbing the nipples to make them firm, but in practice if they are kept soft and elastic, they rarely give any trouble.

In the later weeks of pregnancy colostrum may be found exuding from the nipples. A few drops should be milked each day so that the ducts are kept patent and not clogged by the viscid fluid. It is useful to learn the art of milking during pregnancy, for it may have to be used afterwards to expel excess from the breast after the baby has taken all it wants.

The left breast is manipulated by the right hand in this manner. The first finger is kept straight and pressed underneath the nipple across the breast. The thumb of the right hand is then pushed firmly down to the root of the nipple. This is easily felt if the breast is pressed backwards by the thumb on the upper part of the areola. The nipple is then compressed upon the second joint of the rigid first finger. There is no necessity for force; in fact if gentle expelling efforts have no result, probably there is nothing to expel. In the same manner the right breast should be treated with the left hand. One must stress again that this is done *without any violence* and sometimes it is made easier if the breasts are bathed in warm water and massaged before milking. This should be done at least once every day from the time that colostrum appears up to the birth of the child. The reasons for prenatal milking should be explained to the mother, for by drawing attention to the importance of the breast function, she may become more interested in breast-feeding.

This is not an easy operation if a woman's nipples are retracted or very small. If these bothersome abnormalities are present, it must be pointed out to the doctor quite early in pregnancy because it is possible to improve the most unsatisfactory nipples and in fact make them usable by the baby.

The treatment is a combination of the lengthening of the nipple by the milking exercise that I have just described and also by wearing a nipple shield. There are several patterns of these, but for my own part I have found those introduced by Dr Waller and known as the Woolwich Shields very satisfactory because they can be worn without discomfort. They are fitted inside the brassiere and give the breasts a rounded appearance, but are not obvious. They are made of light plastic material and the nipple is put through an aperture in the shield. The shield is about 2½–3 inches across, circular, and has a dome about 1–1½ inches deep so that it fits firmly around the base of the nipple, which projects into the dome without coming into contact with it. In this way there is a constant action of extrusion of the nipple into the dome. It is not right to wait until the last month or six weeks of pregnancy before wearing these shields. If the use of the shield is indicated, it should be worn from the eighteenth to twentieth week of pregnancy.

I have already explained that when the baby is born and immediately taken by the mother into her arms, she may be urged to put it to the breast. During these first few milkless days the baby must be regularly put to the breast. This stimulates the flow of milk, or the draught, which commences about two and a half to three and a half days after the baby is born. I certainly do not advise giving the baby any prescription before the natural food is available. It has sufficient nourishment in its own body to live comfortably until the milk arrives and not infrequently its desire to take the breast is decreased if it has supplementary or what they call 'pity' feeds before the mother can do this herself.

The Art of Feeding

A mother breast-feeding her baby must be in a comfortable position so that she can relax and avoid strain on her back and shoulder muscles. Many women who sit hunched up with their heads forward peering at the baby, find that within a short time their back is aching from the neck to the waist. It is best to sit in a high-back chair with a pillow across the knees and the baby lying on the pillow with its head level with the nipples. The mother puts one arm around the child with its head resting on her forearm, and with the other hand gently depresses the breast under the baby's nose so that it has a free airway.

If she prefers to lie in bed, she must be propped up on pillows to the sitting position. Some women adopt the habit of lying down on the bed with the baby beside them. This is not only comfortable but enables the baby to take the nipple in its mouth without dragging on the breast.

It should he remembered that if the infant is fed from below, that is to say, looking upwards with the nipple being pulled downwards into its mouth, after three or four months the shape of the breast may be irreparably damaged.

A child does not wish to feed continuously. At first, when it is hungry, it will swallow as rapidly as possible the milk that is pumped into its mouth, but it must have a rest and although it does not relinquish its hold on the nipple, it will cease to take milk for a short time. If it appears to be drifting into sleep, a gentle touch on the upper lip with the finger will produce a sucking reflex.

An infant takes nearly all its feed in the first four or five minutes and if it becomes lazy, it should be taken off the breast. This is done without discomfort to the mother if she lightly compresses the baby's nostrils so that it opens its mouth to breathe.

A feeding mother should be relaxed and alone. Breast-feeding is an occupation which allows of no other interest which may distract from the enjoyment of these few quiet and companionable moments with her child five or six times a day.

Feeding on Demand

During the last few years it has almost become an accepted principle that babies are fed to the clock either three hourly or four hourly. Some teach that until the baby weighs six and a half to seven pounds it should be fed three hourly and if it is past that weight, four hourly. No baby should rely upon a clock, for we know that every infant is a law unto itself which should be studied by the mother.

A newborn baby requires feeding after it has finished digesting its last meal. Some will take large feeds and four or five hours pass before it has a feeling of wanting more. It cries in order to call the attention of its mother to the fact that it is hungry. Others may take smaller feeds or have a more rapid digestion and will cry after three to three and a half hours. The demand in a baby's voice is recognisable from all other cries and a mother quickly learns the difference between the cry of hunger, the cry of colic, the grumble of an uncomfortable nappy, or the irregular bursts-of-pain cry. There are others associated with illness, but mothers must recognise the normal conversational cries of their children.

Demand feeding has many advantages. It is obviously wrong to force a baby to take food into a stomach which is not demanding it and although many will do so, they are more predisposed to attacks of colic or vomiting, than those who accept a meal for which their stomach is ready. On the other hand, it is frustrating for an infant to feel hungry and demand food, and to say so in an emphatic voice, but to receive no attention from the mother from whom it looks for security and food. There is probably no activity more disturbing to the emotional development of a newborn baby than to allow it to lie and cry, hungry or unsatisfied, in a state of frustration and anger. It is not getting what it asks for and it is logical that it should expect its craving to be appeased, but instead, it is allowed to work itself up into a nervous state so that when the clock strikes and the breast is presented to it, it is in no condition to settle down and take its food quietly.

The baby, and the baby only, feels when it is ready for nourishment; and a mother, feeding on demand, soon knows to within a very few minutes the digestive phase of her child.

A five-week baby was brought to me which was on four feeds in twenty-four hours. It was a placid, contented and peaceful child – for the previous twenty-one days it had put on ten ounces a week. The mother already knew, within a quarter of an hour, how long she could be out of the house doing her shopping – she knew that the child would sleep and be cared for by the maid she left in the house. Many, at six weeks, have adopted a five-hour regime, but a high percentage also want feeding after they are a month old, five times a day at varying intervals. Small babies who have to make up their weight quickly will require more meals than the medium-size babies from 7–8.5lb, whilst the big babies from 8.5–10lb may demand to be fed more often because their requirements are greater.

Children nourished in this way are peaceful, calm, colic-free infants who grow healthily and adjust themselves with very little difficulty to their changing environment as the weeks advance.

Rooming-in

When a baby is born at home it is best kept in the room with the mother, where she can constantly see her child and attend to it if necessary, even from the first day. After she has got up from bed and is moving about, that is any time from the second to the sixth day, according to the manner of her birth, she can look after the baby herself, learn its habits and its desires. This close association with the child will make her quick to appreciate when it is hungry or when it needs other attention.

A newborn baby should remain with its mother for she is its best nurse. Even if she is one of those few who are not possessed of great intelligence, she has the maternal instinct which can often overcome many academic deficiencies. I recall that about thirty-five to forty years ago nurseries for all newborn babies were hailed as one of the latest advances in maternity wards. Up to that time it was usual to have the babies in cots either attached to, or standing beside the bed and mother. This change proved to be a most unfortunate divergence from what was then termed the old-fashioned principle of leaving the babies with their mothers. In many hospitals today the nursery system persists and in many, though not all, the purely physical care of baby is very well looked after, but of recent years three important factors have become recognised in relation to this subject. They are the mother-child relationship, the emotional development of the baby during the first few days of its life and the devastating epidemic infections in hospital nurseries that now resist the antibiotics which only a few years previously were so effective. There are, therefore, now many hospitals and maternity institutions which have recognised the advantages of rooming-in, that is keeping the baby with the mother, and have adopted this method of immediate postnatal care. Observations have been made by a large number of hospitals upon different aspects of this treatment. The mental and physical peace of the mother is one of its many health-giving influences. Babies are happier and only cry when hungry or uncomfortable. They develop rapidly the natural sense of security in their mother's presence and mother and child quickly find an understanding of each other's reactions and demands.

The benefits of true rooming-in are not obtained by half measures. Some hospitals refer to its advantages to mother and child in glowing terms, but have a glass house in the mother's room, a viewing screen through to an adjacent room so that the mothers can see their babies but not touch them just when they wish. The nurse can be watched as she changes nappies and organises feeding times. It protects the baby from visitors but too often from mother as well.

The profound importance to the baby of the first forty-eight hours of its neonatal life does not receive the emphasis which many of us would wish it to have. For my own part, I extend that thought to the development of the mother in the first forty-eight hours of motherhood.

The results of a long and intricate investigation of rooming-in by Professor Harvey Carey of Auckland University have just been published. He found that it was an important factor in reducing infection as the mother was the safest person to handle the baby. The research demonstrated that the nursing staff could be a source of danger in spreading staphylococcal infection. Rooming-in meant that as far as possible no one but the mother handled the baby and it had the great advantage that the baby received individual attention. It was fed when necessary and made comfortable when required. The mother ceased to be anxious about her baby and was allowed much more flexibility in ward routine.

The investigation found that 95 per cent of the mothers who had tried both nursing and rooming-in systems were strongly in favour of the rooming-in system at his (Professor Carey's) hospital in Auckland.

He laid stress upon the individuality of babies and the variations of their demands, and his research showed that babies put on weight better under rooming-in and the mother was more confident in handling her baby even though she left hospital a few days only after the birth.

These observations are corroborated by other observers and must be considered seriously for, if the advantages are so great, surely every effort should be made to put this system to a prolonged trial.

Under these conditions breast-feeding had a much better chance of being successful and we cannot overlook the large number of women who had intended and wished to feed their babies who find that they cannot do so in hospital for a variety of reasons. It is one of the many natural functions which can be seriously disturbed by emotional influences and amongst these are the nurse-patient factor. For it is not unreasonable to believe that many nulliparous nurses have a psychological and even physical revulsion to seeing another woman feed her baby. But if we observe for ourselves the babies who are breast-fed on demand and the mothers who feed them by the clock, we shall soon be able to see the difference. This we can do after the mothers have gone home and draw our conclusions from all classes of people. Select, so far as possible, ten babies of the same weight and similar environments, five fed on love milk and the other five on regimented or formula milk. For a time they receive similar amounts of food then one appears to progress better than the other, not necessarily in weight only but in temperament and behaviour. Watch their development at two, five, and nine months. Physically there may not be a marked difference, but one thought will be impressed upon the mind of an understanding observer. This is the stage in life when leaders and followers can be differentiated, when optimists and pessimists are made, when the seeds of evolution or revolution, construction and destruction are sown in society.

The equality of man! This slogan is a tintinnabulation of an empty skull when struck by frustration. 'Madam, you frame your son's future at the breast, not at school – that is the place where we do our best for bottle-fed babies.'

18

The Husband and Childbirth

The question of the husband's attitude towards pregnancy has long been a matter for discussion. That there should be many opinions expressed upon this subject is reasonable, since men on the whole are creatures of definite persuasions. They are not likely to be influenced purely by the merits of a case – that which is convenient or of interest or seemly is more likely to meet with their approbation than that which impinges upon their habits and takes their minds out of the common rut of their daily occupations or their recreations – particularly if it has a flavour of embarrassment or 'unmanliness'.

Not many years ago the idea of a husband being more than proudly, but distantly, interested in the pregnancy of his wife was generally accepted; and in the mid-Victorian era women retired from public life immediately they became 'obviously with child'. The relationship of the father to the family was less intimately companionable than it is today. But there is a change and it is noticeable that during the last two decades husbands have demanded to know more about childbirth.

Over thirty years ago I started a series of lectures for men's organisations because of requests I had received to instruct groups of young and expectant fathers in what I considered should be their attitude and behaviour during the pregnancy of their wives. These talks were given almost entirely to the working classes of the suburbs around London and one of the main features at such meetings was that, after I had spoken, an hour should be set aside for questions and discussions.

It soon became obvious that the ignorance of the average man about childbirth was incredible. At that time I had the advantage of being the father of a growing family of young children and of being closely interested in the problem of the part that the husband should play both during pregnancy and the early months of infancy of his offspring.

Some of the men whose wives had to work, whether they were pregnant or not, expressed very strongly the view that the local nursing associations should organise what they called 'mothers' helps', who would be responsible for many of the domestic duties that normally fell upon the shoulders of their wives. They were concerned for the health of the mother, but at the same time expressed no desire to take upon themselves some of the extra duties that they considered were too much for a pregnant woman.

Others made it clear that the woman of the house was responsible for the provision of food and comfort that they enjoyed when they came home after a strenuous day's work; but many broke down the natural reticence of the Englishman and stated quite plainly what they thought, in some such terms as these: 'I love my wife – she's got to have all the trouble and pain of giving me a child. My job is to go on earning a living to keep the home together whilst she is ill, but I want to do more than that and I don't know how to be of any help to her.'

That attitude of the husband towards the wife was very prevalent and I have no doubt that it was prompted by a deep affection and concern for her welfare. The general trend of my talks was to elaborate this aspect of the husband-wife relationship by giving the men a simple explanation of what went on during pregnancy, how the child develops and the changes that occur during pregnancy in a woman's mind, particularly towards her husband.

I was about to be married when I was House Physician to Sir Henry Head, the world-famous neurologist, and I had the privilege of many conversations with him. This was always a source of great pleasure for his enthusiasm not only in his pet theme but in the art of living stimulated most interesting discussions, which scintillated with observations upon his wide experience of human relationships. Knowing my interest in gynaecology and obstetrics, he turned my attention on more than one occasion to the mind of woman and its activities under different circumstances.

I had no idea at that time that he knew I was contemplating marriage and was a little taken aback when one day he turned to me and said: 'I want to give you some advice and you will be wise to remember it. When you marry it will not be to one woman but to two. The personality and behaviour of these two women will differ widely and it is unlikely that you will remain in love with both of them for many years. One woman is she who lives between her menstrual periods and the other is the woman who is subjected to all the emotional, physical and chemical changes which she undergoes just before, during and after her periods.'

He did not dilate upon the subject but left me with that thought which in a long life of professional association with women has had a profound influence upon my efforts to understand these dual or multiple personalities.

How little of the vast fund of human understanding I gleaned in this particular field was many years later brought home to me. I had been endeavouring to advise a young man who was madly in love with his beautiful Irish wife, but exasperated by her unpredictable behaviour. I did my best, but a few days later received from the lady a magnificently bound book entitled *What Men know about Women*. With a thrill of hopeful anticipation I turned its pages and continued to turn them until I reached the end – every page was blank, there was not so much as a note of interrogation to be found! I sympathised with Thackeray's Mr Brown, who wrote to his nephew: 'Every single woman I ever knew is a puzzle to me, as I have no doubt she is to herself.'

It can be observed, however, that during pregnancy, the menstrual woman no longer being present, a third individual appears within the home, whose activities, thoughts and behaviour need careful understanding and considerable tolerance and unselfishness on the part of the husband. There is, in mitigation of this small burden that he must bear, a change in his own attitude, for pregnancy often intensifies his love for his wife and creates in him an ardent desire to take care of her and attend to her needs and wishes with tenderness and consideration.

The importance of the husband's attitude towards, and understanding of, childbirth cannot be exaggerated. His words and actions, and even the atmosphere in the house that he may create in silence, have a profound effect upon his wife. Her health and happiness during pregnancy, and certainly her approach to labour, will be influenced for better or for worse by harmony or discord that she feels in her husband's mind.

The real joy of childbirth is most frequently experienced when husband and wife have mutual confidence, affection and understanding, and have worked together in preparation for the arrival of their baby.

A man who knows nothing about these things will often sublimate his ignorance in irritability. (He prefers to succumb to the latter than disclose the former.) He may even state dogmatically what is sense and what is nonsense. His urge to take care of his wife, whom he loves very dearly, easily develops into a rigid military-type discipline. Men often formulate domestic principles during their wife's pregnancy and demand that they are meticulously carried out. Rest, diet, exercise, recreation and even personal hygiene are matters in which they suddenly become expert without absorbing any authoritative teaching on the subject. If the doctor does not agree – the doctor is wrong.

This is, of course, a manifestation of conflict in a man's mind. Pride, anxiety and tenderness get horribly mixed up and that is one of the main reasons why husbands suffer so much in childbirth. They need just as much sympathy and help as their wives. The surest way of being of assistance in the cause of peace and confidence, both in the home and elsewhere, is to urge, with quiet but kindly-stern authority, that the husband learns with his wife the phenomena and common sense of this natural human function.

During the last few years I have been gratified to find that the majority of husbands accept this advice and – what a difference it makes to obstetrics!

A stockbroker, who did not come to see me until his wife was near term, and whose interest in her rose and fell with his stocks and shares, asked me resentfully: 'Why should I know all about this – it's her business, not mine.'

I replied: 'Oh, yes, she is excellent and with average luck should bear your baby with little or no discomfort, but – I don't want *you* to have an unnecessarily distressing labour.'

This aspect of the situation appealed to him and in a few days he was adequately informed. He was with his wife when their child was born and it brought to them not only a son, but something else they had never shared before.

But there are men who can never overcome their anxiety and who have no confidence in anyone during labour. They are kept 'downstairs' for they radiate discomfort.

It is quite impossible to make a rule to which all husbands can be expected to adhere. Their variations in temperament are as wide as those of women and their past and present associations and psychological experiences make each man a law unto himself.

Let us, in so far as possible, give a few wide generalisations of the signs and symptoms of pregnancy, both physical and emotional, which will become apparent to an observant and attentive husband.

Conception is a supreme event in a woman's life – it is the beginning of that phase which represents the achievement of her physiological purpose. Conscious and unconscious experiences of her childhood and early maturity flood the vista of her future whilst being strongly influenced by the phantasies of the past. Every impression that she has received of childbirth shapes her acceptance of pregnancy. Each stress and strain that has caused her doubts or fears during those years when every small girl rehearses to her secret self what motherhood must be, find a place in her mind. As women vary in nature so do these psychological manifestations, but even more important are the different aspects of parenthood which arise from such considerations as: 'Is the baby wanted or unwanted?' 'Was it planned or accidental?' 'Is she longing for a child but her husband disappointed that she is pregnant?'

Women develop very early after conception an acuteness of mind and thought which intensifies their appreciation of the words and feelings of their husbands. Although it is not necessary to explore more deeply the actual psychological basis for her reactions, it should be recognised that these are not just whims and moods but real mental states based upon sound psychological deductions.

She may suffer from nausea, which will not only be extremely unpleasant for her, but which should be clearly understood by her husband as a condition which he can assist her to avoid, or, to some extent, overcome. What used to be termed morning sickness, but which now tends rather to come later in the day, is, in very few women, a purely chemical symptom. There are many profound changes in a woman's body which alter the activity of, and the chemical nature of, her internal secretions, but the sickness of pregnancy that is entirely due to these changes is relatively rare; and I believe that in not less than 80 per cent of the women in whom nausea persists to a degree that seriously worries them, it arises as a physical manifestation of emotional states. Husbands should be aware of this, for with encouragement and sympathetic understanding, particularly if accompanied by an honest expression of happiness that they have achieved a potential state of parenthood, they can bring relief to a very considerable extent from this discomfort.

We must not overlook the fact that many husbands go through a stage of alarm when they discover that their wives are pregnant. Some come with their wives upon her first visit to me, and when the lady has gone through to the examination room, they ask me to assure them that she will be all right. Their state of agitation is obvious, and many men have expressed to me a feeling of guilt that they have selfishly caused their wife to become pregnant without even considering the dangers and the pain to which they believe she must assuredly be subjected.

This attitude of husbands who are really in love with their wives is understandable, but could never arise if they had had an opportunity of learning the elementary facts concerning natural and healthy pregnancy and childbirth. What they overlook is that they cannot deceive their wives about their anxious state of mind and all the charm and affection that they show does not hide from the pregnant woman the underlying anxiety of her husband. This is a state of things that should be avoided at all costs. The most healthy pregnancy is that which results from the mutual desire of a man and wife to have a child. Her conception should be welcomed as a victory, not as an affliction, and for her physical and mental health a unity of understanding should bind them together in the closest bonds of their new association.

But a woman does change when she becomes pregnant; in some ways which are quite incomprehensible. She may discover that she has entirely new tastes, particularly for food; and she may eat things which she has previously disliked or, more frequently, dislike intensely articles of food which she had previously enjoyed. Some become pernickety, others voracious.

During the first trimester of pregnancy a woman who has usually been active, athletic and untirable will be easily tired, complain bitterly of the weariness of the flesh, and have small urge either to be entertained or to entertain. This is not an unusual condition and does not indicate illness, for undoubtedly nature calls for a quieter life during the first three months of pregnancy. There are strange changes, too, in her attitude towards her husband, which are quite unpredictable. Some women cannot bear to have him out of their sight, and overwhelm him with their affection and physical demands; others become cold and distant, quite unable to accept with any enthusiasm his wonted demonstrations of affection, and not infrequently the idea of any sexual life between them is repugnant. Such changes should be recognised and tolerated by the husband, who should exercise the art of kindliness and gentle persuasion to avoid any excess of either positive or negative emotionalism.

After three months life becomes easier. Now he should learn with her what the succeeding phases of pregnancy will bring, he should be interested in her diet, her exercise and her antenatal preparation for the arrival of the child. Happily there are many men who are anxious to do this, recognising the value of the enjoyment of this close companionship. They read together books which present childbirth in a pleasant way and which make them realise that they are embarking together upon a natural adventure which has been, throughout the ages, the lot of all mankind and is therefore nothing to fear.

Between the eighteenth and the twentieth week, when the wife has become conscious that the small swelling in her pelvis is no longer an impersonal tumour, and the movement of the child is felt, she tends to become more interested in her baby as an individual. This is a time when the husband should tactfully intensify his interest in his wife, for there is a risk of her becoming too single-minded in her new-found possession to reciprocate his affection. By the twenty-sixth week, she will become noticeably pregnant and should take particular care to maintain her appearance and her posture, and to dress in a becoming manner.

Happily in these days of enlightenment, women are proud of pregnancy and do not retire from the public gaze as many were wont to in the Victorian era. The husband, too, very rarely shows the embarrassment which was not unknown in the time of our grandfathers; he tends to exhibit a laudable pride in her happiness and radiant good health.

Unfortunately, even today this ancient error is maintained in countries in which the misdirected prudery of authorities still exists. A university with which I am well acquainted where there are a large number of women students, many of whom marry before they have obtained their degrees, will not allow a woman who is known to be pregnant to continue her studies as it is considered embarrassing for the young male students! In the same town, where a very high percentage of the women work either in offices or Government organisations, those who become pregnant must immediately cease their employment. This gives rise to considerable worry and many of these young girls will suppress the fact of pregnancy for as long as possible since the money that they are earning is necessary in order to help the husband to obtain and furnish a home.

What manner of mind considers this holy estate, which women are privileged by the Almighty to attain, as a slur upon the social conscience? Fortunately this attitude towards motherhood is rapidly dying out, as, indeed, it must in a world which necessitates that women should work in order to supplement the earnings of their husbands. During the last ten weeks of pregnancy the husband's lot is that of protector and guide for his wife. Her activities are limited and invariably as the weeks creep on he will find it acceptable to his wife if he helps her in the domestic organisation of the house, especially if there are already one or two small children in the family.

By this time he will have been wise if he has learnt with her how the child arrives and the processes of labour by which it comes into the world. He will also be familiar with the exercises that she has performed to make herself physically fit; and he will assist her and even practise with her the art of respiration and relaxation, and at the same time know clearly why these adjuncts of antenatal preparation are so valuable.

Some years ago a busy erstwhile athletic attorney, who had become rather rotund because he had put in too much time at his work and not taken enough exercise, came in to see me with his wife who was about thirty-eight weeks pregnant. She was extremely well and looking forward with absolute confidence to the arrival of their child; he remarked to me: 'This antenatal preparation is wonderful; we do it together and I have not felt so fit for months!' I need hardly say that the arrival of her child was a pleasure both to herself and to those of us who witnessed it. They organised things together for this event and the companionship of pregnancy has been maintained. The signs and symptoms of the onset of labour were familiar to both of them and the transport to the maternity hospital presented no difficulty, whatever the time of the day or night it was required. They appeared to enjoy together a happy, confident anticipation of the arrival of their child and he was there to greet it when it came.

When, finally, labour starts and husband and wife arrive at the maternity hospital, their relationship during pregnancy is made obvious by their behaviour. It becomes almost possible to predict the nature of and the course of a woman's labour by the manner of her entrance to the labour ward. Then the obstetrician in charge has to judge: 'Is this husband one who will be of help to his wife during labour, or will he not only be a nuisance to the attendants but also cause anxiety or even distress to his wife?' The totally unprepared man has no place at the birth of his child. The question that has now occupied so much attention in so many hospitals and maternity organisations – 'Should the husband be present?' – depends entirely upon the husband. If he has assured himself of adequate antenatal preparation and thereby obtained the confidence of his wife, and can be a support to her at that time, then, if she wishes him to be present, he has a right to be with her. If he has not occupied himself to be interested and to have an understanding of childbirth at least equivalent to his wife, he should remain absent until such time as the obstetrician requests him to greet his wife and their newborn child. The question is not, in reality, 'Should a husband be present?'; it is 'Can this husband in particular be of any service to his wife by being present at her confinement?' If the answer is 'yes' then he should be there; if the answer is 'no' he should not be allowed anywhere near her until the baby is born.

Just as pregnancy and parturition bring out the criteria of a woman's qualities, so a husband's behaviour at the birth of his child discloses the fullness of his affection, his fortitude and his philosophy.

I have had many husbands present throughout the whole of their wife's labour; they have stayed with her during the first stage, reminded her of the lessons they have learnt together and assisted her to breathe correctly during the succeeding phases of parturition and relax when relaxation is indicated. They have rubbed their wives' backs when backache occurs at the end of the first and the beginning of the second stage. These men cannot be superseded in the value of their service by the most patient nurse or obstetrician. As labour develops during the second stage and the quiet, purposeful atmosphere of the room creates a calm and peaceful expectancy, the husband, wearing a sterile gown, a mask and a cap, takes his place in the far corner of the labour ward in full view of his wife. If he shows signs of excitement, he is instructed to be quiet and to control his feelings when the reality of birth is witnessed. He understands the difference between physical effort and discomfort; he hears the explanation and admonition of the attendant obstetrician to his wife; he knows that she is offered relief from any discomfort that she may consider to be more than she wishes to bear. He sees the analgesic apparatus ready for her use, but in such cases almost invariably hears her retort that she would not be unconscious at this time for anything. The injunctions of the obstetrician are intended not only for the wife but for the husband; the attendant realises that the doctor's concern is not only to see the child into the world but also to enable these two people to be united in the most wonderful, awe-inspiring experience that can possibly fall to the lot of wedded human beings. There is no drama or play-acting in the full recognition of the magnitude of this event to both of them. The first cry of the child is shared by both husband and wife in almost unbelievable ecstasy and relief from tension. The knowledge of its sex, the wrapping of the infant in towels and the handing it to a conscious delighted woman, presents to the husband a picture of beauty, that he describes in such words as – thrilling, miraculous, mysterious, and so on.

The full evaluation of this mutual experience is difficult to set down in a few words, but it is such that when properly conducted, an association of marriage which is indestructible for all time results.

I advocate strongly that all husbands should make the pregnancy of their wives a heaven-sent opportunity for an association in marriage of the highest level. Men who have been present speak in unmistakable terms of their exultation and amazement – they are unanimous in the sense of 'rightness' of their presence.

To summarise the answers to the question: 'Should a husband be present at the birth of his child?' we must give the replies under conditional headings.

1. Many husbands should be present at the birth of their children. They will have learnt during pregnancy all that is necessary to make them helpful to their wives by imparting the confidence they themselves have in the happy result of her labour.

2. Some men endeavour to learn but cannot overcome their fears for their wives, or their doubts about their own ability to witness the event undisturbed. They should not be present. We sympathise with them, but for their wives' sakes we 'keep them downstairs'.

3. Those who have not been interested, and have not prepared themselves for presence in the labour ward, should not be allowed in. They will bring discomfort and alarm to their wives in most cases.

There are both men *and* women who do not deserve to be present when their babies are born. They have preferred to make no effort to ensure the happy arrival of their child. They employ a doctor to receive or take a baby from their unfeeling body and nourish it on artificial food from an unfeeling teat. They shed their ill-developed parental affection upon the stranger in their midst and never know the moment when two people in the unity of love become conscious of an unmistakable spiritual presence who delivers to them, in an aura of exquisite delight, their new beloved responsibility.

When I write of parents' responsibility I have no intention of producing a dissertation upon the domestic and social conduct of men and women. It would be presumptuous to ape the pedagogue and recite the precepts of the saints to those who never had a hope of being saintly. The responsibility for the children of married parents assumes unity of ideas and harmony of actions. If we start from such altruistic premises, however, we shall draw only false deductions because in nine out of ten marriages it does not happen that way.

A father may have an inquisitive interest and mystified fascination for his unborn child, but he has no direct access to its intra-uterine life and development. His pride, sense of ownership and duty are of himself emotional fantasies and realities only in terms of his wife. His responsibility as a parent during her pregnancy is his wife and so indirectly his child. He contributes most to the good qualities of his unborn child, who contributes most to happiness of its pregnant mother.

The biological law of mammalian reproduction is not only a physical union for it makes provision for the protection and survival of the young. Too much emphasis is put on the procreative urges and activities of man and woman. No one can minimise its importance since it is in a complicated form the irresistible demand for conjugation with a compatible *gamete* as in the single-celled living organisms. This necessity for the maintenance of the species persists throughout nature and so it is in man. The difference, however, is in the growth of the mind. In higher mammals, and it may be in other orders, the *quality* of the young is an important factor in the struggle for survival. Man and woman are no longer subjugated to the simple role of natural selection but, owing to the manner of existence in variable societies, selection has become artificial and to a large extent volitional. There is, therefore, a considerable degree of diversity in the natures of people and this precludes any generalisation upon the responsibility of parents. But certain simple facts are applicable to most young married couples, who, either by 'the inevitability of fate' – the biological urge – or a calculated unnatural selection, have decided to marry and have children. The most important result of these emotional intensities is that, to which ever of the shrewd schemes of nature they ultimately succumb, children are born and the fittest of the species survive.

Mutually well-selected pairs retain, or after marriage develop, a physical and emotional harmony known as love. This awakes in the man a desire for children by the woman he loves and in the woman the physiological preparedness for children and a possessive demand for the soul as well as the body of her man. This is a healthy reaction to the natural and biological law, for it lasts longer and carries assets greater than sexual infatuation and physical satisfaction. For pregnancy sets the course of woman for the fulfilment of herself. She expands her horizons and her ambitions and if healthy in mind and body – the former is all important – she is no longer a woman in love only with a man, she is the mother of her man's child. She needs and expects him to join in her life for the sake of the baby that is their own.

Herein lies the responsibility of a husband to his unborn child. It is a hard saying for a man who has never realised the extent of his obligation to his wife's love, that without any question the mental and physical quality of the infant varies as the direct and indirect influence that he exerts upon his wife during her pregnancy. A high percentage of unnatural births and difficult children are due to the husband's behaviour to his wife during those seven to eight months of development and growth of the baby in her womb. Happily some men seem to have the inborn understanding of a woman's thoughts and need at that time, and others wish to learn how they can be of service to the woman they love and admire; but too many fall back in frustration upon the frail excuse that babies are a woman's job, and many retreat before self-condemnation for the pain she must inevitably bear, because 'he was selfish'.

Husbands must take part in the intra-uterine development of their children and must learn and practise the important role of father. It is the most satisfying phase in the life of a human being, for as the miracle of its construction progresses, the changing tissues, utilised in making the perfect form, may be deflected from the natural course. Therefore the health of the mother is the responsibility of the father of the child.

Let this postulate be examined in simple common sense. A pregnant woman's health has certain manifestations, but first and foremost she must be happy. This demands companionship and interest in her baby and all that concerns it. She can only be happy if her husband shares her hopes and anxieties, her laughter and her waves of fear. He alone can be the safety valve of her unpredictable emotions and accept unmoved the explosions of her love, hate, jealousy, and anger. The storms are usually followed by warm sunshine. But if she is alone and feels, justly or unjustly, that the baby she longs for has robbed her of her husband's love, serious temperamental and emotional states occur which set up local and sometimes general reactions within her body. A disturbed mind will disturb the circulation of blood to certain organs of the body. It will cause a serious deprivation of oxygen supply and some of the vital substances from the glands within the body which are essential for the well-being of the small fetus in the womb.

Therefore throughout pregnancy the husband's part develops with the wife's. He reads and learns with her the dignity, the beauty, and the spiritual advantages of family unity.

To understand he must learn and to be the pillar of strength his wife desires takes time, but nothing can be of greater or more lasting value to each member of the family unit. The best investment a husband can make during his wife's pregnancy is in the shares of his home and family concern. They will rise in value higher and more rapidly than his wildest dreams and pay dividends of which he can be justly proud.

19

Antenatal Education

Objectives of Antenatal Care

One of the most dramatic changes that has occurred in obstetrics since this book was published in 1942 is the approach to the preparation of women for childbirth.

Women have become human beings with minds as well as bodies, and the importance of the influence of the emotions upon pregnancy and parturition has been fully recognised. This is not new and does not constitute a scientific discovery. Neither is it an innovation for over a thousand years ago the attention of those who attended women in childbirth was drawn to the importance of the women's mental condition.

Antenatal care has been carried out to a certain extent by midwives, both male and female, for many hundreds of years. Hippocrates trained women to become midwives and in that training the care of the pregnant, as well as the parturient, was emphasised. The well-being of the body *and the mind* of the pregnant woman has been a recurring theme since Aristotle, three hundred and fifty years before Christ, wrote *The Complete Midwife*.

The significance and value of prenatal observation and care has gradually unfolded with the progress of medical science. In later years, from the publications of Eucharius Roesslin's *Rosengarten* (1513) to John William Ballantyne's *Manual of Antenatal Pathology and Hygiene* in 1904, observations had been made almost entirely upon abnormalities and diseases of pregnancy. In the writings of the past two hundred or two hundred and fifty years, gynaecologists have in general preferred to comment upon the illnesses and defects rather than the normality of childbirth. Here and there, however, we notice that observations are made concerning the woman herself during pregnancy.

Just before his death in 1923, Ballantyne in an address to a Medical Society at Nottingham mentioned six benefits that should be expected from prenatal care. Of these, numbers one, two and four were as follows:

1. The removal of anxiety and dread from the minds of expectant, parturient and puerperal patients.
2. The removal of much discomfort amounting in many cases to suffering.
4. An increase in the number of normal labours and normal pregnancies.

Numbers three, five and six concerned diseases and the stillbirth rate, and maternal mortality. At that time, the influence of fear upon the neuromuscular mechanism and the biochemistry of pregnancy and labour had not been explained. The Fear-Tension-Pain Syndrome had not been enunciated. Today that great pioneer of antenatal care might have included these three benefits under one heading in some such words:

'The increase in the number of normal labours, by the removal of anxiety and dread from the mind and thereby avoiding much discomfort during pregnancy and parturition.'

The objectives of antenatal care are as follows:

1. To OBSERVE the physical condition of pregnant women in order to prevent or diagnose as early as possible any abnormalities or irregularities that may disturb the health of either the mother or child during pregnancy, parturition or the puerperium.
2. To BE FOREWARNED of physical or mechanical factors predisposing to a difficult labour, in order to avoid as far as possible emergent and unpremeditated interference.
3. To EDUCATE pregnant women so that the inhibiting influence of fear may be replaced by understanding and confidence.
4. To INSTRUCT women in the phenomena of labour so that they may interpret its varying sensations correctly and meet its demands with discernment, patience and self-control in order that they may assist the natural forces and not resist them.
5. To TEACH women how to prepare themselves for the birth of the child in a manner which will enable them:
   a. To RELAX when tension will cause resistance and pain, particularly during the inactivity of the first stage of labour.
   b. To have such CONTROL OF RESPIRATION that they can breathe deeply, rapidly or quietly when requested, or to hold the breath when called upon to do so by the attendant.
   c. To be PHYSICALLY FIT to persist in the expulsive effort of the second stage of labour without undue exhaustion.

If these five postulates from *1* to *5 c* are carefully and intelligently carried out, there is no reason at all why any variations from them should be embarked upon.

Objectives *1* and *2* concern the doctors in charge of hospital clinics or the medical attendants upon private patients. They are in the province of purely medical attention rather than antenatal instruction, therefore I shall not discuss them fully because they are described in manuals and texbooks of obstetrics for the guidance of students, graduates and postgraduates.

It is numbers *3* to *5 c*, and their application to the physically healthy woman who is well-equipped to have her baby normally, that I propose to emphasise.

Professor Browne writes: 'Antenatal care cannot be carried out in its full integration without a just combination of all it implies.' Reproduction is a physiological function, not an illness.

The *First Principle* is to ensure good health, both physical and mental, during pregnancy and so minimise the discomforts of labour and the necessity for interference.

Secondly, we desire that childbirth should be accompanied by a sense of maternal achievement and satisfaction, and that the mother-child relationship should be enhanced by pride and pleasure and not tainted by resentment or distressing memories.

And *thirdly*, that the mother should desire and be willing to have more children because of, not in spite of, her experience of childbirth.

To approach such objectives, the mind and the body of the mother must be protected from the encroachment of associations and misunderstandings that threaten from domestic, social and scientific fields. The laws of nature and the advance of science must be balanced in the scales of common sense and each employed with discretion in order to obtain the obstetric ideal. Let us, therefore, take paras *3*, *4* and *5* and discuss the means by which this teaching can be indoctrinated simply and successfully into the minds of all classes of women.

Purpose of Education

It may be asked: 'Why do you lay so much stress upon this "ignorance of the facts of childbirth"; surely everyone knows now, and learns more, about childbirth than they did fifteen, ten or even five years ago?'

This may be the case, but it was brought home very vividly to me one night recently when I had just delivered a woman of her second baby; her total labour lasted for one hour and five minutes. The first baby had been born whilst she was in entire ignorance of all the facts of childbirth. She went into hospital and was immediately given some form of soporific; she was unconscious for twelve hours and regained consciousness in time to realise she was pushing down and then was immediately anaesthetised. Her child was produced with forceps, badly injured, and she herself was severely torn down below. Well, naturally this woman, who came from another country to have her baby here, was a little bit distressed at the rapidity of her labour, but she soon realised that, having learnt and understood exactly what was going on and why, she was not alarmed. Her baby was 8lb, she certainly had a pelvis that could have borne a 10lb baby. The first baby was only 6.5lb and it was not a posterior position so far as the husband could gather from the doctor and attendants. The birth of her second child had been a tremendous joy to her; it was very quick indeed – she had only been in the maternity home a quarter of an hour before the baby arrived. She assured me she felt no pain and was delighted with her daughter.

I came out of the labour ward after the delivery I have just mentioned and found, sitting in the doctor's room, because the other rooms at that time were rather crowded, a woman of twenty-two who was about to have her first baby. She was looking very agitated and naturally I offered her a word of comfort and said: 'What's the matter – you are not in any trouble, I hope?' She said: 'No, but this baby business is dreadful – I don't even know if I am in labour.' So I chatted with her whilst I had a cup of tea and found that she had not been told a single thing about it. She had been away from her parents and alone with her husband, who was not interested. In fact he was so terrified of her having a baby that he refused to come anywhere near when she started labour; her doctor had not informed her of anything whatever, she had had no antenatal treatment and this poor lass sat there literally shivering with fright. She said: 'I don't understand it, I don't know what's going to happen, but everyone says it's frightful. I really do feel like running away.' That struck me as being a most extraordinary thing to happen in 1953. But there it was, she was one of many and I must say I felt in the back of my mind that this charming young woman was suffering so unnecessarily simply because she had placed herself in the care of an obstetrician who had neither the understanding nor possibly the desire to instruct her how to make the whole thing a very much happier occasion.

It is impossible to protect women from the fear of childbirth if they are ignorant of the truth. We do not fear facts, but doubts and uncertainties. Our most tremulous apprehensions arise from anxieties lest the worst may happen. Rumour is more terrifying than assault, ignorance more nerve-racking than knowledge, however bad reality may be.

I am unwilling to believe that the fear of childbirth is a natural, emotional development. Were it so, flight from the impending injury would not only be acquired as a reaction to pregnancy, but some effort would have been made to provide the necessary apparatus of escape. Changes of structure and function are invariably influenced by the necessities of survival. But unlike the fear that Crile describes as protective, there is no neuromuscular machinery which makes flight from labour possible. True fear is the outcome of experience of successive generations throughout the ages, warning the human species of danger, injury or death.

But reproduction is an essential function for the survival of the race. Is it reasonable to believe that the law of nature has gone so far astray that with one hand it prompts, with every wile and craving, women to bear children, and with the other restrains by pain, fear and injury, the natural urge? The fear of childbirth is not an inborn escape from a natural function. It is an acquired demand, arising from personal and environmental association, for the defence against an unnatural state. The unavoidable accidents of reproduction, which occur in all animal life, would not have brought childbirth to its present ill-repute had not man interfered.

How many of the expeditions of this thing we call culture set out from the harbour of ignorance? How many finish deserted and exposed on the rock of knowledge, withered in the sunlight of truth? Culture has been doing its best to destroy the safety and the beauty of normal childbirth for many generations. It has tried hard to demonstrate the wonders of science upon the greatest miracle of nature. It has failed to understand the simplicity of truth and unhesitatingly introduced the complexity of falsehood.

Women have never been taught the rudiments of childbearing; such knowledge was unnecessary when the primitive mind was undisturbed by terrifying associations. No effort has been made to counteract the propaganda of the Middle Ages. Modern science has emphasised the art of obstetrics without calling attention to the fact that there is usually a woman present, as well as a reproductory apparatus.

To the women themselves their bodies are a mystery, and labour an incomprehensible activity too personal and too difficult to discuss. The wonders of reproduction are withheld; the story of the development of a child within the body is only for those who have ears to hear.

What goes on, why, and where and how, are matters of interest to nearly every woman. Very few, for one reason or another, presume to inquire of these things. How the baby starts, how it grows, how it is fed and how it arrives, is not understood even in an elementary way. Woman is therefore robbed of logical reasons for the conduct of her pregnancy. It is much easier to follow a regime if there is some obvious justification for it, but there is no education to assist women to understand the benefits, both to themselves and their babies, which will accrue from careful antenatal procedures. Girls of seventeen to twenty-one years of age are taught every conceivable subject but conception. They become expert in a hundred ways and means of being occupied, of earning a living or of running a house, but how many are trained to prepare themselves mentally and physically for the ultimate achievement of the vast majority of women? The subject is taboo in many places, where its teaching should be enthralling. To thousands of girls of all classes this lore is passed on by hearsay and subjected to all the distortions of misinterpretation. And yet seriously-minded and sensible women long to know the answers to their unspoken questions; they reach out, according to their sense of propriety, to grasp each iota of information that may help to explain some mystery. There is a hush when by accident some sentence falls from the lips of the experienced before the young – the young of fifteen to eighteen years of age! Mothers do not understand; how can they instruct their daughters? Schoolmistresses know of this hiatus in the national education; few of them are mothers. Some of them give elementary chats before the older girls leave school with kindly tact and judicious discrimination. Others rely on the physiology classes of school standard to satisfy youthful curiosity. But those who would most willingly and most competently instruct have told me that they dare not do so because of the antagonism of outraged parents who had heard it rumoured that sex might be spoken of to their daughters.

It is an astonishing truth that this most shocking of all educational discrepancies persists in many of our great girls' schools, not as the wish of the heads of schools, but because of the attitude of parents and school councils. If this is so where the seeds of understanding might easily be sown, what of the enlightenment of the 95 per cent of girls who leave school at fifteen to earn their living? Their education is often only a word of caution and their protection the influence of the home, whatever that may be.

So on the sands of ignorance, has arisen a generation of woman-hood. It is not surprising that many girls crumple either in mind or body. Their foundations give way before the winds and storms of life. If simple lessons in physiology were given at an early age, the truth of reproduction could be more easily disseminated throughout society in all classes and stations of life; it could be taught by those who are able to instill respect and fearlessly speak of its beauties as well as the dangers of misuse. Girls will often value possessions for their beauty and guard them from harm, but when ignorant of both value and beauty there is nothing to lose and if the urge is strong enough, there is everything to gain. This state of affairs must be put right; women must know the elementary laws of reproduction so that the fears of doubt and ignorance may be minimised.

The obstetrician who knows the value of education in the biology of reproduction has to break down false teachings and overcome beliefs born of hearsay. It is pointed out earlier in this chapter how such a state exists and the causes for such lamentable conclusions that women draw regarding childbirth.

When, therefore, the young married woman enters the consulting room, believing, hoping or fearing that she is going to have a baby, the physician's first investigations should be to confirm that she is pregnant; he should then examine her attitude towards childbirth, both personally and generally. Close observation will unmask the true feelings of the prospective mother. We have all known the apparently indifferent women, the enthusiastic, the alarmed, the radiantly happy, the angry and the tearful. From these indications we may well mark out the psychological ground that has to be covered. Opportunity arises at an early visit to ask the important question: 'Do you know, more or less, what goes on? I think you might find everything easier to understand if you had a rough idea of things.' There are girls who hesitate, but not many. Only one has ever said to me, 'I don't want to know anything about it.' But she added, 'I think the whole business is disgusting.' What a picture of her home and upbringing this disclosed!

Nearly all women are interested to learn. Some volunteer the information that they know a good deal; others a certain amount, but, alas, a high percentage own sheepishly that 'they are awfully ignorant about things.' What a host of words 'things' covers in speaking of details of the reproductory function.

The extent to which some of my patients have been unacquainted with the simplest facts is almost unbelievable. Twice in my experience I have known married women who, although well advanced in pregnancy, believed that their baby arrived by way of the umbilicus. On many occasions educated girls had not associated the uterus with the development of the child; they had imagined it free in the abdomen. I was asked by a girl who had just felt her baby quickening, 'Why shall I have such a small baby?' When I enquired why she thought she would have a small baby, she explained that she thought the size of the baby was equivalent to the lump in her tummy and then suddenly became a baby. Women have told me quite seriously that they expected the baby to be about six or eight inches long only when it was born because they could not see how there was going to be room for it to come out if it was any bigger; although they had heard of the normal weight of a baby, they had no size-weight relationship in their minds. I was confronted by a woman who visited me for the first time when she was seven months pregnant. She asked me how her baby was getting air; it was quite difficult to make her understand that although alive and moving, it did not breathe. She had attributed to her umbilicus the ability to provide air for her child.

And so on. These astounding records of ignorance, and many others of a more intimate but none the less devastating nature, are to be found.

I must, however, balance this account by referring to those who come well-informed and happy, inquiring only to learn more detail. Women who have learnt and who understand afford the best evidence of the tragedy of ignorance, for dark clouds look darkest when in the same sky the sun shines brightly.

But happily the last ten years have seen considerable change in the general attitude towards childbirth. In many towns and communities, societies and mothercraft organisations make it possible for young married people to learn; elementary lectures and talks are given by those who are sensible and experienced to introduce the truth of the natural function. In many girls' schools the subject of sex is discussed in advanced physiology classes for the older children, but the development and birth of a child is not yet treated in a manner that emphasises the natural beauty of this desirable accomplishment. But with the dawn of common sense in obstetrics the light of knowledge illuminates the science of motherhood – ignorance gives place to understanding, pride and achievement dispel the pain and anguish of medieval fear and superstition.

It will be noticed that in discussing antenatal education no reference has been made to anaesthesia and analgesia.

It has become the custom in some maternity organisations to describe the various methods of inducing *anaesthesia* or *analgesia;*

different apparatuses are demonstrated and the women are taught how to use them. I have found this introduces a serious fear that the rest of their instruction will be of no avail in labour. If doctors teach them how to take gas as part of their preparation for labour, gas *will be* required to relieve pain which they are expected to suffer. No difficulty arises when analgesia or anaesthesia *has to be* induced – a few words of advice and instruction, and a woman who needs pain relief quickly understands. Since over 95 per cent of women in normal labour neither demand nor desire to use the gas or trilene apparatus, the risk of introducing fear to conflict with faith is unjustifiable.

I have never taught a woman how to use a Minnitt's Apparatus or Trilene Inhaler, I have never instructed a patient in the use of a hypodermic syringe and needle in case she requires pethidine, nor have I ever tied down a pair of hands or legs! These deflections from 'scientific' antenatal and obstetric procedures have not prevented me, however, from eliminating all possible discomfort from normal labour. Analgesia is always available for the women who want it. Pain is the enemy of childbirth, not its natural accompaniment. It is therefore the first principle of an obstetrician to avoid or to overcome by the quickest and safest method any discomfort a parturient woman feels is more intense than she wishes to bear. The means of avoiding pain is the cornerstone of antenatal education, not the necessity for pain and the methods by which it may be relieved.

Instruction

The art of instruction is not easily acquired – good teachers are not didactic demagogues. They must be good listeners. Marcus Aurelius wrote (Book VI, 53): 'Accustom thyself to attend carefully to what is said by another, and as much as it is possible, be in the speaker's mind.' This attitude towards learners enables the instructress to hold the attention of her class.

Expectant mothers must be allowed to ask questions freely and without any fear of being thought ignorant. Many women's anxieties arise from problems satisfactorily solved by a few words of explanation or advice. No question is foolish if, unanswered, it creates a doubt or fear in a woman's mind. The subjects in which pregnant women are interested are fully discussed in other parts of this book, therefore they need not be repeated in detail.

It must be remembered that it is much easier to comprehend elementary facts of an entirely new field of learning if diagrams, pictures and charts are used. A woman can follow descriptions of organs and function if they can be visualised and demonstrated in black and white.

In this way the anatomy of the uterus and the manner in which it receives its blood and nerve supply is explained. By special diagrams, drawn to illustrate the function of the different muscle layers or fibres in the uterus, the influence of their harmony of action and the causes and results of faulty action can be demonstrated. It interests women to learn that the human uterus and the blood vessels of the abdomen provide evidence that we are built to be on all fours, not in the upright stance. The frequent occurrence of piles, varicose veins, and the minor discomforts of pregnancy due to the pressure of the enlarging uterus on the pelvic structures are ailments largely due to faults of mechanism produced by our becoming bipeds without changing our internal supports. It also impresses upon women the necessity for keeping the abdominal muscles in good tone and maintaining the breasts in a shape and position similar to the virgin breast, pendant from the chest when parallel to the ground.

Reference is made to the nervous system and its action. This complicated branch of human physiology may be adequately explained by using the analogy of the telephone exchange. The nerves represent wires leading from all parts of the body to the central exchange which we term the thalamus. Here messages are received and replies relayed. When there is a call for help because of impending discomfort or real pain, protective measures are initiated and necessary action is taken to relieve the organ or part of the body which is in distress. In emergency, the volume and distribution of assistance varies as the balance and integrity of the operator. If the thalamic exchange is well organised it will not misinterpret the importance of the message it receives; but if it is in a state of excitability and anticipation arising from the imminence of disaster, it may well call upon reserves and retaliate in no way commensurate with the severity of the assumed assault. This state of affairs was frequently seen during the late war, based upon lack of judgment and the excessive fear of possibilities which in reality did not exist.

This action and reaction to nervous messages or stimuli can be put into very simple words and generalisations can be made by which the influence of fear upon labour is introduced. I recall a rumour during the Battle of Britain that a vast descent of Germans by parachute was to be expected over a certain area in England. The story goes that as an air battle went on, high in the night sky, a parachute was seen to fall in the middle of a road and a man rose to his feet in view of one of our patrolling cars. The youthful driver, seeking to destroy the invading Germans, accelerated and drove in the semi-darkness straight at the staggering airman, killing him instantaneously, only to discover that he was one of our own brave and well-known pilots who, having escaped from his burning plane, was killed by the hysterical excitement of those whose judgment was warped by the fear of injury. I remember at the time how closely this tragedy was associated in my mind with the series of events frequently witnessed in normal childbirth.

The growth of the uterus and the development of the child from fertilisation and throughout gestation is discussed. Years ago it was unheard of that a woman should wish to see the afterbirth – today nearly every mother who watches her baby born asks me to show her the placenta. This I do and point out the bag in which the infant, now lying peacefully in her arms, developed and became a perfect little human being. I demonstrate the cord and its attachments, and the manner in which substances are filtered from the maternal blood to build not only the body but the mind and nature of her child. The amazing powers of selecting for the fetus at its different stages of growth, the correct food in balanced quantities, and of refusing to admit much, though not all, that might be harmful, makes the intelligent mind appreciate the incalculable genius of creation in all its phases and designs. 'Madam, when man can make one of these, he will have reached the footstool of the Creator; as I hold this discarded mass in my hand, I am humbled by the limitations of science.' Such references and quotations create respect and help to mould the mind to visualise childbirth in its correct perspective. By speaking of the placenta in these terms, the importance of judicious and correct diet and the influence of harmful chemicals which can pass into the baby's blood, can be elaborated.

Reference can be made to prolonged anaesthetics and the excessive use of certain drugs which affect the unborn and newborn infant. This should be done discreetly lest a woman might be led to overestimate the damage to her child should some medication be desirable during the course of labour. I have known women who have believed that their child would be born dead if she 'took chloroform'.

At these classes pregnant women are in a very receptive frame of mind – discretion and considerable tact must be used in order to avoid misunderstanding by exaggeration or understatement. The ease with which a wrong impression can be given more than justifies the allocation of time for questions and discussion.

The bag of waters can be made much of in simple terms. The wide variety of its purposes almost demands mild dramatisation. Our greatest scientists cannot discover how or whence the water comes – some say from the baby, others from the mother, but many believe it to have a mixed maternal and fetal origin. It maintains an even temperature for the baby, it protects it from injury, it equalises the pressure to which the child may be subjected, it allows the fetus to move freely and exercise its limbs in the uterus. It avoids all friction and the umbilical cord floats loosely in a medium which prevents it being compressed or from becoming entangled with the infant.

The dilating action of the bag of waters during labour should be mentioned. Many women become seriously alarmed if, towards the end of pregnancy, the waters leak, and although they are told to get in touch with the doctor at once should this occur, it seldom leads to trouble if wisely treated. Questions will be asked about dry labour, which has earned a bad name – it rarely makes any difference to a straightforward delivery. Nature frequently corrects its own deficiencies; a soft swelling on the presenting part takes the place of the bag and acts as an efficient conical dilator.

The general hygiene of pregnancy often brings to light much that surprises. So many women of all income classes are ignorant of habits and customs which they should have learned and practised from early childhood. The care of the bowels, teeth, hair and skin and even bodily cleanliness have received no attention. These matters must be discussed for they may give rise to disturbances of health. The posture and appearance of a pregnant woman affects her pride and without pride she is unlikely to adopt the correct attitude towards her condition.

All such apparently unimportant matters should be discussed from the point of view that women must associate the necessity for care of their own health with the health of their unborn babies.

There are two simple matters which appear to give many pregnant women a good deal of trouble: the suspension of stockings and the support of the abdomen.

There are two methods of suspension of the stockings during the later months of pregnancy. 1. The abdominal band above the maximum bulge of the uterus to which the suspenders are attached and carried down to the front and side of the leg. 2. The shoulder support which is favoured, is a brace carried for the right stocking over the left shoulder and for the left stocking over the right shoulder, crossing just below hip level.

Abdominal supporting belts are very rarely required by a woman having her first baby and those who have carried out their antenatal and postnatal exercises in order to maintain the tone of the abdominal muscles do not require them for subsequent babies. But some women, particularly those who have large infants or are too fat, develop pendulous abdomens which require support. Maternity belts are usually unwieldy, uncomfortable garments, many of them with complicated laces and fastenings. The general principle of the use of this support is that the uterus should sit in a cup, having no pressure whatever upon it above the level of the navel. The weight of the developing uterus is taken from the hollow of the back above the haunch bones.

More than thirty years ago I devised a belt which serves not only to give comfort to the mother but enables her to maintain good posture; it creates no pressure upon the upper abdomen and does not limit the freedom of respiration. There is no discomfort from distension after a meal, which sometimes occurs in late pregnancy. It is easily put on and adjusted as the uterus increases in size by the employment of two buckles fastened in front, on the undersurface. Suspenders are attached to its lower edge. This type of belt is small and light, meeting with general approval.

As the classes become more advanced, the phenomena of labour take precedence in the discussions and for this pictures, diagrams and my chart of the correlation of the physical and emotional phenomena of natural labour are used. In another part of this book the subject is fully described.

At about the thirty-third and thirty-fifth weeks of pregnancy, two lectures are given. The first is upon labour from its onset to the end of the first stage and the second from the transition to the end of the third stage.

One point is emphasised strongly. Women must co-operate with those who desire to help them for they will by then have been given a clear, though elementary understanding of the task that no one can do for them. Their success will depend upon their effort to become practised and proficient in their preparation for parturition – their achievement will be commensurate with the patience and self-control they exhibit.

Control of Respiration

There are various schools of thought upon the method of breathing and it is an art which has been developed to a very high degree.

Correct breathing is the foundation for good health. We can do without food or drink for relatively long periods and survive; we can vary our diet and our personal habits without any material change to our health; but the intake of oxygen and the output of carbon dioxide persist with regulated frequency many times every minute of our lives.

During pregnancy, when the oxygen intake is dependent upon the correctness of the respiratory function, breathing exercises should have priority over all other physical movements. The enlarging uterus causes discomfort to many women if they are not taught the correct posture and method of breathing that pregnancy demands. It is wise, therefore, to instruct women both in abdominal respiration, that is maximum use of the diaphragm, and in upper thoracic breathing; expansion of the chest, by lifting the ribs upwards and outwards, is made possible by the muscles between the ribs and those attached to the spine and outer surface of the ribs.

In the exercises that are described below the correct method of breathing is explained, and their design is to train women not only for the purpose of muscular fitness and joint mobility, but also in order to facilitate the intake of air and its complete exhalation. I do not propose, therefore, to give any special breathing exercises but rather to point out that, with the performance of the few simple antenatal movements described and an understanding of the importance of efficient respiration, the objective will be obtained.

During labour the control of breathing plays a large part in avoiding discomfort and assisting the uterus to carry out its work. As the contractions of the first stage increase in intensity, respiration becomes deeper and more rapid, sometimes twenty-six to twenty-eight deep breaths are taken in a minute. The reason for this is that the uterus, which is a large muscular organ, requires an extra quantity of fuel to maintain its activity. It uses a great deal of oxygen and has to get rid of the carbon dioxide, the waste product of energy. Since we take in oxygen and throw off carbon dioxide through our lungs, an increased intake and output of air is an obvious corollary to uterine action.

In the second stage of labour, when the expulsive effort is being made, respiration ceases whilst the woman is bearing down, but at the same time the uterus is contracting firmly and the high quantity of carbon dioxide accumulating in the blood is shown by a change in the colour of the face as the contraction persists. The woman may turn swarthy and cyanosed, which is a blue tint under the skin, for blood containing an excess of carbon dioxide is a dark blue-red colour. Therefore a woman must be trained to hold her breath, for by so doing, she can retain in her blood the slight increase of carbon dioxide without distress, and at the same time overcome the desire to let her breath go when it is advantageous to hold it. That is why after each expulsive contraction she is told to take two or three controlled, full, deep breaths, and await the next contraction in a state of complete relaxation. Respiration during relaxation is shallow; the absence of muscle tension minimises the use of oxygen and the formation of the waste products of tension. It also has the effect of allowing complete dilatation of both the arteries and veins in the pelvis, which enables a free intake of all fuel necessary for the low state of metabolism that it produces.

As the head commences to crown, that is, to make the final dilatation of the vulva, it is unwise to allow the expulsive effort of the uterus to be reinforced by the abdominal muscles. At this stage the woman is able to overcome the urge to hold her breath and the baby's head is born by uterine force only, whilst the woman is panting, that is, taking rapid, shallow breaths, in and out, to avoid increased intra-abdominal pressure. In this way the expulsion of the child can be controlled by the assistant and the perineum retained intact. Women should be taught to practise this panting respiration during antenatal instruction and told when to employ it. It has saved many perineums from serious injury and many women from the discomfort of much surgical repair.

The importance of respiration in labour must be fully appreciated by parturient women, by those who teach them and their attendants at labour. During the last few years certain French obstetricians have introduced panting respiration during late first-stage contractions and at the transition. Sometimes it appears to be effective, especially if the woman is closely attended by a nurse who holds her lower ribs and encourages the patient by holding a celophane breathing mask over her mouth. This may or may not have an oxygen supply tube attached. The benefit, if any, from this procedure is not due to oxygen absorption being increased because it is not – but to a disassociation of the mind from her labour. It is an exhausting and undesirable procedure, and offers no advantages over controlled natural respiration.

Relaxation

I have frequently been asked to write more fully upon relaxation in the practice of obstetrics. It has been my opinion in the past that relaxation is a subject apart from obstetrics and must be learned from those textbooks which are intended to set out in full the theory and practice of this most important addition to therapeutics. Edmund Jacobson has written *Progressive Relaxation*; for those who are interested in the subject all will be found in this book that the average student or medical man may wish to know. He has also published a smaller book for the lay reader called *You Must Relax*. This short book has an application to modern life, is easily readable and makes the subject clearly understood. It is a comprehensive addition to our knowledge and teaching upon the subject, and deals with the use of relaxation in the treatment of many diseases and conditions arising from neuro-muscular hypertension.

But in no publication upon this subject do we find reference to its use in obstetrics. In previous chapters I have referred to the causes of tension – mental and physical; and observations have been made upon the influence of the sympathetic nervous system during labour and its relation to the emotion of fear. I have referred to the effect of neuromuscular hypertension, the *Fear-Tension-Pain Syndrome* and the causes of discomfort during labour. It will be understood that relaxation is employed as an antidote to abnormal tension and therefore an adjuvant to the physiological process. All these enemies of natural childbirth are vulnerable to its successful implementation. Fear, tension and pain must be wholly obliterated, for if any one of this trio of evils is active, the other two are almost invariably present.

What, then, is relaxation in the sense in which we use this term? It will be found upon investigation that 'relaxation' has obviously been the cause of great difficulty and confusion to those who have compiled dictionaries. In one I read: 'It is the act of relaxing; state of being relaxed; remission of application; unbending; looseness.' In another: 'The action of unbending the mind from severe application; release from ordinary occupations or cares; recreation; respite; rest; a loosening or flattening of the fibres, nerves, etc, of the body; diminution of firmness or tension, etc, etc.' In a third, a more concise definition is given: '1. A lessening of tension. 2. A mitigation of pain.' But to the man in the street the word means none of these things; he will tell you that it is any form of employment which takes him to the peaceful and quiet recreation which is most apart from his everyday work. But in the medical sense relaxation not only means all these things, but many others as well. I suggest, however, that for the purpose of its application in obstetrics, we consider relaxation to be *a condition in which the muscle tone throughout the body is reduced to a minimum.*

We must remember that physiological reactions and reflexes vary, both in speed and intensity, with the fluctuation of neuromuscular tension. It is a quality which is susceptible to the moods and modulations of individuals and there is a direct relationship between the emotional state and muscular tone. It is also important to consider whether our physical reactions are secondary to our emotional states or whether, as the James-Lange Theory suggests, our emotional states are secondary to our physical reactions. For if we are able to reduce the tone of our muscular system, we know from experiment and clinical observation that the reflexes of the body are diminished in power. We also know that the influence of the mechanism that records sensations arising within the body is much less pronounced in a state of muscular relaxation than in a state of muscular tension. Stimuli arising from the emotional system produce less violent reaction when there is an absence of tension in the muscular system. In fact, Jacobson goes so far as to say: 'Present results indicate that an emotional state fails to exist in the presence of complete relaxation of the peripheral parts involved.' In another place he says: 'It is physically impossible to be nervous in any part of your body if in that part you are completely relaxed.' That is not so clear, but in applying this to obstetrics we can say that if the body is completely relaxed, it is impossible to entertain the emotion of fear. That is the important factor, for if fear is absent, then the overruling power of the sympathetic nervous system is absent from the pelvic mechanism. I must remind you that this eliminates any excess of muscle tone in the circular fibres of the lower uterine segment, the cervix and the outlet of the birth canal. Complete relaxation, therefore, offers the minimum of resistance to the muscles of expulsion in the birth canal. In *Natural Childbirth* I laid stress upon the short but important dictum 'Tense woman; tense cervix'; the converse of this is equally true: 'Relaxed woman; relaxed cervix.' But this is not all; in a state of complete relaxation the sensations of muscle activity during parturition are interpreted in their true sense. It becomes possible to speak of 'muscle-sensation' to a woman who is relaxed; a similar stimulus is interpreted as 'agony' by the woman whose mind is tense with fear.

I strongly urge those who put this method into practice not to associate the dramatic changes which they will notice in their patients with suggestion, mesmerism or hypnotism. *There is no relationship whatever between complete relaxation and hypnotism in childbirth.* I sympathise most sincerely with one who sees for the first time this new experience. I do not hesitate to record that so startling were the results of this teaching when I first employed it in the practice of natural childbirth, that I became suspicious of myself, although I was aware that no conscious effort was being made to influence the minds of my patients by hypnotism. Consequently, I consulted one of our greatest authorities upon these subjects and asked him to examine me and my methods to see whether, by some accident, I was unwittingly employing the use of methods of which I was unconscious. I have never had any knowledge of mesmerism or hypnotism. The examination was most carefully made and I was assured that there was no *relation whatever between the application of relaxation in obstetrics and hypnotism.* Jacobson is very keen on this matter and in his book *Progressive Relaxation* he gives no less than thirty-two distinct points of difference between relaxation and suggestion.

It is important that I should lay stress upon this question of psychical influence. I have had many letters from both doctors and nurses who have merely waived this whole teaching on one side as being 'mesmerism' or 'hypnotism'. A particular case was from the north of England, where a sister who is an expert midwife and who has a thorough knowledge of relaxation and all the methods of natural childbirth, went away from London with her patient because of the air raids. It was late in pregnancy and the patient decided to continue my teaching but to invite a certain well-known obstetrician to attend her when in labour, as it was impossible for me to travel so far afield. In due course her first baby arrived; it was a large infant and although she herself was nearer to forty than to thirty, she exhibited no distress; her child was born completely naturally; the doctor was asked to refrain from giving an anaesthetic and to his surprise met with resistance when he offered it. He had known of the patient for many years because her brother was a doctor also practising in the district and he had heard how nervous she was. When the birth was safely over the obstetrician realised that he had only been a surprised observer and taken no part whatever in the conduct of the case; he was inclined to believe that his patient had been subjected to some mystical influence. The midwife was modestly quiet, but he invited her opinion and asked her to tell him more of those teachings and practices which had led up to this extraordinary labour. She did so and he no longer repeated, as he had at first, 'A kind of mesmerism,' but became interested and wrote at once to hear further of this thing. Had this member of our profession not been of a tolerant and enquiring nature, he would have broadcast that this was a form of hypnosis; the whole system would have been damned in that district, for there is nothing more frightful to the lay mind than the mystical application of psychological influence. Now, however, the young mothers of that district demand to have their babies naturally.

Before we discuss more fully the teaching of relaxation during pregnancy, there are certain other considerations which demand attention. The attitude of woman towards childbearing varies with the individual: some become profoundly introspective; they seem to be examining themselves and their condition every hour of the day; they record the most minute changes in their physical sensations as well as their thoughts. These people not infrequently come to the conclusion that any phenomenon which they do not understand must be wrong. It is not so much that they anticipate evil, but being conscious of the possibilities of abnormality, they search for all kinds of symptoms which might suggest an unnatural state. There are also women who believe that pregnancy must be accompanied by malaise; such things as vomiting, gross frequency of micturition, sleeping badly, losing one's appetite and looking pale and wan are accepted by them as usual and quite ordinary. They move about the community with an expression on their faces which says: 'Behold, I am great with child; I demand your sympathy and your care.' There are also women who are pleased to be pregnant; women who want a child and who devote their time to doing those things that a woman should do when she is about to become a mother. They remain conscious of their condition but find it difficult to alter the routine of their lives. They cannot be bothered to do exercises, but they swing their arms from time to time and walk into the town instead of going by car. They do not like changing their normal and habitual diet; they eat, therefore, what comes, but perhaps they try to eat less or possibly drink a little more water than has been their custom. But their effort to apply themselves to the rules of life is niggardly; they are unwilling to sacrifice for their baby's sake, yet their hearts are in the right place and they are positive mothers as opposed to the others, to whom I might refer as 'negative' mothers. We meet also the enthusiasts: those who swing themselves to the forefront of womanhood; who advertise the fact that not only are they about to have a baby, but that they are doing the most marvellous exercises that were ever invented; they know the books that are written on these subjects; they give up their whole lives to the perfection of their physique for the purposes of motherhood; their diet is most meticulously carried out – each portion is weighed according to their increasing weight; they understand the calorific values of their food; they take certain preparations which, they are told, are 'aids to motherhood', and study all available literature on the modern aspect of maternity. They may be described as the 'plus' women who do everything slightly excessively; they are the enthusiasts whose academic sense of accuracy leads them to believe the theoretical adjuvants to motherhood are more effective than the true and natural spirit of maternity without exaggeration. And finally, we have the born mothers; those who are calmly delighted; those who appear to be able to carry out all the necessary teaching without overdoing it; those who avoid publicity, but who do their job with a stolid sense which in the long run achieves all that nature intended motherhood to mean. These profoundly level-headed women are fortunately in considerable numbers amongst women of all income classes; they are sympathetically astonished at the negative women, just as the plus women are enraged at the attitude of those who do not want their babies. In like manner the negative women envy the natural woman her ability to remain unmoved by these occurrences, whereas they also consider the plus woman to be demented and distinctly a bore.

But, as obstetricians, we must be conscious of what type or pigeon-hole our individual patients fall into and that is particularly important when we commence our efforts to teach relaxation. Now, strangely enough, there are two classes of women who cannot be taught; these 'classes' are, of course, quite arbitrary, but the women who do not want their babies, who are bored by the whole procedure and who feel they are merely doing a duty and are fed up at having to do this duty, very often avoid any practice of relaxation and become antagonistic to its teaching. Curiously, the other class is represented by the 'plus' women; these enthusiasts are active live wires to whom the application of modern science is all-important. They are told the benefits of relaxation, but their reply not infrequently is that it would be quite unnecessary to apply it to them, as they will be able to control themselves when the time comes. They are sure that the whole thing should be conducted in a natural way and they are preparing themselves along natural lines. Very often these women prefer their physical exercises, avoid the careful practice of relaxation and assume understanding without education.

But the majority of women are in the three types that are between the negative and positive extremes:

1. Those who are mildly negative – lazy and casual in the conduct of pregnancy; they have to be kept up to the mark.
2. The real and natural mother to whom all things to do with motherhood are inborn gifts and who have balanced in the exercise of their instinctive activities. They adjust themselves to the new rules of life without difficulty.
3. The slightly positive woman, who is so keen to do everything really well that she has to be restrained and carefully educated.

These types will all willingly submit to being taught relaxation.

Now I am sure it will be readily appreciated by any experienced physician that a rule-of-thumb method of teaching this subject is quite impossible under the circumstances. We have to use our discretion; it would be absurd to ask the negative woman to carry out, in exactly the same way, on the same principles, at the same times of day, those practices which we would invite the plus woman to carry out. If we are to get adequate results, we must balance our demands. I have found that complete general relaxation is the ideal to aspire to, but, on the other hand, it is astonishing how imperfect relaxation may alter the whole course of labour. Possibly an expert like Jacobson might feel that some of our patients were not relaxing at all in terms of what he believes to be complete relaxation. But if he saw a patient both before and after she had been asked to relax by her physician during labour, he would realise what a marked difference there is even if the performance leaves much to be desired. This, I think, is probably accounted for by the fact that a relative state of relaxation is sufficient to diminish the pain of labour – that is to say, to diminish the sensations of labour which are interpreted as pain by the tense woman. I have frequently been told how different the whole thing becomes when the body is allowed to be 'slack,' and if women have tried to learn relaxation and are able to put it into effect, astonishingly gratifying results are obtained. We know that complete relaxation, in terms of expert practice, is unusual during pregnancy; we do not demand it, because those of us who are experienced with women know that if we demanded it, we should rarely get it. Our objective is to help each woman to become as efficient as possible in the art of relaxation. The quality of performance varies widely; the most conscientious efforts may either appear to be of no avail, or result in excellent performance. Not infrequently the former type finds difficulty in applying herself to any teaching whereas the latter is more mentally alert and quick to learn. The discomforts of labour vary inversely as the woman's ability to relax, for this accomplishment is usually the concomitant of a state of confidence and intelligent equanimity which allows the ever-changing phenomena of parturition to be correctly interpreted without loss of self-control.

20

Preparation for Labour

I have been asked at what stage in pregnancy instruction in this practice should be started. There again there is no rule of thumb; if there is the slightest tendency to nervous symptoms in the early months of pregnancy, such as morning sickness, salivation or persistent frequency of micturition, I embark on the early lessons of relaxation at once, providing that there is no retroversion of the uterus or bladder irritation. The effect upon nervous symptoms is very marked in some cases and certainly worthwhile in all. If a woman is perfectly healthy and begins to feel as she should, healthier and happier than ever before, I do not commence instruction in relaxation until the baby has quickened. There is a reality of pregnancy at that time which somehow seems to make a woman anxious to do these things which, having confidence in her educator, she is told will be of assistance both to her and the child. She is anxious very often to acquire calm; many women believe that their own mental outlook and nervous condition will have a marked effect on the baby during its development. There is certainly some evidence which suggests that they are correct in this assumption, but it is very difficult to be quite sure. What I mean is that the best babies are those who, for the first three months of life, just eat, sleep and have their playtime during the late afternoon. They are automatic little human beings growing into more mature life without hesitation and apparently without questioning the rightness of their own conduct; such children are born to mothers who have practised most successfully the art of relaxation; it may be that some mothers have good babies anyhow; we cannot tell. Certain weight is, however, added to this possibility when we realise that another observation points in the same direction. The troublesome, sleepless, 'green nappy' babies, who are querulous and windy and who do not seem to know what peace means, are frequently the children of negative women who have not practised relaxation and calm during pregnancy or labour. These babies are often born anoxaemic because of anaesthetic and sedative drugs given to the mother. The most frequent and serious cause of ill-health and death of newborn babies is the deficiency or lack of oxygen immediately before and after the moment of birth.

It is upon such considerations as these that the teaching of relaxation is commenced about the time, or just after, the mother is conscious of the quickening of her child. Most intelligent women can be taught in the remaining months sufficient to enable them to get very good results from their efforts. I fully realise that those physicians who teach progressive relaxation for the purpose of cure in other conditions – or, should we say, cure of pathological states – require six months to obtain good results. In pregnancy I have seen the most excellent results after two months of teaching and practice.

But whenever this instruction commences I would call most serious attention to the manner of approach that a physician makes to his patient upon this subject. I have been met sometimes with the argument: 'Why should I practise this relaxation that you speak of? My mother did not do so and she has never heard of it, and she has come through her pregnancies safely.' And again: 'But I have no time to do these things; I can just do a few exercises in the morning, but after that my day is one long rush, and I cannot undertake to do anything else.' Therefore, I suggest to obstetricians who propose to introduce this subject, that they speak of the necessity for a certain amount of rest whilst the woman is carrying her baby, even if it is only for half an hour in the middle of the day, either before or after she has washed up the lunch things if she is a housewife. It should be pointed out to her that physical tiredness is likely to become embarrassing in the later stages of pregnancy if the habit of rest is not made in the earlier months. It is usually possible to persuade a mother-to-be that a rest of half an hour before or after lunch becomes an easy habit and the majority will conform to this suggestion. Frequently I lay stress on the necessity for their becoming relaxed after they are in bed at night or of putting into practice those things which they have been taught before they go to sleep. I dare say that this is not very effective, but it does seem to ensure that one of two things occurs; either they practise and carry out the teaching or they go to sleep soundly and well. This appears to be rather a poor compromise, but it is better than nothing.

When instructing in relaxation we must be careful not to make a mystery of it. It should be treated in a perfectly common-sense, practical manner, and if possible made interesting to the woman so that she understands the 'why' and the 'wherefore' of what she is being taught. I cannot allow this opportunity to pass without telling of one experience that I had in the teaching of relaxation. I was invited to attend a lecture given to midwives by a lady who had become keenly interested in this matter and who was an instructor in one of the teaching centres of the University of London. I had a note from the matron of the hospital at which the lecture was being given inviting me to attend, as she felt that I would be able to supply the answers to certain questions that might be asked afterwards. I felt it was rather a busman's holiday, but, on the other hand, I was curious to know how this teaching was being conducted, particularly by one of whom I had never heard and whose work had never come to my notice. This was nearly five years after my first publication on this subject. The lecture itself, as such, was perfectly all right in an elementary way, but the entertaining part was after the lecture, when she called from amongst her audience a protégée whom she had brought with her and who was trained in relaxation. An examination couch was hastily brought into the room and the model flung off her ordinary clothes, under which was revealed a gym tunic. She leapt on to the table like a well-trained fox terrier. She lay rigidly, with her legs stiffly extended and her arms by her sides; she was then demonstrating, we were told, a position of tension. The induction of relaxation then commenced to take place. Now the lady who was 'inducing' the condition of relaxation proceeded to explain that the first essential was to get controlled, regular, deep breathing. That is, of course, all right in its way, but she herself then proceeded to rise up on her toes, raise her arms and hiss with inspiration, at the end of which she said 'H'in,' and then as she let herself go, her body rippled down over her patient, expiring with a loud huff to the tune of 'H'out.' This went on with increasing fervour, strange noises, strange rippling movements of the body which appeared to be as elastic as a skilled ballet dancer. Her fingers, tendrillous and long, quivered above the prostrate form of her victim; her piercing eyes gleamed brightly and gazed deeply into those of her patient; her mouth moved feverishly, as if she were muttering the formula of some ancient incantation. This ludicrous performance was an effort to induce what we were to believe was relaxation. A colleague of mine who was sitting nearby turned to me and raised his eyebrows; someone sitting behind me slid over my shoulder a piece of paper on which was drawn a witch's tripod with a steaming pot under it. That was the general impression this lady gave us. There was very little real instruction; it was rather like a conjuror putting a small ball of tension into a hat and bringing out the silk handkerchief of relaxation. There was nothing to teach us how it was done although the model appeared to be quite skilful. I was introduced to the lecturer afterwards, who said how nice it was that medical men should at last be taking some interest in the subject of relaxation during pregnancy. She hoped that I would try it and gave me her name and address, so that should I find any troubles she would be only too pleased to assist me to get better results! I assured her most conscientiously and most sincerely that she had been of far greater assistance to me than she realised. That was indeed true; I had seen a practical exhibition of how not to deal with women; a practical exhibition of what not to do when endeavouring to instruct in relaxation. No one is likely to impart wisdom by appearing foolish.

Even today we have to beware of those who aspire to teach, never having learnt. One of my most unhappy dilemmas is to find an adequate reply to the women who meet me or write to me, that my principles have failed, because they had been to antenatal classes and lectures and learnt everything but had the most distressing labours. As I write this in the Year of Grace 1953, I received a letter from an expectant mother who had read this book. She was attending antenatal classes and lectures at a hospital in a well-known university city: 'Our first lecture as mothers of first babies was given by the maternity sister and consisted of advice on the use of the gas-air machine for the "eighteen-hour stretch when labour would be unbearably painful." Furthermore, she promised (with a sincere effort to be comforting) that we would, none of us, be required to "endure more than two hours in the second stage, as instruments would then be used"!' Happily this is unusual when senior hospital sisters lecture, but many times I have tactfully enquired for more details and found similar reprehensible notions being propagated. The classes have been physical training, conducted by those who had little or no knowledge of obstetrics and no labour ward experience. The gentle art of education in the elementary rudiments of childbirth was not employed and many had been cheerfully told in 'lectures' that labour was easy and without any discomforts; others kindly informed them when the pain was too bad they would be doped. This so-called antenatal work is often carried out as an addition to the incomes of those practising physiotherapy or even beauty culture!

Through such organisations the approach to childbirth as a natural or physiological function is being misrepresented and a high percentage of failures earn a bad name for procedures which have been improperly employed. Relaxation is incompletely taught and its use as an adjuvant to normal labour is not explained. Most of the attendants, though possibly good 'obstetricians', are not familiar with the technique they are expected to follow by their patients.

Positions for Relaxation

A hard, flat mattress is the ideal support for a relaxing woman, but since this is rarely available in these days of soft comfort and spring beds, the floor with a thick carpet or folded rug should be used. This is usually available and needs no preparation. Two small pillows or cushions from the sofa and a warm cover if in a cold climate, complete the outfit.

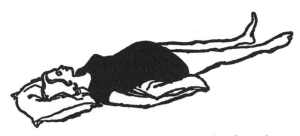

There are three positions for relaxing upon the floor during pregnancy which are: on the back, and the right or left lateral. It must be noted, however, that many women who are more than eighteen to twenty weeks pregnant have considerable difficulty in being comfortable if they lie upon their back; but since some can relax in this position between eighteen and thirty weeks, I will describe the method.

Lie on the back with the head on a thin cushion, the arms by the sides about eight inches to one foot from the trunk, the fingers open and the hands and elbows resting loosely so the whole weight of the upper limb from the shoulders to the fingertips is taken by the floor. Clenching the fingers, arching the wrists or raising the shoulders are common beginners' mistakes. The legs must lie straight from the hips with the feet about six inches apart, not crossed and falling naturally outwards upon the heels. The trunk or torso must be kept as flat as possible on the floor. One of the difficulties of this position is found in the woman who has pronounced or prominent buttocks. It is almost impossible, in such cases, to loosen the muscles supporting the spine unless either the shoulders are raised or the knees are pulled up. A small cushion can be placed in the hollow of the back, but in my experience this is not a satisfactory position for a pregnant woman. Later on she will be taught how to relax on her back when the trunk is raised at an angle of 45 to 50 degrees to the floor or the bed; in that position with a pillow under the knees complete and comfortable relaxation can be obtained and is particularly useful in the second stage of labour.

The better positions, however, for a woman to adopt in the later months of pregnancy are 'the right and left lateral'. This is not generally recognised. In practice it is of considerable importance and of proved value during the latter part of the first stage of labour. There is one small difficulty that may have to be overcome, for a number of pregnant women are astonished that they should be asked to lie with any weight upon the baby in their uterus. When the explanation of the manner in which the baby is protected by the bag of waters is given, and the fact that the weight is not directly upon the baby, their minds are set at rest. The *right lateral position* is adopted by lying upon the right hip, with the front of the chest turned prone upon the floor. The right arm is behind the back and the left arm is loosely extended. The head rests upon the pillow facing either to the right or left, whichever the subject finds more comfortable. The right leg is fully extended and the left leg, bent at the knee, is raised up to a right angle or even less to the chest. A cushion is placed under the left knee. The equivalent position is adopted for the left lateral position. The illustration shows the ease with which this posture can be sustained. In the later months of pregnancy when the abdomen is large there is practically no pressure upon it as the weight of the body is taken upon the right hip and the drawn-up left leg. The equivalent position is adopted for the left lateral position.

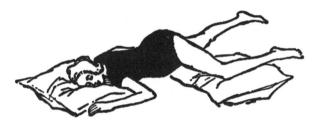

You cannot be conscious of relaxation unless you are conscious of muscle tension. When we speak of muscle tension in this sense we refer to the muscles attached to the bones of the skeleton, that is the skeletal muscles. These are under the control of the will, can be tensed or relaxed, with practice, by order of the mind. The involuntary muscles of the intestines, blood vessels, heart, lungs and so on, are not directly concerned with this exercise although complete relaxation profoundly influences their activities.

Instruction is given in a quiet voice, slowly and clearly:

'Take a deep breath through an open mouth; curl up the toes and tense the muscles of one leg ... (short pause) ... release the breath slowly, and relax the whole limb. Compare in your own mind the feelings of tension and relaxation.'

This exercise is repeated, followed by the other leg. The instruction is then extended to groups of muscles allowing them to become alternately tense and relaxed. And so one works through the whole body, recognising the sensation of tension in a muscle and its absence in relaxation. This applies not only to the arms and legs, but to the trunk, the abdomen and the chest. When relaxing the abdominal muscles particular attention should be called to the muscles about and within the pelvis. Special care should be taken to instruct women in the tensing and relaxing of the muscles of the pelvic orifices and will be explained when antenatal exercises are discussed. The muscles employed in breathing are described.

A word about the forehead. The wrinkled brow must, of course, be avoided. Relaxation of the face as a whole is extremely important and I am quite sure that any woman who is capable of relaxing her facial muscles will go through labour with the maximum ease that the absence of tension makes possible. It must be remembered that a woman does not look her best when her face is relaxed; I always point this out and tell her that I have no desire that she should look her best just then; I want her to be her best. I find that it is probably the most difficult part of the body for a woman to relax; it may be because they depend upon the expression of the face for their basic personality and for much feminine finesse. A few women have definitely refused to allow their faces to become relaxed in my presence; they have been self-conscious and have promised to try when alone in their room. If a woman is wearing false teeth, it is wiser for her to remove them rather than try to relax her face with them in the mouth. Many dentures are not absolutely safe without some support from the facial muscles; we do not like to see them half in and half out when the muscles of the cheeks and jaws are relaxed! Women must be taught to relax the muscles around their eyes, cheeks, mouth, and, in particular, the eyelids, and if they are really good triers, the eyes too. The cheeks and jaws relax quite easily if the subject is properly instructed, and after a time she who acquires relaxation of the face finds it very much easier to eliminate tension from her whole body. It is extraordinary how quickly the average woman is able to relax once she understands muscle tension, but it takes considerable practice before she becomes expert. At each successive class the technique is improved.

The detailed instruction of differential and general relaxation is too big a subject to include in a chapter, but if more information is sought,

I recommend that the books I have already mentioned should be studied. Above all, I urge the use of common sense; human understanding is the asset of a good teacher. Some people endeavour to induce this state by the quiet repetition of persuasive clichés such as: 'Now you will find that you are breathing quietly, regularly, slee-ee-pi-ly' or 'Now you are sinking through the floor and soon you will have that beautiful feeling of alienation from all the troubles of life.' That sort of thing is not required. Relaxation is a practical, volitional acquisition of a physical state. *There is no necessity whatever to employ any fads or fancies in its teaching.*

The Performance of Relaxation

After this series of exercises has been carried out, the women adopt the most comfortable position and if they feel cold, they are covered with a rug. The curtains are drawn and the instructress moves without ostentation amongst her pupils to test or assist their relaxation. She does not ask them to let their minds become a blank; she knows that when physically relaxed their minds will take care of themselves. Several patients have told me it is very difficult for their imaginations to become quiet; all the events of the day are vividly recalled directly they try to relax. This is, of course, an indication that their relaxation is incomplete and, therefore, they should not be urged to avoid thought in any way, because the avoidance of thought is one of the most active mental exercises, They should be urged, rather, to concentrate upon their relaxation, to practise it more thoroughly, trying to recognise what groups of muscles are remaining in tension. It must be remembered that no emotional state can be present if there is real physical relaxation of the body. This may be accepted as a fact and will probably be best appreciated by those medical men who can bring themselves to practise this invaluable aid to good health, particularly people who work hard at all times of the day and night.

Residual Tension

The difference between lying limp and neuromuscular relaxation can he recognised by observing indications of residual tension. It can be diagnosed by listening to the breathing of a woman; any irregularity is evidence of imperfect relaxation; a flicker of an eyelid, movement of the eyeballs in their sockets behind closed lids, the restless shift of a finger or toe, or an uncontrollable swallow, all demonstrate the presence of residual tension of which the woman herself is unaware. If, in the silence of the relaxing class, the instructress makes a sudden slight noise, she will notice those who react immediately or even violently to this auditory disturbance. It is further evidence by which the presence of residual tension may be detected. The physician makes other tests which in antenatal classes are not really necessary; for instance, the pulse rate, certain nervous reactions and reflexes and the manner of respiration are means by which we can estimate the degree of relaxation. We aim at training women to relax to the elimination of residual tension, but at the same time realise, without trying to persuade ourselves to the contrary, that the instruction received at the antenatal classes is insufficient to obtain that desirable state in all pregnant women. Those who do overcome residual tension are usually the perfect obstetric patients, providing they have no disproportion between the size of the infant and the pelvis, and the baby is lying in the anterior vertex presentation. Select such a patient for demonstrating physiological childbirth to maternity nurses, medical students and postgraduates, who wish to learn of these procedures. The experienced accoucheur will realise, however, that no one can prophesy with certainty the conduct of any woman in labour, but we can detect those who appear to be likely to do well.

Many women will go to sleep soon after they become relaxed, but it is the most restful form of natural sleep there is.

I was invited to visit the Antenatal School of Instruction organised by my wife in order to observe certain methods being used and also to discover, if I could, to what extent the relaxed women showed any signs of residual tension. The room was darkened and quiet; I entered without any unnecessary noise, the instructress met me, and although speaking quietly it was in a normal voice. I walked around the women, some of whom were in the left lateral and some in the right lateral position. They had then been relaxing for about ten to fifteen minutes. I sat in a chair and watched them individually and although several had obvious evidences of incomplete relaxation, which was not unreasonable since they had only attended four classes, I was astonished at the sleepiness of those who were not asleep. As I sat there in the peace of the room it came to my mind how easily anyone who was not initiated might have presumed that these women were being subjected to some form of hypnosis. When given instruction, they reacted slowly but accurately and it reminded me of the dictum of Edmund Jacobson, referring to relaxation: 'No university subject and no patient ever considered it a suggested, hypnoidal, or trance state, or anything but a perfectly natural condition. It is only the person who has merely read a description who might question this point.' I talked for a short time with the instructress and left the room. I learnt afterwards that only two of the class knew of my visit.

A note upon this instructress at the school is of considerable importance, for it demonstrates the advantage of having the authority to teach. She is a highly qualified physiotherapist, twenty-two years old, of pleasing appearance, quiet manner and voice and a retiring disposition. She was trained in every aspect of antenatal work including the application of physiotherapy to obstetrics by my wife, particularly the approach to, and understanding of, the mind and emotions of the expectant mother. After she became pregnant she continued to take her classes at the School of Instruction, be present at deliveries, and direct postnatal exercises. She was absent from the school only one working day until her baby was born. Just nine months ago, on a Friday, she took her classes as usual; the next day she did her weekend shopping and called at my consulting rooms about midday to tell me that she had the early signs and symptoms of labour – I examined her and agreed. She went to the maternity hospital and at 4pm that afternoon I delivered her of a full term 7lb son.

It was a perfect example of natural childbirth entirely free, she assures me, from any discomfort; each phase and changing sensation of her labour was expected and recognised; everything she taught was demonstrated by her. Her relaxation was exemplary, her amnesia was deep and her reception of her son, holding his arms as he emerged from her *uninjured* birth canal, was a joy for anyone to witness. I turned to the matron who was present and said: 'Why, oh why, were not ten thousand obstetricians here?' That is a remark I have frequently made after a natural labour.

Instruction in relaxation is an important adjunct to physiological labour, but at the same time women feel acutely that childbirth is a private and domestic affair. The authority of these ladies is not established by an immaculate uniform or a domineering presence. The high standard of their knowledge and efficiency is not reflected in the friendly or homely atmosphere of the school. A stranger might have difficulty in telling pupil from teacher! Their authority emanates from an unshakable faith in the truth which they impart to others; they have a pattern to impress upon the minds of women who have been afraid. It is the memory of their own experiences, when, in an aura of indescribable joy, they saw their babies born and knew the blessings of a natural birth. They demand that all women shall learn to achieve this happiness; my wife and this young teacher-mother have a prerogative to which I can never aspire. No woman ever turns with scorn to them, as they do to me, and say: 'It's easy enough for you to talk!'

Physical Fitness*

And, finally, we come to the consideration of the place of physical exercise in pregnancy. There are certain fundamental facts which must be clarified. Largely influenced by the justifiable incursion of the physiotherapists into the realm of antenatal preparation, the advantages of this aspect of the training have been overestimated and its real value in pregnancy and parturition misunderstood. We must not allow excessive enthusiasm to give the impression that obstetrics is a new branch of the robust growth of physiotherapy; this science is employed mainly to improve the general health and deportment of expectant mothers – it is an adjuvant to the implementation of certain obstetric procedures, but the birth of a child in healthy young women proceeds quite satisfactorily without any prenatal physiotherapy.

There is greater discomfort in childbirth amongst women who have led sedentary lives than amongst those who live and work out of doors. We must 'consider the lilies of the field, and how they grow; they toil not neither do they spin'. There are still many women who rarely exercise either their minds or their bodies and bear their children with greater difficulty and more frequent interference than the peasant woman at the plough. The office worker tends to have more trouble than the fisher-girl, the farmhand or the riverboat woman. In all forms of higher animal life reproduction takes place in the environment that ensures the female may be as fit as possible to give birth to, and nurture, her young. The survival of a species depends largely upon the bodily and mental state of its individuals – it is women of low-grade health who profit most from a judicious use of physiotherapy.

The benefits derived from exercises are the same whether a woman is pregnant or not. When they are undertaken seriously the physical condition rapidly improves and a sense of well-being takes the place of dullness so frequently found amongst people who live in lethargic, comfortable and somnolent inactivity.

Certain movements associated with the mobility and flexibility of the muscles and joints of the pelvis are valuable during delivery and

---

*'There is no reason why a woman should not have an even better figure after she has borne a child than before. It is unnecessary to become fat and ungainly because she is a mother.' *Introduction to Motherhood*, G Dick-Read. Heinemann.

others assist in the depth and control of respiration. When we visualise the course of normal labour we realise that the first stage must be without muscular effort on the part of the woman and the second stage may require an hour or two of physical effort to help the uterus to expel the first-born infant. In a multiparous woman the expulsive stage may be completed by a few contractions of the uterus and these, in a well-conducted labour, are not necessarily reinforced by the skeletal muscles of the mother.

Any instruction in regulated exercise is good because it enhances the efficiency of both mind and body. Of itself it has very little, if any, influence on the mechanism of labour. Without the correct mental attitude towards parturition no amount of physical training will enable a woman to have her baby naturally. In fact, some of the most difficult labours I have attended, which should have been straightforward, have been those of muscular and lissom women without any antenatal instruction. Years ago, after some unhappy experiences I remember wishing that ballet dancers and Centre Court Wimbledon 'types' would cease to honour me with their request to deliver their babies because they so frequently had trouble! These women, of magnificent physique and as fit as racehorses, were often nervous and highly strung. Most good athletes have hair-trigger emotions and almost instantaneous reactions to stimulus; they are quick-thinking and apprehensive, having learnt to rely upon themselves for personal success. Since a more understanding approach to the education of childbearing women has been acquired, these ladies have become excellent subjects and are a pleasure to attend.

Some of the most perfect labours I have witnessed were of women with groups of muscles below the waist partially paralysed without any disturbance of sensation. They had suffered from polioencephalitis and their crippled bodies, which they swung from the hips on crutches or walking sticks, could not be physically trained. Women with education without exercise do better in labour than those meticulously prepared and skilled in physical culture, but without education in childbirth.

I am anxious therefore to write of this aspect of antenatal preparation, fully recognising that although it is beneficial for many women it is not essential for normal childbirth. A healthy woman who takes sensible exercise either at her work or recreation, can obtain all the advantages aspired to by learning the general principles of physiological reproduction and understanding the course and conduct of labour. The athletic woman or one previously expert in physical culture may wish to elaborate the movements described below. It is agreed those I advise constitute the most elementary practice of physical training, but it must be remembered that very few women who attend these classes have ever previously performed regulated and controlled movement of their limbs. The important observation is, however rudimentary this physical preparation may appear to be, it has been proved beyond all doubt sufficient for the purpose of its employment. Anything more than sufficient has been shown by experience to make no difference to the course of labour; anything less than sufficient deprives a woman of advantages she might so easily enjoy if she were in a better state of health.

There are many methods described and teachers have, in their publications, assumed some originality in systems carrying their names. The majority of these have been devised by representatives of various colleges of physiotherapy and I feel that there are two serious omissions in these works. The first is that the authors are not trained midwives or obstetricians – none of them has attained the degree of the Central Midwives Board or similar organisations. They may have had some labour-ward experience, but few have learnt the significance of the psychosomatic phenomena of natural or physiological childbirth. This serious deficiency in obstetric understanding has been clearly manifested by the unhappy results obtained when the efficacy of physiotherapy has been exaggerated at the expense of the more important principles of antenatal instruction.

Secondly, there is nothing new in the principles of physical exercise since Per Hendrick Ling, the greatest pioneer of medical gymnastics, who was born in 1776, laid the foundations upon which all schools of physiotherapy have grown. His name is too rarely mentioned by the authors of new works upon this subject.

I have endeavoured to adapt, for the benefit of pregnant and parturient women, the advice of Ling to those who desire to attain the maximum efficiency of both body and mind. My conclusions have been drawn on the one hand from my obstetric experience and on the other from an enthusiasm for athleticism and physical culture since early boyhood. From this I have learnt the evils of both excess and deficiency; it is by results that we are best able to judge.

Exercises

These exercises are done slowly, with each movement controlled, strict attention being paid to the co-ordination of respiration and muscular action. All the exercises are simple and no strain is required to do them satisfactorily. They are all performed with an easy rhythm, correlating breathing and movement, without holding the breath – with one exception, Exercise 6.

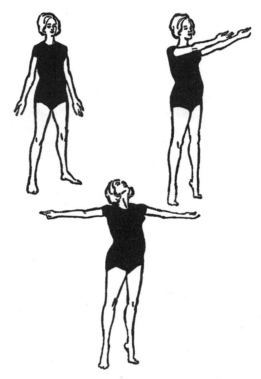

Exercise No. 1
This is a respiratory exercise. Stand with the feet comfortably apart, the hands at the sides, palms to the front. Raise the hands in front of the body to shoulder level, at the same time rising on the toes. Swing the arms outwards, throwing the head slightly backwards. Complete this movement during deep inspiration, slowly resuming starting position with expiration. Repeat six times.

Exercise No. 2
For loosening the knees and hip joints, toning up the muscles of the

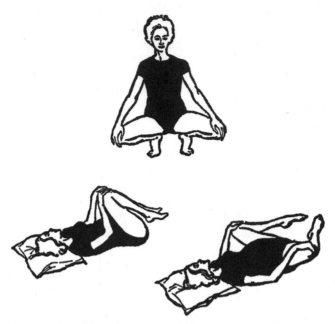

leg and stretching the adductor or riding muscles on the inside of the thigh.

This exercise is to facilitate the best position for delivery of a child, for in this position the pelvic diameter is enlarged. Rise on the toes, sink down to the position of squatting or sitting on the heels. Place the hands on the knees and stretch the legs wide open, keeping the back upright. Rise to standing position, dropping the heels. If the balance cannot be retained at first, with one hand hold on to a support. Repeat five times.

Adductor stretching is very important. This exercise can also be done whilst lying on the back with the knees flexed, allowing them to fall outward and the hands to press them widely apart.

Exercise No. 3
This loosens and mobilises the lower spine and pelvic joints. It prevents and sometimes relieves backache.

Assume position, the hands about shoulder width apart, the knees approximately eight inches apart, the back hollow, elbows slightly bent and head well back. In this position take a deep breath. Tuck the head between the arms, raise the back, at the same time straightening the arms, and pull the buttocks inwards, allowing the breath to be expelled as the back arches. Resume position and do this *six* times, slowly and firmly.

Exercise No. 4
This not only loosens and mobilises the pelvic joints, and the articulation of the spine, but facilitates a free and controlled deep breathing exercise. Kneel sitting on the heels with the hands on the knees, which are fully flexed and about a foot apart. With the back straight take a deep breath in, bend forward, breathing out until the elbows and arms are flat upon the floor in front of the knees. Breathe in as the body is raised to the original position and complete the movement by pressing on the knees with hands, hollow the back and lift the chin. Return to normal position and breathing. Pause and repeat eight times.

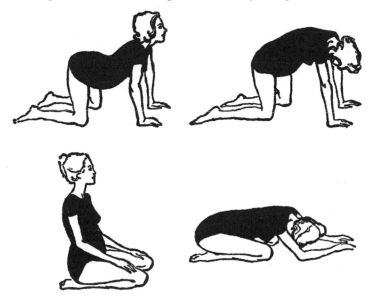

Exercise No. 5*
For straightening muscles of abdomen and thighs. Lie on the back. Whilst breathing in, raise right leg without bending the knee, as high as it will go comfortably. Lower it slowly to the floor during exhalation. Do the same with the left leg and repeat alternately six times each.

Raise both legs together, bending the feet up rather than pointing

*EDITOR'S NOTE: This exercise is not recommended today. *Vide* Françoise Freedman and Doriel Hall, *Yoga for Pregnancy*, Cassel,1998, Wendy Teasdill, *Yoga for Pregnancy*. Gaia Books, 2000

the toes. Lower legs slowly to the floor. Legs up, breathe in – legs down, breathe out. This may be difficult at first but with practice it will become easier to perform without strain. It is an excellent exercise for pregnant women. The intervals between the repetitions should be longer than in less strenuous movements.

Exercise No. 6
For tensing and relaxing the muscles of the front of the chest. This exercise increases the circulation to the tissue under the breasts and appears to enhance the establishment of adequate lactation. It differs from the others in that it is also used for training in holding the breath.

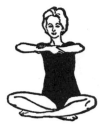

Grip firmly behind the wrists. Push the skin up the forearm, thereby tensing the arms and the muscles of the chest. Relax and repeat. The breath is held in inspiration whilst this is done ten times, taking about ten seconds. This time is gradually increased until the breath can be held comfortably for twenty seconds, which is of considerable aid in the expulsive stage of labour, when a contraction may last for ten to sixteen seconds without a remission allowing expiration to take place.

Exercise No. 7
Tensing and relaxing the pelvic floor and sphincters. This is different from Nos 1–6 as it is performed without any visible sign of movement. I describe it last because it is, in my opinion, the most important of all antenatal and postnatal exercises and requires some explanation in detail.

The anus, the vagina and urethra are three orifices of the female pelvis. The anus is the end of the bowel, the vagina, of the birth canal, and the urethra that from the urinary bladder. The adoption of the upright stance throws, by force of gravity, an immense strain upon the muscles that support the floor of the pelvis and close the orifices.

As the uterus grows, the blood vessels multiply in number and increase in size. If the tone of these muscles of the outlet is below normal standard, inconvenience arises. A desire to pass water frequently is not uncommon in the early months of pregnancy and if the sphincter, that is the muscle that closes the urethra, is weak, urine may leak, particularly if extra pressure is exerted, such as laughing or moving suddenly and quickly. Similar defects may arise in the anus; fullness is complained of and uncertainty of anal control. Piles, which are varicose veins of the anus, develop and secretion from the anal mucous membrane may cause discomfort and irritation of the back passage. The vaginal orifice is sometimes subjected to pruritus and soreness from a mucoid discharge that occurs during pregnancy and laxity of the supporting tissues.

It has been found that if these muscles of the pelvic floor and outlets are exercised and kept in tone, the troubles I have alluded to occur less frequently, indeed, in most women having first babies they are avoided.

The exercise is performed as follows: Concentrate on the anus; its movements are more easily appreciated than the other muscles, though they are all supplied by nerves from the same source. Close the anus firmly until the sensation of drawing it up into the rectum is felt. There is no necessity to move the legs or buttocks, it distracts attention from the important area. When the anal sphincter is closed and retracted, the vaginal sphincter, the levator ani, a large internal muscle, and the sphincter of the urine outlet are also tensed. Each orifice is surrounded by fibres of muscle arranged as a double figure of eight, therefore all three outlets are closed by what is virtually one muscle. Squeeze up the anus as tightly as possible, hold for a definite pause and relax slowly. This should be done twelve times at least, and twice a day. It can be done at any time and anywhere; no one else knows what is going on and many of my patients in the war-time shopping queues in England occupied themselves whilst waiting by doing this exercise!

I advise it as an antenatal preparation of the pelvic outlet because it not only prevents some minor discomforts, but facilitates restitution of the stretched and dilated orifices to normal after labour. Those who have assiduously practised this exercise justify its use in many ways. Prolapse, or feeling of insides dropping, does not occur unless the birth canal has been injured by an operation. Piles are avoided or rapidly improved. Control of the anal outlet is not faulty and stress incontinence or leaking of urine rarely occurs. The feeling of firmness underneath has a marked influence on a woman and she moves or stands in a confident posture. Controlled activity of the vaginal sphincter and the static tension of the pelvic floor are assets of considerable domestic value. Coitus can be performed satisfactorily to both husband and wife. Instead of the too frequent complaint that after a baby a woman, so far as intercourse is concerned, is uninteresting, I am told from time to time of the improvement of the natural marital function.

This exercise is a panacea for many ills and should be taught and performed regularly or even habitually, by all women – I can add advisedly, whether pregnant, post-parturient or just woman!

Postnatal Exercises

After the natural birth of a child a woman gets out of bed the following day and moves about. On the third day the instructress in postnatal exercises calls upon her and starts breathing exercises, both abdominal and upper thoracic. Movements for the arms and legs can be begun on the fourth day.

Concentration must then be placed upon exercises for the abdomen and muscles of the chest. The immediate adoption of good posture is important; so many women walk about after labour as if they had been seriously ill for a month – we see them in maternity hospitals after an uncomplicated parturition, stooping, hanging on to someone's arm and staggering rather than walking. This postnatal assumption of malaise is, in most cases, a psychological demand-activity, and an entirely uncalled-for condition in a healthy woman who has been properly cared for. She should be a happy, upright, easy-moving person with the bloom of health and expression of happiness on her face which is the prerogative of young mothers.

I do not advise postnatal massage as a routine. It is generally thought to be the simplest way to get rid of the extra fat that may have been laid down in the tissues during pregnancy, but experience over a number of years has not led me to believe that massage is of any service to the normal healthy woman providing she carries out the instructions stated above. There are cases of very fat women, or those who for some reason are unable to do postnatal exercises, when massage may be prescribed, but they should be looked upon as pathological conditions and treated as such by the doctor in charge.

I advise women to exaggerate their posture for the first few days, to tuck their abdomen well in and carry their shoulders well back when they walk, with head and chin up, breathing in such a manner that the chest expands and fills below the collar bones. This slight exaggeration of posture enables rapid reabsorption to take place in the softened articulations around the pelvis and lower spine, with the minimum risk of discomfort from backache. They are taught the evil of sitting with hunched shoulders and poked chins when feeding the baby; the baby comes to the breast, not the breast to the baby.

During the seven to ten days that women stay in the maternity hospital, they can be given a good start in postnatal exercise technique. But when they return home with the baby, maybe other young children, the husband and the home to look after, they may not find time to set aside even half an hour a day for their own personal benefit. If it is difficult to continue the full course of postnatal therapy, in order of precedence, a few exercises and deep breathing should be sufficient to ensure good carriage of the body. Relaxation must be persisted in, for it is an adjuvant to breast-feeding. As I have written before, the mother feeds her baby 'with her mind through her breast'. She should be relaxed whilst the baby is at the breast, with her mind at rest and her body free from tension. If she has the opportunity for relaxation during breast-feeding, does her breathing exercises, and continues the habitual performance of the pelvic tensing and relaxing described above, she will be laying the foundation of good health and happiness for herself and efficient breast-feeding for her newborn infant.

21

Antenatal Schools of Instruction and their Organisation

The purpose of the antenatal school is to offer to women the opportunity of having their babies naturally with the minimum of discomfort and unnecessary interference in attaining the most glorious of woman's achievements.

Education and preparation for childbirth is not a substitute for the essential routine medical examination by a doctor during pregnancy.

Teaching must be simple and understandable to all types of women, covering the four essentials:

1. *Education*
2. *Correct breathing*
3. *Relaxation* and
4. *Exercises* concurrent with breathing.

These simple and interesting components of childbirth education cannot meet with full success if partially carried out by instructress or pupil. The best results are obtained when the same approach and procedures are used by all who teach, examine, attend, and deliver women. Teamwork in home and hospital avoids many unnecessary misunderstandings and mistakes.

Included in the teaching is simple anatomy, the functioning of the womb and its muscles, personal hygiene, care of the breasts and skin, proper support of the breasts and abdomen (where necessary), care of the hair, teeth, fingernails, feet, and clothing, diet and mothercraft and the principles of postnatal care.

Instructresses must have a wide knowledge of the principles of natural childbirth and an ability to teach. Labour-ward experience is desirable, though not always available. Experience has shown that women, quite naturally, make better antenatal teachers than men. Women who have had their babies naturally are often excellent teachers; midwives and physiotherapists must be trained in the natural childbirth procedures to obtain good results. Classes should be conducted in a friendly way without regimentation or a display of authority but with quiet companionship. Keen concentration on the work gives women the confidence to ask questions and to do their best to become efficient.

Pattern and structure of the school. Three rooms are required, one for teaching, one as a changing room (divided into cubicles to allow for two persons to a cubicle) with a washbasin and toilet, and a small anteroom for secretarial and office work. In the main room, the floor should be covered with a soft rubberised or similar material and an accurate weighing machine is kept in this room for weight checks at each attendance. For other equipment allow one mat, one small blanket and two small pillows per pupil (the latter with loose covers allowing for easy washing), with the following diagrams:

- The Dickinson-Belskie Atlas and the Eva Schuchardt diagrams.
- The Grantly Dick-Read Correlation Chart and diagrams of uterus.
- Illustrations from *Childbirth Without Fear* and/or illustrations from *Introduction to Motherhood*.

Classes. Ten classes in a course including two lectures on labour which husbands are encouraged to attend and which take place between the thirty-second and thirty-sixth weeks. Classes commence at eighteen to twenty weeks' pregnancy, eight pupils at a time but not more than ten for one instructress. They should be within four to six weeks of the same period of gestation so far as possible and experience has shown that it is preferable and makes a happier class altogether if the multiparae and primiparae are not segregated. Mothers attend once a fortnight and the class lasts approximately one to one and a half hours, and progressively covers the teaching set out above.

In this way, under the organisation of two instructresses, an antenatal school can be efficiently run maintaining four classes a day, or three during the day and one in the early evening so that women who work during the day may attend after office hours, i.e.: 9.30pm to 11am, 11.30am to 1pm, 2.30pm to 4pm and 4.30pm to 6pm or 6pm to 7.30pm. The lectures can also be held in the evening if this is more convenient.

It is understood that routine clinical examination will be carried out by the doctor in charge of the case or the staff at the hospital which the patient attends. Women should be encouraged to attend the classes.

When women visited the school of instruction for the first time, record cards were filled in giving all the relevant data, age, weight, etc, and the history of previous births. Their attendance and weight were noted each visit and certain other observations, at the discretion of the instructress, might be inserted which were of importance both to the doctor or the hospital at which the woman was to be confined. This included any inability the woman might appear to have either to absorb the teaching or carry out relaxing or exercises. It was of interest to record also her blood grouping and rhesus factor. This last was of purely academic significance so far as the school was concerned. Finally the date and weight of the baby at birth were recorded on the card and any postnatal instruction if she received it from a member of the staff. The doctors of private patients were informed from time to time of observations made which were likely to be of assistance to them in the conduct of pregnancy and labour. Such classes of instruction can operate in provincial towns and urban areas.

The administration of larger maternity organisations may make it difficult to adhere strictly to the pattern of the smaller schools of instruction, but the basic principles of this system need not be altered. Classes are being conducted successfully in private homes, village halls and great hospitals.

Arrangements can be made for the classes to hear the gramophone recording of a natural childbirth or see the 16mm sound and colour film of three natural births entitled *Childbirth without Fear.*

I have described the administration and the manner of conducting the antenatal school which my wife organised and directed. She has been familiar with and closely associated with my work for just on twenty years and incorporated all the main features of the teaching gradually evolved in thirty-five years of trial and error by myself. There is no claim to perfection or finality, but the results were so uniformly good that, with the exception of caesarean sections but including abnormalities of presentation, only 5 per cent of the pupils received anaesthesia or manipulative delivery.

It is not only the delivery of the children according to the procedures believed to be in keeping with the design of the physiological mechanism and function of human reproduction that justified the principles in which those who attended the school were instructed. The physiological state exhibited by the mothers has been such that childbirth means to them one of the most gratifying achievements that is within their power to imagine. The incidence of unbearable discomfort was so low that on four occasions only did women in uncomplicated labour elect to use the inhalant analgesic that was always available. Sedation to the maximum obstetric advantage, from the point of view of the baby as well as the mother, was never withheld and if there was evidence of emotional disturbance which was likely to cause inhibition of the processes of labour, pethidine was used.

These women wished to breast-feed their babies and with few exceptions were successful in so doing. Many of them with babies aged only thirty months or less approached their second pregnancy and labour in a spirit of confidence and happy anticipation that had to be seen to be believed.

The babies born of mothers who attended the school earned the reputation of being what is known as 'good babies'. They did not have the digestive trials of the weaned infant and colic was a relatively rare accompaniment of breast-feeding. They regained their birth weights, on average, within ten days of birth, which was two days fewer than the previous series of over five hundred consecutive cases, the statistics of which I published in *The Lancet* on April 30th, 1949. So far as was possible, these babies spent most of their time with the mothers, who fed them when they demanded food. The ease with which the newborn infants adjusted themselves to neonatal life strongly suggests that the mother-child relationship established at the time of birth is a valuable means of eliminating the element of friction and irritability that we used to see so frequently twenty-five or thirty years ago. The women who are taught that it is the baby who makes the mother have a different approach from those who believe that the mother is ready-made and the baby, after birth, is entirely dependent upon her skill and knowledge for its well-being. We teach that the newborn baby knows much more than the mother gives it credit for and one of her first duties is to learn the language that it speaks, the indications of its varying cries, so that she may meet its demands without making a series of errors which give rise to discomforts and frustrations in the infant.

At present antenatal preparation is voluntary, but the enthusiasm of expectant mothers for knowledge and their belief that childbirth should not be an illness are clearly demonstrated by the numbers who seek admission to the classes.

Supporting this common-sense attitude of the women is the rapidly increasing desire of young husbands to learn of childbirth. Today we live in a changing world and nowhere are the mutations of social development more acutely felt than in the homes of the people. Domestic service is an honourable occupation of the past; it fades before the fascinations of factory routine and the attractions of more personal freedom and often better pay. The husband's place in the home is no longer that of wage earner only; he is a helper, interested in those things which concern the survival of his family unit. A pregnant wife and a newborn baby demand his attention and he desires to be of greatest value to those who need him as the duties and responsibilities increase. In some towns there are classes for the instruction of husbands in this new sphere of activity. They learn the art of companionship and care of their wives during pregnancy and understand by reading and discussion with them the training that they undergo to make childbirth the happy, healthy, yet monumental, mutual accomplishment of their ambitions. One of the greatest assets of a husband is the love and confidence of his wife during pregnancy and labour. It is frequently the unshakable foundation upon which a stable family unit stands firm when others fall.

Although this work is spreading with almost incredible speed across the face of the earth, it must be protected from profiteers. Its purpose must remain pure and unsullied by the siren song of proselytes or politicians and its presentation must be perfected by experience.

The indifference of many of the senior and authoritative members of my profession to the teaching of the natural and physiological approach to childbirth is more damaging than the vituperation and loud voices of smaller men, who can hardly be expected to appreciate the significance of hope, comfort, health, and even happiness of child-bearing women as important factors in the progress of human society. They remind me of the Grey Lurie, a crested bird of fine feathers, who screeches 'Goway' when anyone approaches. He lives on other people's fruit. Schools of instruction are wanted by women, and what women in the mass want they will get in due course. Obstetricians will either lead or follow.

Another factor which makes it difficult to meet this demand is the shortage of fully trained and experienced teachers. Schools for teachers of antenatal work must be organised on a large scale. The physiotherapists have done their best in many places to train instructresses, but their obstetric experience is inadequate, for they are not always accorded the cooperation of obstetricians and labour ward sisters. This deprives them of the ability to speak with authority upon one of the most important aspects of the subject.

Organisation, upon a wide scale, of schools in which women are instructed in the art and science of childbirth is essential to the maintenance of modern social structure. Every effort should be made to establish and perfect them wherever children, the arbiters of the future, are born into this world.

22

In Conclusion: Thoughts Addressed to the Rising Generation of Doctors

As this imperfect collection of observations is concluded, it may well be asked of me, 'Why have you written this book?' There is no more exacting task and no occupation more thankless than the public expression of heretical views. Our profession welcomes those new shoots that spring from the paternal bole and serenely bloom on the sustenance that flows directly from the parental source. But green things that appear in unorthodox shapes have little hope of survival unless they bear fruit before they are noticed. A contribution to medical literature should be the result of experience and meditation, for without experience it is unconvincing and without meditation it is presumptuous.

It is twenty-five years since I published my first series of observations and outlined the theory and practice of natural childbirth. That teaching has borne much fruit and so I write more fully, hoping, not without justification, that more of my medical brethren may be persuaded to give this method fair and prolonged trial. I am not prompted by a missionary zeal that seeks to proselytise the obstetric world, but only to invite attention to bare and irrefutable facts. Much that has been written is controversial, but whether the anatomy, physiology, neurology or psychology concerned in the function of parturition is accurately or inaccurately stated, the composite parts of this theory have dovetailed so satisfactorily that practice made upon the assumption of their truth has succeeded beyond the most optimistic expectations. This success cannot be denied; it has survived the most exacting examination; therefore, the foundations upon which it is built are probably sound in general principle.

The health of a new teaching or new approach to any branch of medical science depends largely upon the criticism of the author's colleagues. It is only human that emphasis may be laid by the original observer upon some aspects of his work which others consider to be unimportant and, conversely, matters which appear to the writer to be of little consequence may become the basis for considerable discussion.

It must be accepted, therefore, that opponents to natural childbirth will appear from time to time with arguments which require answering and ambiguities which must be clarified. It is not necessary to specify either complaints or differences of opinion; no serious dissension has arisen, but on the other hand the ubiquity of this teaching and its principles, not in any one country but throughout the world, detracts from the weight of suggestions which antagonise its employment. Furthermore, the large majority of seriously-minded obstetricians unhesitatingly concur with the general principles that have, in one decade, been responsible for reducing the fear of childbirth wherever they have been taught.

The Fear-Tension-Pain Syndrome and its significance has been generally accepted as the foundation upon which a fuller understanding of parturition has arisen. It is neither intended nor expected that medical men and women who have become established in the profession largely upon their skill and ability in the employment of past orthodox procedures, will suddenly change their opinions, discard their routine and occupy their time in learning that which may destroy the concepts upon which they have relied from youth. In defence of the doctrines they uphold they will naturally search closely for justification of their views in order to establish the right to continue their habitual practice.

There are also branches of our profession associated with childbirth such as psychologists, gynaecologists, pediatricians, and anaesthetists, etc. I have received considerable complaint that natural childbirth nullifies all the benefits which have been obtained by research in analgesia and anaesthesia. That is to say, the work done by many of our foremost anaesthetists, in order to discover the least harmful reagents to both mother and child in labour, will have been of no avail if only a small percentage of women either require or demand pain relief!

The pediatrician will find the provision of formulae for baby foods and the constant attention upon the newborn will be necessary only when some pathological condition prevents the woman from breast-feeding her baby. Gynaecologists have already discovered the birth canal requires much less attention after labour conducted naturally than after the use of forceps and deep episiotomies. Some psychiatrists believe this method invades their field and introduce arguments which suggest that because of this assumption they should have a closer association with obstetrics than in the past. Many obstetricians have given their reasons for believing that the law of nature is at fault and modern scientists have provided safer and better means for the reproduction of the human race than the Creator!

We must sympathise with those who meet with factors complicating the work to which they have been accustomed, but, at the same time, our attitude must not countenance wide departures from procedures which bring obvious benefits to the mothers and children of our time.

I do not mention here the large number of contributions to the lay press upon this subject. Such opinions are expressed with all honesty by those whose association or experience have led them to be either for or against this teaching. But one outstanding fact remains that over twenty years ago when I published my first book, *Natural Childbirth,* I received immediately many adherents to these tenets. Since then there has been no record, either published or privately communicated to me, of a medical man or woman having seriously applied this approach to childbirth, who has turned back to the orthodox procedures because my teaching has proved to be faulty. One or two have publicly denounced their use of these methods because they could not withstand the assault of tongues. Such success produced rumours amongst their colleagues.

It is, therefore, to the youth of our profession that I appeal; to those who have just qualified and to those who are about to qualify. It is for you to join in the battle against fear and pain. In the march of this great and noble science of which you have become worthy soldiers, you must not call a halt and sit serenely complacent where your seniors leave you; soon they will retire and hand on to you the leadership; you must progress to further objectives, to a higher attainment and to perfection within our science.

Nearly fifty years ago, Sir William Osler wrote, 'The pains and woes of the body to which we doctors minister are decreasing at an extraordinary rate and in a way that makes one fairly gasp in hopeful anticipation' (*Aequanimitas*). Each one of you has it within his power to observe carefully the phenomena of labour; each one of you has the birthright of investigation. Do not accept the conservative teaching of a past generation without careful examination. For the most part, such teaching will stand scrutiny and will be proved correct in general principle. But from time to time you will be amazed at the inadequacy of the evidence upon which accepted principles are borne. Be critical of culture; look long and carefully before you accept its tenets; take notice of the subtle ways and means by which youth is robbed of its power and its inborn genius. Be accurate in your deductions and delve deeply into the details of each succeeding problem. Analyse your observations and do not be slow to ask 'why'. Develop an inquiring mind; seek guidance and advice whilst you have around you those competent and willing to help you. There is no reason to be humble in your questioning, and certainly no justification for aggression in your differing. Learn from your mistakes, for if you seek honestly the truth, the errors that you make will be of service in your search. As you scramble from one pitfall to the next, you will gain strength and experience. The borderlands of the realm of knowledge are shrouded in a mist which is not penetrated by the earliest efforts of the beginner. As he gains a greater foothold within those realms, so the mist clears, until he finds the vista of unending possibility, the existence of which he had not previously envisaged. There is no such thing as knowing all. Cowper wrote:

> *Knowledge is proud that he has learned so much,*
> *Wisdom is humble that he knows no more.*

If, therefore, you feel humble because of your limited accomplishments, recognise that in humility alone lies the true urge and goad to further progress. If you have read the preceding chapters of this book, I do not ask you to accept one written word, but rather to recognise the possibilities of the theory and practice which I set before you. When occasion arises, try to apply these principles; you will fail before you have learnt to carry them out in detail, but soon you will succeed in such a way that the teaching will appeal to you as being worthy of further application. I give you the assurance that you will succeed if you persevere. I know that if you strive manfully you will find in obstetrics a new life, a new science and new benefit to humanity. More frequently the thought has passed my mind: How will you take success? How will you balance in the scales the gratitude of the women you have attended with the criticisms of those who do not believe? I urge you to be discreet in your pronouncements; keep your successes quietly to yourself; you should never be the source of propaganda. Discuss freely with those who would discuss with you, but do not try to persuade the disbeliever. Remember that he has no practical experience with which to justify his intolerant attitude. Neither is it possible for you to persuade a woman who has had a painful labour that her pain was unnecessary or a misunderstanding. She has had pain and she will tell you that she had a very clever doctor in attendance. Woman cannot be persuaded by mere man, but only by members of her own sex who will quietly differ from her and smile, with added satisfaction, at their own experiences.

You cannot persuade a daughter that her mother knows nothing of childbirth and there are not many mothers who are either in a position to, or willing to, teach their daughters that labour is a painless, happy thing. You cannot persuade many a doctor that the cries and groans of his patient might have been prevented had he understood the phenomena of labour. These people and many others will either laugh at you or be angered by your opinion. Let women speak who have borne their children naturally and who know the truth. Sit silently and listen to the experiences of those who have given these practices a fair trial – those who have worked until they have understood labour. There you will hear no adverse criticism or dissentient note, for now the volume of these voices, rising as the roar of breakers borne on by the sea breeze, is heard wherever women meet. Spokesmen of the disbelievers who but a few years ago had many listeners, retreat before the inevitable torrent of established facts. Be tolerant, for they are just and honest with few exceptions. They have only known painful labours because they have not been aware of any teaching that can mitigate suffering without endangering the health of mother and child. Why should they accept the opinion of a young man when they have learnt that women whom they attend in labour suffer pain?

Yes, you who set out with high ambitions and ideals for the improvement of the art and science of obstetrics will meet with unexpected and exasperating difficulties. The teaching and training of your student and intern days will fit you for all emergencies. Academic foundations are invaluable and must be soundly rooted, for it is from them that the high standard of your work results. For my own part I have found the greatest opposition within the ranks of our own profession, but I have not had any desire to shield myself from insinuation, however invidious. The inviolable sanctuary of truth, well proved in the fires of long experience, is not likely to be shaken by the assaults of ignorance. For those who have not seen this natural childbirth cannot speak of it with authority. The criticisms of those who have not practised it are indeed empty. What would we reply to one who said, 'The works of Plato are not worth reading because I cannot understand Greek.' We would say, 'But listen to him in a language you can understand.' From Phaedrus, Euthyphron and Lysis you may learn something of the beautiful, of holiness and of friendship that you have not known before.

I have tried to put in simple words the friendliness, the beauty and even the holiness of childbirth, but its magnificence can only be felt by those who have learnt to read in the original this masterpiece of the Creator. Your shield and buckler will be hard work and quiet determination. Resolve to be patient for by the results of your work you will be known. Men often value themselves by what they know they can do, forgetting that the world only values them by what they have done. Do not be disturbed by gossip; it is a doctor's lot to be subjected to the whisperings of those who do not know him. Anonymous critics are those who hide behind high walls and throw mud or bouquets, according to the disease from which they suffer, at those who march along the high road of freedom. Whether you are flattered or bespattered, pass on; they will not be allowed to meet you face to face. Beware lest word or look betrays resentment at the work of others. Unless we are in a position of authority, we have to watch tragedies that may well make the blood of him who has been more fortunate in his training boil with indignation. It is unlikely that you will escape the scorn of the Urban District Icon, who has been raised to his pedestal by the adulations of his devotees. He wears a white coat and an ingratiating smile. The orb of omniscience rests lightly in his rubber-gloved left hand and in his right he holds the sceptre of his own opinion. An oriflamme, emblazoned with licentiates, waves with modest clarity in his autogenous breeze. He is protected from the light of nature by a canopy of self-confidence, which also serves to ward off any insidious attacks of truth. You will hear his praises sung; his genius with the forceps; the neatness of his stitching after labour; the convenience of his inductions and innumerable caesarean sections.

But let your practice be founded upon the judgment of the intelligent, and your reputation upon the honest opinion of those who are in the best position to judge. Above all, your own personal satisfaction will raise you to a different plane; your work will be in a different cause; you will not be numbered among the 'Gehazis who seek only the shekels'. Your belief is not in today, but rather tomorrow and those distant tomorrows which will bring nearer to man his ultimate heritage. Your faith is in the law of nature; your science an adjuvant and not an impediment to its implementation.

But medicine is a science of opinion and opinions differ, not only in diagnosis and treatment but in philosophy and ideal. In obstetrics you must form your own philosophy without fear and observe with equanimity the ideals of those about you.

The privilege of attending women in childbirth is far greater than

you are taught to realise. The public applaud the genius of skilled surgeons; famous physicians are beloved and respected for their healing
power; great gynaecologists are both surgeons and physicians within a
limited field. Their lives are given up to the noble work of succouring
the sick, curing the diseased and mending the broken. The advances
that have been made in these sciences have earned the praise and gratitude of the world. The stern course that an ever accelerating life has
set for the human race leaves many casualties by the wayside. Those
who come of stock ill-suited for the struggle break down and need
attention; the mental equipment of a high percentage of the people
of today is inadequate for the task imposed upon it; it shows signs of
stress; it requires adjustment and support. The physical manifestations
of disease, surgical, medical and gynaecological, are frequently the direct sequelae of functional derangements of the nervous system.

So the casualties of living are the first call of the medical profession.
But obstetricians do not work among casualties; their work is primarily among the supremely healthy members of the community. They
watch over and improve original models from the great factories of
human life; their responsibility is to improve the stock and render it
fit to meet the new demands that modern communal existence makes
upon each succeeding generation.

Surgery and medicine are mainly concerned with repairs, patch-
ings and renovations. The less efficient the stock in terms of survival,
so much greater is the demand for medical service. Since when have
repair shops been more important than the production plant? In the
early days of motoring, garages were full of broken down machines,
but production has been improved; the weaknesses that predisposed
to unreliability were discovered and in due course rectified. Today it is
only the inferior makes that require the attention of mechanics. Such
models have been evolved that we almost forget the relative reliability
of the modern machine if it is properly cared for. This is not only due
to the use of better materials, but also to more complete knowledge of
construction. Education and research are the essentials of progress,
particularly in child production. This does not depend upon parturition only. The mother is the factory and by education and care she can
be made more efficient in the art of motherhood. Her mind is of even
greater importance than her physical state, for motherhood is of the
mind and the body is usually subjected to the mental processes, unless any gross abnormality exists. There is a vast territory around and
about maternity which is still unexplored. If there is anything in these
pages which has not been previously observed or practised, it is culled

from the fringes of this waste of potential enlightenment.

Each stone which has been turned in search of explanation has revealed a rock, beneath which rests a hidden truth. Every fresh endeavour to perfect the art of natural motherhood has impressed upon me the magnitude of our task. It is with envy that I look upon the students of today. A hundred paths lie open, inviting them to walk unhindered to the granaries of greater knowledge, demanding only that they shall bring back such store as will be profitable to their fellow creatures. There may be found the solution to innumerable problems. They will take to women the knowledge that dispels the fear of childbirth, by perfecting the already flourishing organisation of education of mothers, preparation for the arrival of the infant and care of the newborn. They will be able to attack the calamitous absurdity of our social system, which prevents thousands of our best women from having the families they crave for because they *have not the money* necessary to feed, clothe and educate more than two children. A race dies out if families average only two. Untold millions are found for wars, rearmaments and social services every year. How much is allotted to the defeat of our most insidious enemy, the canker that destroys the family life of the people. 'Too little money.' Every week and almost every day I hear the same disgruntled remark, 'We simply cannot afford any more.' The allowances from taxes are inadequate. The young mother of today watches her childless friends; their cost of living and their responsibilities are less in every way; their clothes, their recreations and their entertainments appeal to her as the price she pays for her children. No, she cannot have any more or she will never be able to go anywhere or do anything. And so at an early age an affectionate, happy couple with one or two children adopt contraception as a financial necessity. 'Better than poverty and all its devastating anxieties,' I am told, and I cannot disagree. It is not healthy recreation, in this life of rush and turmoil, that I disagree with. It is not – under these circumstances – contraception that I quarrel with, but relative poverty, particularly in the middle classes. Look closely into the homes of those who struggle to keep and educate two children, those whose job depends upon their appearance of affluence. Behind the scenes you will find financial strain, real poverty, self denial, and, at an early age, contraception and all its mental stresses and physical disappointments. It is the spirit of home life and parenthood which suffers. Love itself is starved and often blamed for its own decline. When love goes, anything may go, but worst of all the most glorious gift of womanhood remains inhibited and immature. The spirit of motherhood is never fully developed; our social system is gradually crushing the most powerful force for real goodness that is known to the human race. Here indeed is a problem for the rising generation of obstetricians; make it possible for healthy married women to have all the children they want; make it profitable and one of the main causes of domestic unhappiness and social unrest will fade into thin air. Give us back the Victorian mothers of seven and ten children, and we shall again be swayed by the quiet but irresistible goodness of true motherhood.

Leave the bugbear of overpopulation and world shortage of food. I have flown over millions of acres, well-watered and luxuriant with fruit and foliage, land so fertile that vast hordes of animals survive upon its untended provision. Here, where the immutable law of nature maintains a balance of species, is an offering to man to utilise the earth for his own survival. Let those who are responsible for the food of the people apply themselves and their riches and the adjuvants of modern science that the human race may continue. This will be possible only when men cease ranging their sullen armies to hurl the wealth and lifeblood of our youth into the wilderness of impotent waste. In the meantime let obstetricians strive to increase and improve the human stock by caring for the mothers, whose children will be fitted to design and to create a new world. Man's knowledge only sees so far, but wisdom opens vistas of a great beyond.

Human nature has not changed since the days of the Psalmist. The man who has a 'full quiver' and adequate maintenance is the peace-loving worker whose presence in the community is an influence towards moderation and reason. But should his home be in jeopardy or his hearth in danger, he knows no fear but flings himself into the fray with the violence of desperation. Is it for his own comfort or for his childless wife he fights to the death? Is it in the cause of justice among the nations or is it for children who crowd in his small cottage and climb upon his knee? Whence is the power in a man's arm? Let fathers of families answer and husbands with good wives who mother their growing sons and daughters. The phylogenetic development of man has equipped him physiologically and mentally to fight for the protection of his children and their mother. Perhaps that is why peace-loving men who are forced into battle by an aggressive enemy fight with such fury that the professional gladiator is amazed.

Amongst the mothers of large families we find the grand old ladies of our race whose calm yet forceful personalities radiate strength and attract affection. How many of the greatest men in history will unhesitatingly ascribe their success in life to the influence of their family life and home?

Therefore, the student of today has the very foundations of society to investigate; in his hand lies the power to wield a mighty weapon in the cause of progress within the human race. I do not extol the art of motherhood without a sincere belief that it is a force of incomprehensible magnitude and worthy of the highest place among the major considerations of our time. Millions are spent each year on educating children, a high percentage of whom have suffered the strain of unnatural birth, whereas a few thousands a year spent on educating mothers might eliminate *ab initio* the congenital conflicts of the mind of which Freud has written, and the injuries within the brain to which Crile and many other workers in that field have drawn attention.

If a fraction of the amount now spent upon the so-called education of children up to the age of fifteen or sixteen were allocated to the instruction of youths and maidens in the elementary knowledge of their primary biological functions, much misery and discontent would be avoided. Such teaching to girls is becoming more desirable with each generation. Respect and reverence for motherhood are the natural reactions to sensible instruction in these matters. The early years of maturity are cleansed from those doubts and fears which spring from ignorance. The adventurous voyage of marriage in a ship made seaworthy by education and understanding is more likely to survive the rough waters of life than that which is fitted out in ignorance for joy trips on calm blue waters only. No one is more aware of this than the obstetrician from whom young married women seek advice.

I am persuaded that our work should be that of physicians to women. No girl should leave school without the direct or indirect influence of our teaching; no young woman should enter a factory to earn her living, or be presented, or 'do' her debutante season, without adequate knowledge. We should be prepared to discuss the problems of those about to marry, as well as the most intimate details of marriage, with those who come to us for help and advice in times of trouble or difficulty. Conception, pregnancy and parturition are our accepted spheres of activity, but they depend for their perfection to a large extent upon earlier training. And after the puerperium our lot should be to continue in the personal contact we have made during childbirth and to be an oracle to whom reference can be made during the years of recurrent motherhood. Here is more than enough for the mind of one individual, yet in these few phases of womanhood a physician holds the lifeline of civilisation.

Today, antenatal clinics are doing, in many places, magnificent work in preparing women for labour. The home life and economic conditions of women of the poorer classes are investigated and no effort is spared to make motherhood a joy and not a burden. You will have to ask yourselves whether the middle and upper classes, who pay for private attention, receive the same standard of care and attention as 'hospital' folk. Whatever your reactions to the discoveries you make concerning the practice of obstetrics in all classes of society, bear in mind a wide and philosophical attitude towards its ultimate value to humanity. Aim high and bravely; dare to aspire to new standards. Today the world passes through the ordeal of conflicting ideologies. The combat is not of peoples but of philosophies. The grim hosts of materialism have combined to overthrow the spiritual forces of life. You of the rising generation of scientists will be called upon to make some sense of the universe and you will be unable to do so without a belief in ultimate purpose. Sir Arthur Keith wrote, 'I cannot help feeling that the darkness in which the final secret of the universe lies hid is part of a great design.' Frances Mason edited a book called *The Great Design* (Duckworth, 1934). In this collection fourteen renowned scientists, each writing in relation to his own subject, state clearly their belief in a power greater than science. They are convinced that a spiritual influence exists as a reality and not an assumption. It is from the order and precision of natural phenomena that this deduction has been made by men whose genius has enabled them to penetrate the mysteries of nature more deeply than their contemporaries.

As obstetricians, you will be in constant association with the most beautiful of all natural functions; it is not just the assistance of women in childbirth. If there is design in the universe, and if that design is of spiritual force, then the birth of a child must be an incident of spiritual importance, for it is the production of a new vehicle for elements of that force which will fulfil the purpose of the universe. This brings us near to Goethe's rumination that 'the whole purpose of the world seems to be to provide a physical basis for the growth of Spirit'.

Surely there is a law which enables a woman to bear children in the knowledge of her inestimable privilege. The importance of motherhood must be worthy of much greater attention than it has yet received. The organisations which will instruct and educate, as well as train mentally and physically, the mothers of tomorrow, is only one of the great responsibilities that rests upon your shoulders. Howard Haggard, in the opening sentences of his book *Devils, Drugs and Doctors* (Heinemann, London, 1929), writes, 'The advances and regressions of civilisation are nowhere seen more clearly than in the story of childbirth.' Today we stand on the brink of a new world; it is unlikely that the future will depend upon money and personal power. The fundamental urges of masses which have found truth and hope in social enlightenment must be accepted as necessities of racial progress. Motherhood is the common denominator of international relations; it is the one mutual possession which is shared both in body and soul by women of all races, creeds and colours.

From my contact with men and women of all classes, I have been led to believe that it is for homes and families our people will cry out. The demand will be for parenthood and reward for their work adequate to provide for children in health and happiness. The greatest force behind the peace and prosperity of a nation emanates unseen and unheard from the mothers in their homes. Samuel Taylor Coleridge wrote in *The Three Graces*:

A mother is a mother still
The holiest thing alive.

The health of mothers and their babies should be the first consideration of an obstetrician. The injuries inflicted upon both mother and child have results which influence whole communities. I do not refer to gross and obvious lesions only, but to such things as pains and fears; nights of horror and vivid memories of agony which scar for all time the mind that should be fortified by the beauty of its first sweet thrill of mother love. In my library there are thirty-seven volumes, each leather bound and stamped in gold, 'Mother's Letters. From 1905 to 1941'. These manuscripts of indescribable beauty are not to an only son, for I was number six of seven children born in nine years. Schooldays and Cambridge, the London Hospital, the Great War, are recalled and reviewed in terms of sympathy and understanding, admonition and advice. Betrothal, marriage and parenthood are discussed with me in words of which Madame de Sévigné might well have been proud. Year after year this fount of mother love has poured its influence into my life and still, at eighty-six, this grand old lady filled me with pride when I read her views on 'things of today', written in the light of long years of quiet observation and deduction. A few years ago, when her eldest child died at the age of fifty-six, she wrote, 'Now that she has been taken to rest at this early age, I think back upon the noble self-sacrifice of her life, but my mind seems to rush past the intervening years, and I recall most vividly of all the cry of my first-born child as I held her in my hands a few moments after her birth.' At over eighty years of age, that sweet initiation into the great masonry of motherhood still shone so clearly above all other lights and shades of her daughter's life, that she added, 'It seems as if it were but yesterday.'

There is no logical reason to presume that the influence of one mother is exceptional. It is my belief that I quote an example only from many thousands. There would be many more with each generation if this great source of power were fostered and nourished by the obstetric physicians of today. The science of obstetrics should no longer be considered the bread and butter of young consultants until and only until a gynaecological practice is established. It should not be the rather boring but relatively profitable necessity of a busy general practitioner. It must be recognised as an invaluable adjunct to the health and happiness of humanity.

I express to you only my personal opinions and offer for your consideration certain aspects of our calling which should raise the obstetrician to the highest place among the builders of our future race. I have just received a brochure from the Parents' Association called 'Civics', in which I read these words: 'Our ultimate goal, therefore, lies far beyond our present transitory life. While we must live this present life for others, fully and actively, we must also try to make contact now with the higher wisdom and beauty, as yet only partially revealed, which lies beyond.'

You must make your choice now and to your innermost self lay down the principles upon which your future will unfold. There are many paths leading to the rock of a physician's calling. Along the well-worn roads thousands pass, blindly following the lead of orthodoxy, pushing and jostling in a throng which steadily advances with the years to a comfortable plateau called mediocrity. Here men gird themselves with mental and material armour, and search the descent to old age for respectable nooks and crannies where they may rest and watch the sun go down. It is possible to decorate a well-selected nidus with an accolade, so that those who pass by may whisper to their friends, 'Behold!'

There are also the untrodden paths which require not only youth, but freedom and fortitude. Those of you who seek a new truth must blaze a trail of your own. The jewels of our science lie off the beaten track. Press on in danger; with the risk of failure you have the urge to persevere. You will clamber among landmarks accepted by your forbears as immutable. Accept nothing, for under each established fact is the foundation of a new future. Gold is hidden in the solid vein of quartz. Climb up along the precipice that leads to no plateau, but only to higher peaks from which you can look down and see the truth you have uncovered on your way. You need no social armour in your isolation; seek no comfortable haven of rest; sharpen your axe, respike your shoes and struggle on, conscious always of the vision of youth, guided by the hand of experience to a greater reward than public recognition.

Pioneers pass on unheard and unlamented until the trail they blazed is followed by a few who have believed. At the end they are discovered where their life's work finished, mourned only by the wild flowers of the wilderness they loved.

Appendix

The Autobiography of Grantly Dick-Read

These pages have been compiled from the many personal experiences about which Grantly Dick-Read wrote, scattered through his books and letters as well as Childbirth without Fear, *so there is some repetition from the previous pages. They give us an understanding of the man as a person that few of his contemporaries had.*

During his life he was an enigma to many people. He was a far-seeing man who looked beyond the immediate. He observed details in the natural world around him that escaped the attention of others. He looked back through the centuries in search of wisdom and forward into the future of the human race.

As the years passed, his goal in life focused increasingly on one essential purpose: to make this world a better place in which to live, through happier mothers and homes. As he grew older he became increasingly outspoken in his views, in contrast to the timidity of his earlier years. The fact that he was right did not increase his popularity among his colleagues!

Yet it was not arrogance that drove him on, but an inner anguish over so much needless suffering that he had found clues for overcoming. It was the anguish similar to that of another prophet, who cried, "There is a fire burning my bones, and I cannot keep silent!"

Early Impressions

In my library there are thirty-seven volumes, each leather bound and stamped in gold: *Mother's Letters, from 1915 to 1941.* These manuscripts of indescribable beauty are not to an only son, for I was born in 1890 as the sixth of seven children. In these letters, school-days and Cambridge, the London Hospital and World War One are all recalled and reviewed in terms of sympathy and understanding, admonition and advice. Betrothal, marriage, and parenthood are discussed with me in words of which Madame de Sévigné might well have been proud. Year after year this fount of mother love poured its influence into my life and still, at eighty-eight, this grand old lady filled me with pride when I read her views on things of today, written in the light of long years of quiet observation and deduction.

There is no logical reason to presume that the influence of one mother is exceptional. It is my belief that I quote an example only from many thousands, and there would be many more with each generation if this great source of power were fostered and nourished by the obstetric physicians. The science of obstetrics must be recognized as an invaluable adjunct to the health and happiness of humanity. From earliest childhood, since as far back as my memory reaches, I have devoted nearly all my interest, and most of my energies, to this cause.

When I was a small boy, I delighted in hearing my sister play "The March of the Gladiators." Many evenings before my bedtime she would sit at the piano and play it to me, until "old Ellen" came to take me up to bed. One night I sat by her, listening and supremely happy, when three revolver shots rang out from the woods at the bottom of the drive. Then I heard that "old Ellen" had been shot dead by the soldier she had been going to marry.

For the rest of my life, one phrase in that tune, if ever I am forced to hear it, brings back to me the chill of horror, the agony of fear, and the inconsolable anguish that I suffered that night. "The March of the Gladiators," by association, ceased to bring me pleasure, but was a conditioned stimulus for violent emotional disturbance – so much so that, ten years later, when I was in medical school at Cambridge and it floated across the campus to my room during lunch, I suddenly felt sick and had to leave the table, only realizing afterwards that it was a reaction to an almost forgotten emotional state. This experience later helped me to appreciate the negative emotional reactions of a woman to any mention of childbirth, if she had unhappy memories concerning it.

As a child I was very happy and fortunate to spend at least six months of the year at our Norfolk home, which was a farm, where I became acquainted with nature and enjoyed it far more, I regret to say, than I enjoyed the society of my older brothers and sisters. I got to know my animals, the cows, the pigs, and the horses. I sat with my bitches when they had their puppies, and caressed Topsy when she had her kittens, those natural things children do under the happy circumstances of such an upbringing. I spent much of my time on my own because I believed so unquestionably in the miracles of nature – they were all mysteries to me of absorbing interest. I sought the loneliness of silent places where only naturalists really find companionship.

On one occasion during my obstetric practice in later years, a nursing student remarked to me: "We have only had normal cases lately, but Dr. X is coming in later on this afternoon to put on forceps. The woman has been in labour two and a half days – we think she is an occipito posterior. It should be quite interesting."

"Ah, splendid," I replied to this lady, who though a student was a potential mother of tomorrow, "very interesting. I expect the woman is getting interested by now!"

Of course it is exciting to see the abnormal, and necessary for training, but must the normal and natural be considered dull? It is only in these cases that any beauty can be found in obstetrics. The simple, straightforward performances are the perfect initiation into motherhood; surely here is the field for observation. Each constituent of the ordinary is so extraordinary when understood. It is so in nature, in every sphere, one of its great fascinations. It is more thrilling to watch an avalanche crash in a cloud of snow to the bottom of a ravine, to hear the roar of its thunderous progress and witness the devastation in its path, than to lie on the edge of a Norfolk marsh. Yes, more thrilling – until you have looked quietly and closely into the reeds.

Here as a boy, prone on the grass, I observed the peaceful beauty of nature as its constituents gradually appeared. Silver fish lit up the shallow water, great swallowtail butterflies flitted decoratively from ragged robin to wild flower; small cotton tufts revealed the newly hatched cocoon; each wee spider was a thrill as it set out on its great adventure. I heard the moorhen call and hurry her fluffy offspring past my observation post as a bittern boomed in the distance.

At every turn of the eye the simplest form of nature is found to be full of excitement and fresh beauty to the quiet, respectful observer. As we look more closely, the treasure-house opens fresh doors of wonder until we become absorbed in the perfection of simplicity and the magnificence of the ordinary. I have continued to do this so often during my life that the intrusion in these marshes during the past several years of foreign bodies in smelly motorboats is equivalent to disease attacking the peacefulness of natural beauty. The thought of these disturbers brings resentment; they are not interesting. They upset the natural order, and are unheedful of the beauty around them.

In all observation of a natural state, the more concentrated and penetrating it becomes, so much the more is found to observe, to understand, and over which to marvel. Many people think the Norfolk marshes dull. They abhor the silence, so they bring radios and tape recorders and regale the voices of nature with ragtime. These are the same people who love to be on the Jungfraujoch with me and count the roars of avalanches and say, "Stupendous!" while I say, "Dead ends falling off dead beginnings." These are the type of people who also find normal labour dull, but who are thrilled with a forceps operation, a postpartum haemorrhage, or a face presentation. If only they would look closely into uncomplicated labour, observing every change in the mind and body of their patient, how much they would find of absorbing interest, and how all-important the harmony of nature would become!

One day in 1907 I made my first observation upon the pains of childbirth. There were a number of cottages on the Norfolk farm, and I had discovered that when a woman in one of the cottages had her baby, it was an anxious day of woe and sadness. The maids climbed up at our windows to see when the doctor galloped past our house on his horse. My mother went quietly down the drive to the cottage with a basket on her arm in which was a chicken or jelly or something she was taking to Maria, Mary Anne, Robina, or one of the others.

I questioned my mother about this, and she told me that it was a dreadful thing to have a baby. This didn't make sense to me, for as number six of seven children born in eight and a half years, I thought my mother looked awfully well to have gone through seven really dreadful experiences in such a short time! But, owing to the peculiar nature of my extremely pious and religious upbringing and my observations on the marshes, I turned to her and said something that was probably the stepping-stone that changed the course of my whole life. "That's not true, Mother! It must be man who is making the mistake, not the God of nature in Whom you have taught me to believe!"

After an awkward moment she said to me, not unkindly, "I think you must realize that these are things you should not discuss. You are much too young to understand. But in time, perhaps, you will realize what a serious thing it is for a woman to have a baby."

For years her answer troubled me, and prompted me to keep my thinking on the subject to myself, but inwardly the direction of my thought had been determined. I had learned by this time that the Creator uses neither the words nor the methods of human beings to obtain results more magnificent than our greatest scientists can ever aspire to. It is an essential law of nature that all species should be reproduced in the safest and easiest manner possible. Two of nature's greatest laws are the law of reproduction and that of the maintenance of the species. If either fails, we all fail.

Sir Thomas Browne's statue stands in the marketplace of my own home town. It was there he lived and wrote the famous *Religio Medici* in the seventeenth century. From the time I was a boy one of his most famous statements has remained in my mind: "Nature does nothing in vain." I have learned nothing new from the work and writings of man. Man's discoveries, innovations, creations, and cleverness are only nature opening a little wider the window through which all knowledge will, in time, be found. Nature separates the apple from the tree. We must learn to work in harmony with the law of nature if life on earth is to survive.

In the following year, 1908, I started my medical career with these impressions already forming in my mind. But my sense of discovery and adventure soon brought me face to face with inflexibility. My chiefs were more rigid and less approachable than any senior staff is today. Their noses were so long, it seemed to me, that when one looked down his at the junior who was inquiring, he became an indistinct object that could not be clearly focused. His questions were an even more distant blur upon the horizon of the great man's dignity. The answer I received in the classroom was, "My dear boy, we are trying to teach you, and before asking questions you don't understand, I suggest ... etc., etc."

Fortunately, because of my love for sports, I soon learned to appreciate the reality of blunted noses against my boxing gloves. Some of the owners of these previously haughty noses became my lifelong friends. Strangely enough, it was here by the ringside, on the playing field, on the football field, the tennis court, or golf links that my chiefs, off duty, approached their juniors without restraint. Here I learned that they were men of great accomplishment and human understanding. They were people who could laugh at themselves more readily than at their colleagues, and whose hands were always outstretched to receive the grasp of a man who needed guidance and help. A little later on I began to realize that long noses were only lifted as a means of self-protection, protruded when difficult situations or even more difficult questions threatened the proprieties of orthodoxy.

It was my good fortune during the years of my training to have been under the able teaching of Professors Shipley and Gardiner,[1] John Baxter Langley, and Thomas McCall Anderson at Cambridge. I revelled in the study of zoology, biology, and physiology because of my hobby of natural history. The notions and ideas upon the birth of the young of any phylum, class, or order that I saw or studied filled me with wonder and curiosity. It was not inherent discernment that drew me to this research, but a resentment that the law of nature should be held responsible for such injustice to women.

I was also privileged in having such men as Rivers[2] and M.D.W. Jeffereys as my professors for my courses in anthropology. In the years 1908 and 1909 I often sat with one or two of my friends on the floor of Professor Rivers's rooms at Cambridge, drinking tea and eating biscuits with him, while listening to much that was fascinating, interesting, and almost terrifying to us undergraduates, as he related the experiences he had had in his life of pioneering work in social anthropology. And Professor Jeffereys had spent thirty years of his life as a government official in East Africa before retiring to a university appointment as senior lecturer in anthropology. From these men and others I learned that we must not draw deductions from small premises!

In 1910, while still at Cambridge, I spent considerable time in collecting varieties of colour associations and the visual patterns of numerals. This was especially interesting to me as I have, among other peculiarities, a certain form of colour blindness. Later I persuaded some of my musical friends to record the forms and colours connected with sound. We found that, with practice, definite types of colour patterns were consistently associated with the characteristic works of different musicians. Here, in musical works, we discovered that the mind of the creative genius not only conveyed clear and unmistakable pictures to us by sensuous auditory paths, but imprinted them on our memories as well. When these pictures were reproduced in mental imagery behind closed eyes, they aroused again in our minds the musical patterns, airs, and harmonies that they represented. Dvořák has painted the simple pathos of the Negro slave; Tchaikovsky has unveiled the panorama of tragedy and woe; Handel has opened our eyes to a great celestial choir massed upon white clouds beneath the azure dome of heaven, flinging its song of praise across the amphitheater of illimitable space. Thus I found that sights, sounds, and associations, real and imaginary, imprinted themselves upon the human mind, moulding and influencing its present reactions to past experiences.

These observations later raised in my mind the question concerning what mental picture might be within the mind of a woman in labour, and how this might influence her actions at that time. But I still kept such thoughts and impressions to myself, unable to find anyone with whom I felt free to share. Once I mentioned my loneliness in a letter home, and my mother replied: "I know that you are lonely; it is possible that you will be for many years. But we are close together in spirit and you are never alone, for God is with us both."

During my four years as a medical student at Cambridge, on only one occasion did I gather courage to ask specifically about pain in childbirth. I was watching one of the experiments by Professor Langley, in his study of the sympathetic nervous system. In this instance the nerves to a cat's uterus were being stimulated with nicotine, and I asked, "Is it possible that these sympathetic nerves have some bearing upon pain in the uterus during childbirth in a human being?" Professor Langley looked up sharply, and then, after a moment's pause, said, very quietly and very slowly, "Yes – yes, that is indeed possible." That is all that was ever said on the subject.

In 1912 my internship began at the London Hospital. It is situated in the heart of the East End slums in an area called Whitechapel, where fifteen hundred to two thousand patients passed through the outpatient department every day. It was an exciting and a busy time for me. On the surgical side I felt that I was dealing with real science, and on the physician's side with humanity, which interested me even more. But nothing so far turned my interest so close to excitement as gynaecology and obstetrics. When I first arrived I had not yet seen for myself what childbirth was really like, but felt that at last I was on the threshold of discoveries that would help answer the troubling questions in my heart and mind concerning it.

Among the women I attended at Whitechapel there was one in 1913 whose casual remark had a far-reaching influence on me. The whole picture made an indelible impression upon my mind, although at the time I had no idea that it was the seed that would eventually alter the course of my life.

I had plowed through mud and rain on my bicycle between two and three in the morning down Whitechapel Road, turning right and left, and innumerable rights and lefts, before I came to a low hovel by the railway arches. Having groped and stumbled my way up a dark staircase, I opened the door of a room about ten feet square. There was a pool of water lying on the floor. The window was broken; rain was pouring in; the bed had no proper covering and was kept up at one end by a sugar box. My patient lay covered only with sacks and an old black skirt. The room was lit by one candle stuck in the top of a beer bottle on the mantel shelf. A neighbour had brought in a jug of water and a basin; I had to provide my own soap and towel. In spite of this setting – which even at that time, near the turn of the century, was a disgrace to any civilized country – I soon became conscious of a quiet kindliness in the atmosphere.

In due course the baby was born. There was no fuss or noise. Everything seemed to have been carried out according to an ordered plan. There was only one slight dissension; I tried to persuade my patient to let me put the mask over her face and give her some chloroform when the head appeared and the dilation of the outlet was obvious. She, however, resented the suggestion, and firmly but kindly refused to take this help. It was the first time in my short experience that I had ever been refused when offering chloroform. As I looked at her, I saw an expression on her face that showed she hoped she hadn't hurt my feelings by refusing the offer.

As I was about to leave some time later, I asked her why it was she would not use the mask. She did not answer at once, but looked from the old woman who had been assisting to the window through which was bursting the first light of dawn. Then, shyly, she turned to me and said, "It didn't hurt. It wasn't meant to, was it, doctor?"

For weeks and months afterward, as I sat with women in labour, women who appeared to be in the terror and agony of childbirth, that sentence came drumming back into my ears: "It wasn't meant to, was it, doctor?"

That young woman doesn't know what a tremendous fund of comfort and happiness her casual but purely honest cockney remark has made to the women of the world. So it is from the seeds dropped unknowingly and in unexpected places that the greatest trees may grow.

Not long after successfully completing my final medical examinations at the London Hospital, I was called into military service, as World War One was raging. Dejected, I wrote home that "I had hoped my life would be in the reproduction of the human race. I don't want to be called on now to attend to those who are mutilated, and watch them die!" But England was at war, and, like countless other young men, I had no choice but to serve my country. I was attached as a doctor to an ambulance unit, and soon sent overseas to Gallipoli.

I do not lightly recall my most hideous hour; it was in August 1915, shortly after we had landed at Suvla Bay. My watch upon the beach began at 2 am. On the edge of the mud of Salt Lake, crystal-coated and faintly glistening in the brilliant starlight of a moonless sky, was my first-aid station. Some three hundred badly wounded men were lying shivering in the cold night air; the fierce heat of the day had fled with the fading light, and in a few hours men's breath was frozen on their beards. To those who were in pain I gave the maximum dose of morphia; rifles and bayonets used as splints required adjusting; tourniquets had to be released and reapplied. Water was scarce, but some could ill afford to be left without their share of our meager supply. The monotony of this round was depressing, for there were no ships' boats to take the wounded off the beach. From time to time, Death seemed to reach down from the empty spaces and seize this man or that, and, on each round I made, a carcass lay where but a short time past I had heard courageous words of patience and gratitude.

I sat to rest upon a mound of sand from which I could hear any call from my stricken flock, and wondered if the living knew that their silent neighbours had passed on. It became so still that only the breathing of the sleepers could be heard, and suddenly I became aware of utter loneliness. I thought afterward that some instinctive warning brought that strange desire to fly. In fact, such an impulse was unthinkable, but in theory at least I was reacting to an undefined fear. I had not many moments to wait for the explanation: from only a mile across the bare lake, on Chocolate Hill, a rifle was fired, rending the stillness so unexpectedly that I started and became alert. It was followed by a sound of war that still rings in my memory, more terrifying than the bombs of World War Two that are bursting nearby as I pen these lines, falling close enough to rock the lamp on my table.

It was the sound of a bayonet charge: the lights leaped from beyond the hill; the shrill yells of madness and bloodlust mingled with the wild whoops and screams of victor and vanquished. A few revolver shots, and soon the lights died down. The stillness was a thousand times more intense after that mad quarter of an hour. I knew our line was feebly held by tired and battle-strained troops. I peered into the distant blackness, wondering who had won. Had the Turks broken through, and should I see the gleam of steel and the fire of mad eyes looming up from the darkness?

I would have given anything within my power to have had a trusted companion with me, even if only to ask him who he thought had won. But I was alone, and that sickening doubt wore down my vitality. I stumbled, tired and frozen, around my patients; my hand shook as I held the water bottle to their lips; my eyes turned unwillingly, but half expectantly, to the black mile that stretched to Chocolate Hill. My mind ran riot, and I suffered agonies of apprehension and fear. Not long after, dawn broke in gray and purple lines across the hills. The doctor who was to relieve me came with the first rays of the sun, and he asked me about the night. I gave him my report, and he looked at me and said: "You look worn out. What's wrong?" He was an old Cambridge friend of mine, and my answer was: "I have never known before how frightful loneliness can be."

The landing on August 6th, several days earlier, with its hail of fire over our heads, had been the reality of slaughter; but it was not so fearsome as that lonely night on which I died a hundred deaths. Later on I was in many battles – on the Somme, at Ypres, Arras, Amiens, and Cambrai; Bourlon Wood, Farbus, Flecquière Wood, Fampoux, and a dozen others where there was ample reason to be afraid – but I never suffered so acutely in any of these as when I learned that night what loneliness can mean.

Perhaps that is the reason why I shudder when I pass the door of those wards where women lie alone, enduring the first stage of labour with no understanding of what is taking place, fearfully imagining what greater agonies may await them.

One day while still at Gallipoli, a shell burst over me and I was seriously injured. Some time later I regained consciousness enough to discover that I was on a hospital ship, a converted cattle boat, bound for Malta. There I was taken, along with the other wounded survivors, to the Blue Sisters Convent for medical care. As I sit with women in labour, I not infrequently remember those dark days in 1915 when I arrived there, blind in one eye and with clouded vision in the other, almost completely paralyzed below the waist, weakened by dystentery, my pulse at thirty, and with a raging fever. The surgeon would have removed my injured eye if he had not been so pressed with caring for those he thought more likely to survive. As the weeks slowly passed I longed to live, yet at the same time wished that I could escape from life.

I recall the horror of those sympathetic visitors who brought me flowers I could not see; told me to cheer up, I should soon be home. "Remember how lucky you are to be alive," was their parting comfort. It made my whole body burn with agonizing tension; my head throbbed and uncontrollable twitchings came into my legs; my spine felt as if it were torn in two at its fractured vertebra. I perspired, and had I been able would have yelled in a wild mixture of pain and fury.

One of the sisters came in after they had gone and saw me alone in my trouble. I had been given a room to myself. She was a tall, stern-looking woman of some fifty years whose features I could not clearly define. She took my hand in hers and stood silently beside me. After a time she knelt beside my bed, and in broken English said: "I will stay with you. We will be peaceful, you in your way and I in mine."

Can I ever forget the miracle of that understanding? My back relaxed and ceased to torture me; the uncontrollable spasms left my legs; my clouded eye seemed to clear, and before I sank into my first long sleep for weeks I saw her head bowed and her eyes closed as she sought in her own way the peace that swept over me.

We may all have our own way of bringing peace to women in labour, but it is in the end a balm of restfulness to a tired mind – a mind that has no energy to withstand the irritations that intensify its discomforts.

I finally recovered enough to be sent home to England for further rehabilitation, fifty-six pounds lighter than my usual hundred and ninety pounds. Determined not to remain a lifelong cripple, I co-operated fully with the hospital program of heat and massage to restore feeling to my legs. Grimly I exercised my useless legs day after day and week after week, until gradually co-ordination began to return.

Because of the great shortage of doctors on the battle front, I was sent back to active duty in foreign lands soon after regaining the use of my limbs. This time I was attached to a cavalry unit. One of the things that occupied my mind during quieter hours was the weighing of the reactions of the men around me to danger. I described my reactions in long letters home:

'I am not pretending to like shells nor to pose as a fearless fire-eater. I know well enough how I loathe it all. The excitement for me is the fight between body and mind. Instinctively I should run away, fly to cover although the shell is nowhere near. But of course one doesn't. I have that instinct more or less under control. Then comes the fight to stand still, to continue dressing a wounded man; not to start or jump but to continue talking, eating, writing.

People will confound and muddle the terms "fearless," "brave," "heroic," "gallant." The fearless man cannot be brave, he has no physical fear (and there are such). He has no battle of the mind versus body. He can be heroic or gallant – but never brave. The only brave man, to my mind, is the one who is afraid. That sounds like a paradox. But the man who cannot breathe because of fright, who is pallid, whose legs shake and whose voice quivers, who feels death at his very throat, at whom each shell is personally aimed, but who yet forces his legs up the embankment, who sees men fall back dead and wounded, who forces words of encouragement through his teeth and leads the first wave over; that is the man.

He is the man who has all the glory for me. He is the best fighter, fighting as no other man can, because suddenly the bonds of fear become loosened and the whole tense physical strain relaxes into an overwhelming reaction.

It is no honour to be fearless; it is a gift. To be brave is more than glorious. If I won honours or died, I could wish for nothing less than for it to be said of me, "He went fearlessly into his duty." That is no praise! It is but making light of an arduous duty. Let it be said of me: "He was afraid, but went because it was his duty." Then honour is earned.

I am afraid. I have not won so far because I have not yet had a severe test compared to many. I am not brave, and that does not apply only to war. There are many things at home around which the same conflict rages. What I want you to do for me is to send me the thoughts to win on. And if I am not here to write, you will know that I have won. . . .'

But I learned more on the battlefield than just from observations of myself and the men around me. It was during this time that I witnessed several women having their babies in the most natural and apparently painless manner. But I also saw those who suffered pain and to whom the birth of their child was an experience horrible to remember, and weighed in my mind what it was that made such a difference. I learned more that was to be of service to me in obstetrics than I would ever have learned had I remained safely in England.

On one occasion a young woman approached the trench and asked for a doctor. The soldiers brought her to me, as she was obviously very pregnant. I had sacks hung up at the end of the dugout and placed her on a stretcher there, while the orderlies on the other side of the improvised screen continued dressing the wounded men who were being brought in. I examined her and found her well advanced in labour. She seemed to be having no discomfort at all. Soon the baby appeared and all was well. She seemed oblivious to the noise of war all around us, sat up on the stretcher, laughed, and took the child in her hands at once.

Four British soldiers came to carry her gently away on the stretcher, rather than the usual two. I could not forget the look of joy on her face as she was carried off with her new baby. She probably would have walked away had the soldiers permitted her to do so. If this is childbirth, I thought, how can childbirth be compared, as it is, with the pains and agonies and hopelessness I see among the wounded men who are brought down to this very same place where this child was born?

One day I had been off the base playing polo, and on my way back to camp came across a Flemish woman leaning against a bank in the field where she appeared to have been working. I tethered my horse and walked over to her to see if anything was wrong, telling her both in French and in English that I was a doctor. She spoke only Flemish, but indicated with gestures that she was bearing a child. She did not in any way appear to resent my intrusion. With the recurrence of the contractions, which appeared to me to be out of all proportion in their strength to those of the average European woman, her face became set, not with pain or fear, but with an almost stern sense of expectancy. I sat down and smoked a pipe and waited, knowing enough of this people's customs to realize that no interference would be welcome.

Within a short time a child arrived. It is possible that during the last ten minutes her expectation almost became apprehension. The child appeared when she was in a half-sitting position. She smiled almost immediately. I felt then that my presence was unnoticed. For some minutes the child lay on the ground and cried, and then she took it in her hands. After a time its yells were all that could be demanded of a newly born baby, and I observed that the cord was already like a thin white string. She took this in her fingers, about six inches from the umbilicus, and neatly severed it – whether by tearing or with her long nail I could not see. She wrapped her baby in the cloth that was around her own shoulders and then looked at me and laughed. It may possibly have been five minutes later when contractions recurred, and with minimum effort the afterbirth arrived, certainly with minimum haemorrhage, for there was none that I could see.

I left her then, hastening into the village on horseback to see if any of her people would come to help her home. They appeared unconcerned and shrugged their shoulders, so I galloped back to where I had left her. I met her walking back to the village, carrying her baby.

The spirit of joy, the spirit of happiness and pride at the arrival and sound of the child, appealed to me. I had never seen a cord so rapidly anaemic. The separation of the placenta and its expulsion all appeared to be carried out under the influence of the joy that the mother was experiencing. For the first time it entered my mind that this joy was not for nothing, and that this perfect physiological process could not be an accidental occurrence. My visions of postpartum haemorrhage, blue babies that would not breathe, uteri that would not contract, and placentas that would not separate, all seemed entirely foreign to this exhibition of labour, conducted more efficiently than I had ever visualized in my most ambitious moments. Elation, wonder, tenderness, and the pride of creation appeared to combine in a great storm of pleasing emotions, and under their influence the birth of a child had been perfected.

During the war I was transferred from my unit to the Indian Cavalry Corps, as deputy assistant director of Medical Services. One of the black-bearded Indian officers noticed one day how tired and jumpy I was after having cared for the wounded under fire and losing several men. He approached me and politely asked if he might demonstrate how he and so many of his people overcame tiredness. He explained in great detail how to achieve complete muscular relaxation. Afterwards, on many occasions I recovered from the stress of my duties by relaxing completely on the little broken-down sofa in my quarters, breathing deeply and quietly as he had taught me.

As the end of the war approached I gave many thoughts to my future, and wrote home how I felt about it:

'I am not suited to be a general practitioner. My object is not to become popular. It would be madness for such a man to settle down in suburbia. It is far better for him that he should aim at a position where the work matters more than the pay he receives, where the service to which he is called is not constantly and obviously in view, where he is not overloaded with the various social and domestic impediments which have spoiled the work of more than half of our good men in the provinces.

. . . Some months ago I was thinking about things, just sitting quietly with my feet on the table, trying and managing to pick holes in myself. Then I turned and picked up a *New Testament* and read, for no reason at all, *James*. I just seemed to drop on to it and came upon some rather startling phrases when you remember the trend of my thinking. I know that service and not self-aggrandisement is the only life one is justified in living. I *know* it. That is the great subconscious influence governing and guiding the whole trend of my thought, and then I read it as if I had been arguing with James himself: "To him that knoweth to do good and doeth it not, to him it is a sin." That is plain enough, is it not?'

Again I was injured near the front – playing football! Some of the men and I were enjoying a bit of recreation on a stretch of open land just beyond reach of the German shells. I was returned to England with a broken leg, shattered by a swift kick in the shin from one of the men who had been aiming at the ball. But I recovered before the Armistice was signed in France. I was reassigned as a brain surgeon in a hospital at Le Havre, meticulously taking shrapnel out of wounded heads.

When eventually the war ended in 1918 I returned to the London Hospital as the senior resident obstetrician, overjoyed to be back in obstetrics. I got out all my old papers and research notes on childbirth and began going over my developing theories again. Here in the hospital I found the same contrast occurring that I had seen on the continent of Europe. Most women seemed to suffer greatly, but here and there I met the calm woman who neither wished for anaesthetic nor appeared to have any unbearable discomfort.

It was very difficult to explain why one should suffer and another be free, apparently, from pain. There did not seem to be much difference in the actual labours; they both had to work equally hard; the time factor was not markedly different one from the other. Perhaps those who had suffered had slightly longer labours on an average than those who had less discomfort. In those days we did not know the mechanism of pain as well as we do today, and a good deal was overlooked that certainly would not have passed unnoticed in the light of our present teaching. It slowly dawned on me, however, that it was the peacefulness of the relatively painless labour that distinguished it most clearly from the others. There was a calm, it seemed almost faith, in the normal and natural outcome of childbirth.

So gradually my mind was influenced by these observations to investigate the part played by the emotions in the natural function of reproduction. Was the nature of the labour responsible for the emotional state of the woman, or was the emotional state of the woman to a large extent responsible for the nature of her labour? Which was primary and which secondary? Could it be that fear of impending pain actually set in motion those factors that caused pain?

Fear is not necessarily abnormal; it is a natural protective state. In the presence of danger, fear engendered by knowledge is the stimulus that prompts escape according to that which threatens. For example, we slow down, if we are wise, when passing through dangerous crossroads. There is, however, an exaggerated state of caution. As students at the university we heard many stories about the "height of precaution," like the decrepit old gentleman who always wore the armour of a first-class wicket-keeper when he went out to play croquet.

In childbirth, fear and the anticipation of pain give rise to natural protective tensions in the body. Unfortunately, the natural muscular tension produced by fear also influences the muscles that close the womb and thus delay the progress of the labour and create pain. What I was witnessing in the labour wards of the hospital convinced me of the truth that this aspect of childbirth held. The Whitechapel question still came back to me: "It doesn't hurt. It wasn't meant to, was it, doctor?"

Now at last I knew that I had found an answer, and that answer was "No. It was not meant to hurt."

Prophet Without Honour

It was my good fortune to serve as house physician under Sir Henry Head for a time after my return to the London Hospital. He is one of the great pioneer neurologists whose writings have helped form the framework for the later rise of the branch of science known as psychosomatic medicine. He demonstrated that somatic or physical changes may occur as the direct result of psychological states. I had the privilege of many conversations with him. These were always a source of great pleasure, because of his enthusiasm not only for his speciality but for the art of living. This stimulated most interesting discussions filled with observations upon his wide experience of human relationships.

Knowing my interest in gynaecology and obstetrics, he turned my attention on a number of occasions to the mind of woman and its activities under different circumstances. The obstetric orthodoxy of the day required the mother to be drugged into unconsciousness during labour and birth to spare her from "suffering." Nothing is more to be abhorred. The forceps deliveries of normal babies – blue and flabby babies who will not cry, babies drugged and anesthetized – were common pictures in current practice.

As senior resident obstetrician I began probing deeply into my patients' backgrounds, hoping for more clues, observing their state of mind. I sat for long hours at their bedsides in labour, seeking to ascertain the strength of the relationship of fear and tension to pain. In every spare moment I searched through every textbook that might provide a clue. I could not relax until I was satisfied that I had found an answer.

And then, in 1919, when I was nearly thirty years old, I gathered together my conclusions from my copious notes into a manuscript painstakingly written out in longhand, hoping eventually to have it published. I had had no one with whom I could share my views freely, but finally I gained courage to present it to my three obstetric professors for their evaluation. They were kind men, and accepted the manuscript graciously.

For some time there was no response. But finally I was called in to meet with them and given their decision. "Look here, old chap," the spokesman of the three said quietly. "The truth is we think you really ought to learn something about obstetrics before you start writing on the subject."

Deep in my heart I had known that this would be their reaction. Although my thesis still contained a great deal of orthodoxy that I had not yet discovered could be discarded, it still represented a major change from current obstetric thinking. "All right. I'll learn," I told them. Returning to my room I buried the manuscript and notes deep into my trunk and went for a long walk alone through the grey, dismal back streets of the East End slums. I never brought up the subject again while at the London Hospital.

When the time came for permanent appointments to the hospital staff to be made, I was passed over, much to the astonishment of my fellow classmates. This meant I had to leave my loved work in obstetrics and go into general practice after all.

Soon after entering general practice, in partnership with an elderly physician in a small town away from London, I married, and in due time our first child arrived. I was not permitted to be present, and was found, when informed of the child's birth, reading the daily paper, apparently calmly– except that the paper was upside down! This, I regret to say, was true, for every obstetric abnormality I had ever seen was, to my knowledge, occurring upstairs.

A few years later, in May 1926, I entered into a clinic practice with three other doctors so that I could devote my time completely to obstetrics. The idea of specialists working together from a single clinic was such a new concept in medical circles that what we had done was not well received. A wave of resentment among the doctors who heard of our action set in, and one of them reported us to the ethical committee of the local division of the British Medical Association. They investigated us, but eventually ruled in our favour.

Now at last I could concentrate fully on my speciality, continuing to apply my theories to my patients, perfecting my methods both from their comments and from my own observations. On one occasion I had spent three hours with a girl of nineteen, and just at the beginning of the second stage of labour she assured me that everything was fine. She had learned how to conduct herself and her labour, and everything was going extremely well when her mother tiptoed into the room. Wearing an agonized expression on her face, she went to the other side of the bed and took her daughter's hand. She stood there during the next contraction, and then, with tears rolling down her cheeks, whispered, "Darling, if only I could bear some of your agony for you!" Fortunately, by that time my patient had transferred her confidence to me, because she smiled at her mother and said, "Yes, it must be painful for you to watch. Now please go." I added in a stage whisper, "Yes, please go."

I shall never forget the harassed, agonised expression on the face of another nineteen-year-old girl whose doctor had sent for me. The labour had been slow, and the mother-in-law – a perfect example of one of the major pests of parturition – rushed dramatically into the driveway and flung open the door of my car before the chauffeur could leap from his seat. She tugged my arm and cried, "Come, oh come quickly. They are killing my daughter. Save her!

Save her!" I ceased to be popular when I looked down upon her and asked with a smile, "From whom?"

The scene upstairs was one of tribulation and turmoil. The girl, uncovered from the waist downward, was biting a towel that had been stuffed into her mouth. When I entered the room the towel was taken from her mouth, and she flung a tired arm across the bed to me and said, "For God's sake give me peace!"

There was nothing abnormal in her labour except its conduct. Each contraction had been a signal for loud shouts of "Push, shove, pull, hang on!" Pressure on the abdomen alternated with the raising of the left buttock to see if the child was appearing. Nurse, doctor, and even mother-in-law gazed at the inoffensive outlet in an agony of anticipation. But the cervix was not fully dilated. It was suggested that they were all very tired; I advised a large brew of tea – down-stairs, away – and a cup of tea for the patient and myself upstairs, weak and warm. In one hour a normal second stage had produced a healthy baby. A few whiffs of gas just at crowning time, for she was still very alarmed, and peace reigned. The pitiable request of that girl, tortured by the turmoil of her parturition, "For God's sake give me peace!" embedded itself in my mind and left an indelible impression of the power of calmness and confidence.

It had become obvious to me long before this that the first place to strike in eliminating pain was at the cause of tension. An aphorism was already imprinted on my mind: "Tense woman – tense cervix." All obstetricians know the effect of a tense cervix: pain, resistance at the outlet, and the innumerable complications of a prolonged labour, with probably an operative finale. I believed the cause of tension to be fear. Restoring a measure of confidence to this badly frightened young woman had released tension enough to produce the baby without difficulty within a short period of time.

However, the fear of childbirth originated from so many sources and from such high places that the whole scheme of society would have to be altered if the attack were made at the source! It was equally obvious to me that those who had suffered were very unlikely to refrain from saying so, and even less likely to preach that their suffering was unnecessary. It was also rather difficult to go around saying that the Bible and the Prayer Book did not really mean what they said on the subject! The Prayer Book had not been altered since 1662, and contained the special service known as "The Churching of Women." The following is from the Prayer Book of my grandmother, to whom this service was read many times:

'Forasmuch as it hath pleased Almighty God of his Goodness to give you safe deliverance, and hath preserved you in the great danger of childbirth; you shall therefore give hearty thanks unto God and say …"The snares of death compassed me round about and the pains of hell gat hold upon me. I found trouble and heaviness, and I called upon the name of the Lord … I was in misery and he helped me…. Thou has delivered my soul from death."

Oh, Almighty God, we give Thee humble thanks for that Thou hast vouchsafed to deliver this woman, Thy servant, from the great pain and peril of childbirth.'

And finally, I came to the conclusion that it would not be much fun to shake a theory in the face of my contemporaries in the attempt to persuade them that all our greatest obstetricians were wrong, and on no account should anyone believe what they were saying! It appeared to me to be rather like a flyweight squaring up in the corner to not one, but a dozen professional heavyweights.

It will be seen that the correct line of procedure was not obvious. On the other hand, I must own to a profound affection for my theory, and that, combined with a modicum of quiet pigheadedness that always stimulates a Norfolk man to discount odds, prompted me to get on with it without further "quavery mavery." Thus I began making an effort to educate women in the facts of childbirth during their pregnancy, in addition to striving to calm their fears during the labour itself. I soon received encouragement, for many women instinctively felt the truth and disbelieved in the necessity for suffering.

At first this did not appear to be enough, for too often, as soon as labour began, the exaggerated receptivity of the mind to all forms of stimulus, both physical and psychical, swept aside their good intentions. Some method had to be found to overcome this main weapon of the enemy, which was muscular tension.

So the practice of physical relaxation that I had learned from the Indian officer during the war was introduced. I had my patients learn to relax well, applying it during the last four or five months of pregnancy for health reasons. Again in labour they were to relax all muscle tension. It was found that when the muscles were flaccid, the mind remained at rest. More gratifying than anything was that the interpretations of the sensations experienced during labour were not invariably that of pain.

Relying almost entirely on this simple, Oriental method of muscular relaxation, in a short time I was more astonished than my patients. In the absence of turmoil, anguish, and misunderstanding, many of the phenomena of labour appeared in their true light. After not more than two years the results of the application of these procedures had not only established my own belief but – what was more important – the large majority of the women whose labours had been conducted in accordance with them had an entirely new attitude toward childbirth.

It was during this period that I began including the husbands in antenatal education, encouraging them to learn and to be with their wives during labour and birth. Our clinic practice was prospering, and my file of case histories growing. Each time I returned from attending a birth I carefully recorded all details of the case, the woman's attitude, and my own handling of the labour and birth, including my mistakes.

By 1929 evidences and experiences in homes and hospitals satisfied me and a large number of patients that the effort to learn and follow the untarnished physiological pattern of normal childbirth was acceptable to nine out of ten women who knew there was such a procedure. I began preparing a book on childbirth, working from my 1919 manuscript and compiling material from the massive library of case histories that I had been building. I did most of my writing at night. Now for the first time since my mother's rebuff to my boyish question during my teen years, I ventured to bring up the subject to her again by letter:

My work has led me to a line of thought which I believe will become of tremendous importance to all women one day. It is to the end that motherhood in the normal case is not a painful and terrifying proceeding but one which is without pain and beautiful beyond all other experiences.

Since the work has developed, a large number of women have testified to the truth of the teaching. Without any anaesthetic and with no pain or discomfort they have learned the joy of natural motherhood. To have had children has been their greatest happiness and the act of childbirth has been the most wonderful experience of their lives.

Now you will agree that is a work which may justifiably enthuse any man. It is a service which it is more than a privilege to render. If motherhood can become a painless joy, how great a change in the whole nation. That is my ambition...

But behind my enthusiasm is the drag – opposition to my greatest useful-ness. Again my old enemy, professional jealousy, is working slowly to take away from me what might make me so worthwhile to others. But this time I say: "*no*! It is too big to give up." It is my only justification for being alive at all.

And so I go on firmly, quietly, certainly. Perhaps in the end the Prayer Book will be altered ... and there will just be a simple thanksgiving that a woman has, by God's grace, been admitted to the joy and wonder of mother-hood and all the marvels of childbirth – God's greatest miracle.

You will keep this confidential to just us, won't you? It has been so nice to write this; so grand to have you still there, so many years after my leav-ing home, to pour out my whims and my grouses, my ideals and ambitions, knowing that you will understand and sympathize.'

By 1930 my manuscript was completed, and I chose as a title the words *Natural Childbirth*. Before submitting it to a publisher I first showed it to one of my personal friends, Dr John Fairbairn, who was at that time one of Brit-ain's finest obstetricians. He returned it to me later, thanked me for letting him see it, but then added, "Look here, my boy" (He still called me "my boy," even though I was over forty!), "you aren't really going to publish this, are you?" I told him that I hoped to.

He said soberly, "It will ruin your practice, you know. Ruin it!" I asked him why, and he replied, "*Because it's true*, my boy. It's true. But it's a truth which will not be accepted by our profession. If you can stand having that sort of trouble, go on; but if not, then my advice is that you should give it up." He patted my arm, and left.

In the months that followed I submitted the manuscript to one publisher after another, all of whom rejected it, some without comment, some with for-mal "regrets". Finally, two years later, William Heinemann (Medical Books) Ltd accepted it for publication with certain reservations, upon the recom-mendation of Dr Johnston Abraham, a well-known London surgeon who was one of their directors. A letter from them in October 1932 stated:

'We have now received the report from our reader on your manuscript and while he considers it an extremely interesting work, full of valuable ideas, he does not think, owing to the fact that you have no definite obstetrical appoint-ment and are comparatively unknown, that it would have any commercial value for a large sale.

If you like, we will be pleased to publish it at your expense with the proviso that as soon as we have sold a sufficient number of copies to cover our cost, the money will be returned to you and a royalty paid on subsequent sales. We shall only print 1,000 copies to start with and probably 500 will have to be sold before the cost is covered. If this idea appeals to you, will you be good enough to let me know and we will send you an estimate for same.'

It was nine months before the book was ready for publication, but in 1933 *Natural Childbirth* was published, and not only did the subject become controversial but the author "a controversial figure"! At first the book was received with gentle kindliness, more like sympathy, by my colleagues in obstetrics. The first reviews were surprisingly favourable. When my friends heard what I had found off the beaten track, they listened politely – much too politely for my comfort.

After the initial fairly favourable response, the reaction set in. My clinic partners dissolved our relationship, bringing against me charges of unprofessional conduct. For a year my professional life hung in the balance. I could not legally practice until the charges were resolved. Ten months later the court cleared me of every charge for lack of evidence, and I was free to open a practice on my own.

But it was difficult to find patients. At first I did not understand why, until someone informed me that I had been anonymously reported to the General Medical Council for advocating cruelty to women! Husbands called me on the phone to cancel appointments for their wives. Pregnant women hurried past my door like scalded cats. But in spite of it all I was satisfied to be nobody with something special, rather than somebody with nothing.

On the advice of friends, I applied for a chair of obstetrics that was vacant at one of the universities. My application was rejected. During this difficult period my health became affected. The old war injuries in my back and legs caused increasing pain and paralysis. I was able to get around with difficulty by using walking canes, but could only manipulate stairs to reach my patients by dragging up on hands and knees.

But encouragements as well as discouragements began coming. Eventually my practice began to grow again, prospering far more than it had in group practice. I maintained a second office on Harley Street in London during part of each week.

I began receiving an increasing number of invitations to lecture on obstetrics. In 1933, before the Ninth British Congress of Obstetrics and Gynaecology I read a paper that I called "Prophylaxis of Fear," using that name to explain how to prevent the pain of uncomplicated childbirth. I was invited to address religious gatherings as well as medical groups, in which talks I laid stress upon the family and the importance of the husband's role. Among the addresses I made were to two conferences of Catholic priests in 1936, one in March on "Psychological Aspects of Maternal Welfare", and one in July on "Maternal Happiness", explaining the importance of the husband for a woman's good childbirth experience.

I was invited to contribute a chapter in Professor Francis James Browne's textbook, *Antenatal and Postnatal Care,* which was published in 1935. Apart from my own book, this was the first time that either the practice of relaxation during childbirth, or the thesis relating to the cause of pain, "The Fear-Tension-Pain Syndrome," had ever been published and widely circulated in the medical world.

From America a letter of encouragement came from Joseph De Lee, Emeritus Professor of Obstetrics at the University of Chicago, dated June 29th, 1936:

'I thank you for the book [*Natural Childbirth*] which you have kindly autographed.

I had already been reading the book, having obtained one of the first copies that came from the press. I agree with you to a very great extent on the thesis which you have therein set forth.

It may interest you to know that I loaned your book to Dr Paul de Kruif, who made rather extensive references in some articles that he wrote for the *Ladies' Home Journal*.

I will incorporate some of these ideas in the next edition of my book on obstetrics, which will probably be finished some time in 1938.

With best regards ...'

These encouragements made me eager to complete a more comprehensive book on the subject. Dr Johnston Abraham assured me that Heinemann would publish it, and Dr Browne kindly offered to read the proofs.

When De Lee's book came out in 1938, he wrote: "It will take several thousand generations before we can train women back to the state which Grantly Dick-Read speaks of as 'Natural Childbirth.'" Because of his comment, it seemed best to prepare my new book as a teaching book addressed to women, and once again I spent long nights poring over my notes, and writing. I am sure that, had this great obstetrician lived, he would have modified his opinion concerning the ability of women to learn, for he set up an experiment using a hundred of his former students to examine the procedures. At the end of the experiment he announced the principles as sound and wrote asking if I could hurry along the completion of the new book. A few weeks later he died without having seen it.

My growing practice and lecture opportunities made progress on the book slow, but I learned from these as well. I was lecturing one time in a large county centre. There were a number of medical personnel present, as well as two or three hundred practicing midwives who listened appreciatively to my observations. The matron, whose brilliant career at a London maternity hospital justified her appointment to a large county maternity organisation, rose to speak. She spoke with simplicity and a charm of manner that accentuated the sincerity of her revelation:

"I feel it is the moment to disclose a secret. For a long time after I became matron I failed to understand why so many women asked to be looked after by the nurses and not by the medical men who attend the hospital. I was constantly embarrassed by the situations which arose, and finally decided to inquire why the request was so frequently and so urgently made. The reply I had was astonishing: 'Because the doctors all make us have chloroform whether we want it or not, and the nurses don't.' "

The matron in another maternity home told me, "The more I see of this natural childbirth, the more I am persuaded that education is what really matters." I asked her frankly if there was any obvious difference in the conduct of labour in my cases from those of other obstetricians who also practiced there. She said, "Yes, in your technique, but the outstanding difference is in the women. They seem to know their job before they start. They understand why relaxation helps and why it prevents pain in labour...."

Two brilliant and progressive headmistresses of large girls' schools in England became persuaded that the teaching of elementary biology and anatomy should be extended, in the higher classes at school, to human structure and reproductive function. It was believed that confidence in discussion would make it easier for girls to have a balanced acceptance of womanhood upon leaving school. But before introducing the subject they felt it necessary to obtain the opinions of the parents of the three hundred girls in one of the schools, as a guide to what the reaction would be in all the others. The response was prompt and dogmatic. If, under the guise of biology and physiology, the parents said, their daughters were to be introduced to the subject of sex and reproduction while still in school, they would be removed immediately!

The tremendous need for such training was brought home very closely to me when one of my own daughters, at the age of seventeen, made these remarks in her weekly letter home: "Jenny's mother is going to have another baby; she is terribly upset about it and awfully worried because her mother told her it was absolute hell. Isn't it too frightful for her?"

It was near the end of the term, so I did not reply in any controversial manner, but neither did I waste any time at the beginning of the holidays in introducing my daughter to the opinions of those who not only entirely disagree with Jenny's mother, but who would have liked to tell her of the infinite harm this effort to gain the sympathy of her daughter had done. To my own child this was an example of the hearsay with which sooner or later all girls become familiar, even in those schools where it is not a frequent subject of conversation among the girls themselves.

One problem that frequently confronted my patients was the unhappiness of the other women in labour. One of my patients was very comfortable and progressing well toward second stage when the loud cries and moans of a woman in labour from a neighbouring ward floated through to the peaceful room in which we were situated. My patient hastily grasped my hand, looked appealingly at me, and said, "How unnecessary it is that she should suffer. Can't you go and help?" I said that I was indeed grieved, but it was no business of mine to interfere uninvited with other cases. I assured her that the chances were the cries were not of suffering, but of fear, and under the influence of narcotic drugs. About an hour later, from the ward on the other side, groans obvious to me to be those of a woman in real pain came loudly across the passage. In a few minutes we heard clearly the crescendo of her screams for help. This was extremely disturbing to my patient, who said, "Surely that is not another?"

I explained to her that a perfectly competent doctor was attending her, because I had gone out to see whether she was asking for help that could be given by me. This went on for an unhappy quarter of an hour and I was afraid it would disrupt the harmony of my own patient's labour. But she proceeded quietly, saying, "I am not having any pain, why should they?" Some time later her baby was born perfectly.

Two women medical students were present at her labour. They had asked to see how natural childbirth was conducted. I was as much interested in the expressions upon their faces as I was in the normal, peaceful birth that I was conducting. Their mouths opened, and, in silence, their eyes opened wider and wider. They looked at the woman as though she were mad or demented; they failed to understand that she was speaking the truth. They had, each of them, seen and conducted many labours, but did not realise the importance of certain simple phenomena of labour that can only appear under these conditions. As I came away after the birth, one of them commented, "It's perfectly simple to have a baby like that. If that is what obstetrics means, there is nothing in it." I replied, "Exactly. Obstetricians are essential to deal with the abnormal – they should not complicate the normal."

When I stopped by to see my patient later, she asked about the two other women whose babies had been born that same night. I told her in plain words that all was well with them, but did not tell her that one of the women had been deeply anesthetized for an hour and a half, her child extracted by forceps, and a large tear of her perineum repaired. The other one had had her perineum repaired later in the night. I kept for myself all thoughts, and merely left her with the knowledge that they were two mothers with two babies.

All this did not endear me to some of my colleagues! There were those who encouraged and helped, but there were others who not only disagreed, but continued to make a number of untrue accusations. The most frequent and most damaging of these continued to be that I did not allow anaesthesia or anything else to relieve pain. This accusation was brought to my notice by a doctor whose wife wanted me to attend her. He had read a book in the medical library that stated that I would not give anaesthesia. I knew at once the book to which he referred. It was popular with medical students because it was short and easy to read. The author never corrected the statement, although he knew full well that it was a deliberate falsehood. My teaching on this has always been clear: (1) no woman should be allowed to suffer; (2) analgesia must always be available for the woman to use if she needs it; (3) analgesia is to be administered according to the clinical indication and the judgment of the attending physician.

One lady wrote and told me my name should be struck off the medical register; such inhumanity was unbelievable in our enlightened age. Society whispered that I sat and watched women writhe in agony. A doctor who had intended to invite me to attend his wife wrote and explained that he did not think I was quite good enough as an obstetrician.

Another startling accusation was that there was some kind of mystic quality I possessed that made the good results possible, but of course other physicians were not so endowed and could thus be excused from even trying to achieve the same results. Others dismissed the results as a kind of personal hypnotism. Frankly, when I saw myself in the mirror in the morning, I hesitated, for one brief moment, before even considering this distinction!

I had considered hypnotism in my early research, along with anaesthesia and every other means of relieving suffering, but had dismissed the thought of learning to use it. Why hypnotize when education and understanding give better results? Hypnotism only hides the phenomena of normal labour behind the ephemeral curtain of disassociated consciousness.

It is true that I possessed one personal quality that helped make the good results possible. But it is a quality I share with tens of thousands of other doctors the world over. It is said by psychologists that in the subconscious mind of woman there are but two types of men: those who injure and abstract from her and those who protect and give to her. The first of these is the materialization of cruelty, and the second the personification of kindness.

There is no more definite division of men than that which is found among the attendants upon women in labour. For, without any question, some by their presence alone stimulate the normal neuromuscular activities of parturition, and others, in spite of the utmost sympathy, appear to cause delay and suffering. In short, there are "motor men" and "inhibitory men" in obstetrics.

An example of the sympathetic yet inhibitory physician is a medical man I once overheard try to encourage his patient. "Ha, ha. Cheer up, old girl. You've got to go through hell, but I'll go anywhere with you, so keep smiling. Ha, ha!" Then there are others who inhibit because they are prompted by the impulses necessary for the perfection of the work *they* have to do during parturition.

Fortunately there are many others who are truly activated by motives of kindness and human understanding, willing to assist the woman in her work of giving birth and to let her be the "star" of the show. These I characterise as "motor men." One of the many accusations made against me was that I was a "motor man," but this I did not mind.

One thing I would never do was to induce labour unnecessarily or hurry things along for my own convenience. We still hear of normal cases having the membranes ruptured early or the labour induced in some other way, so the physician can get the case over in time to do this or that. We still hear of anaesthesia and forceps being employed to assist in the maintenance of a social program, and even for the purely selfish motive that it is the quickest method. Obstetricians are sometimes busy men, but there is no reason why busy men should not be good obstetricians! I have frequently been told, "But my dear so-and-so, I simply do not have time to do all this. There are other things to attend to, and other things to be done."

For three years in succession my summer holiday was planned for three weeks, giving ten days clear at each end from any booked dates for births. Each year from ten to fifteen days of that three weeks had to be sacrificed to infants who insisted upon remaining *in utero*. It is not surprising that my family had a poor opinion of obstetrics as a hobby! To invite friends to dine was to precipitate a labour during dinner, and to fulfill a long-standing promise of a family evening at the theatre was practically impossible. The special days of the school term when the children looked forward to a visit from their "baby doctor" father were frequently days of disappointment.

Late in the summer of 1939 I had finally been able to take my family for a short two-week holiday at the beach. On the last Sunday, we were all in church when the pastor made the announcement that war had been declared on Germany just a few minutes before. We hurried back to our home, which was only twenty-five miles from London, only to find it filled with evacuees. Our first air-raid warning came quite soon after, and, in the absence of any proper shelters, the women and children hurried to the cellars in which we have the boilers and furnaces. I stayed upstairs to make tea for the "party," feeling that bomb splinters upstairs were preferable, should they arrive, to a nightgown party in the cellars with females and boys.

My practice on Harley Street in London was gone. My big car had to be put away for lack of fuel, though two small cars were still available for my local practice. During the Christmas holidays that year war and peace were strangely mingled. I sat in my study after an air-raid warning was over one day. Suddenly the irregular zoom of an airplane, quite low and coming toward the house, attracted my attention. I listened and, as I did so, there was a loud, shrieking rush of a heavy bomb seemingly howling past my window.

Within a few yards of the house I found myself at the raised edge of a crater sixty to seventy feet wide and about twenty feet deep. The cottages near were blasted to a ruined, dusty mass of rubble. All of us, including a nurse who was staying with us, worked like Trojans to find some traces of life. By pushing my arm in the rubble I came upon a small hand. It had a pulse, firmly and surely beating.

Hurriedly working my way up the arm I gave directions to the others to clear away the debris from the face to which the hand belonged. Soon the mouth was free, and then the head and shoulders. A little more clearing and I pulled the child out by the shoulders. He was a boy of about twelve, who soon recovered consciousness and was taken away by the nurse.

I delved again and found another hand and arm – but this time, no pulse. The body was quickly pulled out of the wreckage. Together we worked rapidly until all were accounted for, some dead, some surviving.

That evening my daughters gave a previously planned party for about twenty couples. The evening went well. We had no near bombs that night, and at 3 am the last guest went out into the darkness, cheerful, war free, and contented. So life and death lived side by side.

Inwardly I had decided to burn my new manuscript. I was fifty years old, and although my teachings had become known throughout Europe and in America, they were still unacceptable to the majority of medical men in my own country. Besides, no one knew when this dreadful war would end. I gathered up the chapters that were finished, and the notes, and stuck them into a far corner of the library.

Babies keep coming in wartime, too. A doctor's wife had come to the maternity home in labour. As her baby was born, the labour ward was shaken by the concussion of guns and shells; the first cry of the baby was in concert with hordes of German airplanes going over the maternity wards. I looked at the maternity supervisor and we wondered what might happen next. The Blitz was at its height, but the mother, who had been very nervous of these things, took her small child in her hands and played with it with all the utter carelessness of joy that only this occasion witnesses. It was an extremely pretty picture.

But as I stood and watched these two, still the German hordes went over our heads; the roar and thrum of their engines, the crash of guns, the bursting of shells, and from time to time the bursting of their bombs seemed to make the picture of peacefulness in that labour ward unreal, ephemeral, or a figment of the imagination. It was the permanent record of humanity at its best, and overhead were the emblems of humanity in its most primitive barbarity.

I think perhaps I shall never forget this series of events. In the immediate presence of childbirth there was no thought of fear within any mind in that labour ward. Our work was the privilege of those who assist in laying the foundations of a fuller life, and our thoughts were far beyond the activities of those who seek to destroy. When I went out, having put on my tin hat and placed my gas mask beside me in the car, and drove the three miles home through the Blitz that was harassing the countryside, I was possessed of a sense of elation that here indeed is the true calling of an obstetrician.

Man Without a Country

There were bombs and many deaths in those days. It may have been despondency or frustrating incredulity that men, so gloriously born, could be such fools that made me lose all faith in purposeful writing. But my wife Jessica rescued my original manuscript from being consigned to the flames. She found it, unfinished, discarded in the corner of my library. She placed it before me on my table, asked me some rather pointed questions about myself, and finished by saying, "Don't you realise? That is what women have been wanting for centuries!" So, thanks to her encouragement, the book was finished.

In 1942 William Heinemann published *The Revelation of Childbirth*. It was a more complete book upon the principles and practice of natural childbirth than the one I had published nearly ten years before, its thesis tested and perfected during the decade between. It was followed in 1943 by the publication of *Motherhood in the Post-War World*.

The early reviews of *The Revelation of Childbirth* were not discouraging. The British medical journal, *The Lancet,* spoke of it as "this rather 'Through the Looking-Glass plan,'" but ended by saying, "The book is simple, kindly and often brilliant."

The reviewer in the *British Medical Journal* said:

'This book accuses the medical profession in general and the consulting obstetrician in particular of gross mismanagement of all cases of normal pregnancy and labour. . . . In spite of all this, no one can doubt Dr. Read's sincerity and the book contains a message to all who work in the field of midwifery – namely, that the physical condition is considered at the expense of the psychological and that neglect of the latter frequently converts what would have been a normal physiological function into a pathological process.'

The *Journal of the American Medical Association* advocated that "this small volume should be read by every obstetrician and every student in the physiology of reproduction."

But some of my colleagues, for whose academic attainments I have great respect, argued: "You assume too much. This is not proved – this is not strictly scientific. We disagree with your neurology and your psychiatry is misleading, therefore you must be wrong."

My reply has been, with all humility, "Yes, of course," and I have returned to the labour ward to be greeted by happy women with their newborn babies in their arms: "How right you are, doctor, it is so much easier that way." Frankly, if there is a whole series of academic flaws in my argument, I cannot be too seriously concerned, for its practical application shows clearly that "it works" with considerable success. My thesis was evolved from observations made by the bedside, not in the laboratory.

Reviews continued to pour in from all over the world, nearly all of them favourable. Natural childbirth became the topic of many lively discussions from Canada to Australia. Requests for translation rights began to come in from several foreign countries and were granted. A request came from Harper's in New York to publish the book in the United States, and it was thus that in 1944 *The Revelation of Childbirth* was published in the States, under the title *Childbirth Without Fear.** ·

At first the book followed a course in the United States similar to the original publication of *Natural Childbirth* in England eleven years previously. It brought new thoughts from an unknown pen and introduced theories upon the pain of labour that appeared at first sight to challenge the validity of much that was considered basic orthodoxy. It did not die, however, but survived in spite of small support from the obstetric field. It was neither obstetric nor academic perspicacity that gave it security, but women, from whom letters began arriving in increasing numbers, thanking me for making possible the beautiful births of their babies, and often relating by contrast previous unpleasant childbirth experiences. Many thousands of similar letters have swelled my files as the years passed.

As the war came to an end, invitations to lecture in other countries increased. Among the invitations was one from the United States that arrived at Christmas time, 1946. The president and board of directors of the Maternity Center Association issued a large number of tickets for a meeting at the Academy of Medicine in New York: "Dr Grantly Dick-Read of London, England . . . comes to this country to discuss for the first time on this side of the Atlantic his concepts of natural childbirth. . . ."

Over twenty-five hundred medical personnel were present, an opportunity greater than I had ever had in my own country. The kind reception and interest in the United States overwhelmed me, although not all agreed with my beliefs.

While still in New York I was invited to attend a meeting of the senior obstetric specialists in the city. They gathered once every two weeks to discuss problem cases or current difficulties. I had gone as a spectator, but after the first case had been reviewed the moderator turned to the hundred and twenty or more medical men and women and said, "And now, since we have him here, we'll use him, and he can spend the rest of this session telling us all about his teaching and explaining to us how it works." I need hardly say that before such an illustrious audience, to be thrown unprepared into an hour

---

* *Childbirth Without Fear* was published by the staple trade department of Harper & Bros., which was under the direction of George W. Jones for about twenty-six years. The book sold slowly at first, but by the early 1950s had reached a sale of 100,000 copies.

When the sales of a book reached this figure, it was the custom at Harper's to have a copy hand bound in leather for the proud author. Grantly Dick-Read was in South Africa at the time, and he and Mr Jones had not yet met. Mr Jones had the book leather-bound as was the custom, and shipped to South Africa, "expecting the letter of burbling gratitude authors usually send on such occasions. He was deflated but also amused by Dick's reply, 'Thank you for the handsomely bound book. However, I wish to point out that there are 3½ million babies born every year in the U.S., and I think you have merely scratched the surface.'" When the doctor returned to England he and Mr Jones became firm friends, and remained so until Dr Dick-Read's death in 1959.

By the mid-1960s the book had reached a sale of 275,000 hard-bound copies in the United States, and a million copies throughout the world. It has been translated into many other languages.

and a half's lecture and discussion might well have been an ordeal. But again, there was the same spirit of friendliness in our differences of opinion, and we had many reasons for good laughter.

Toward the end of the afternoon a brilliant psychiatrist and scholar, who stood well over six feet, suddenly strode to the foot of the platform and addressed the moderator in a furious voice: "What sort of nonsense is this? Are we supposed to believe his ideas?" He turned on me. "Tell me, sir, could I pass a coconut through my anus without pain?" There was a pause while we all collected our wits. He pressed his question: "Well, doctor, what have you to say to that?"

Fortunately, the gods visited me hurriedly and fairly. I apologised politely that I was unable to give him a definite reply. "Because," I added, "I am not familiar with the orifice!" His anger turned to friendliness, and the perspiration dried off his forehead in the good humour that followed.

I found that some senior gynaecologists who teach abnormal obstetrics disagreed with prenatal instruction of women. "It is better for us if they don't know anything about childbirth, and anyway, it is our job, not theirs," I heard more than one say. That is the war I have referred to of *man against woman*. There existed a demand that women be kept in ignorance of the truth of childbirth, so that they would be unquestionably submissive to the recommendations and demands of the orthodox obstetric profession. The women did not know that this submission might expose them to routine interference and physical injury, without any clinical indication that could justify such assaults upon their bodies.

I was proudly told by a gynaecologist, before a gathering of colleagues at another meeting, that 75 per cent of his women were delivered with instruments. The labours of 85 to 90 per cent of his patients were surgically or medically induced to have their babies at a time convenient to all concerned. He said also that no woman was allowed to be either sensitive to the sensations of labour or conscious when her baby was born. "No human being," he exclaimed vehemently, "should be allowed to suffer this appalling agony." All women having their first babies were operated upon by having the outlet of the birth canal cut open to make it wider, and he did not advise women to breast-feed their babies. It was an unnecessary call upon their time and it made them tired; social and domestic routine was disturbed and formula feeding gave better results.

He refused to listen to argument or discussion. "I have used my methods for twenty-five years," he said, "and I see no reason to alter my ideas."

I asked him if he was interested in cerebral palsy. He was not – it was the pediatrician's business. Had he read the results of the recent wide-scale investigation and the report that medical authorities believe that over 70 per cent of these disabled children had been crippled by interference at birth? He replied that there was undoubtedly a lot of bad obstetrics, but what could be done about it? I pointed out that there were thirty thousand new cases in the United States every year, making a total of one and a quarter million – did he not think that the natural or physiological method might be worth a trial in this fight against the tragedy of so many maimed babies?

He replied that with all respect he must tell me that there was no such thing as natural childbirth. It had ceased to be a physiological function; culture had seen to that, and civilization must be blamed for the diseases it brings with it.

Did he know that 10 per cent of all the children of low-grade mental development were in their sad plight because of meddlesome obstetrics? He found the evidence difficult to accept and preferred to leave the cerebral trauma children, epileptics, and the results of birth-oxygen starvation to the experts. He was an obstetrician.

Had not the obstetrician a great responsibility to the nation as well as to the parents and homes? "Yes, certainly, most important," he said. And so the conversation finished.

Only twelve weeks after returning from the United States I gave a course of lectures at the Clinique Tarnier in Paris, in May 1947, at the invitation of the late Professors Brindeau and Lanteujoul. I mention this to demonstrate that the general acceptance of this work resulted in a large number of invitations and requests to lecture. I lectured in French. It was at these lectures that the late Dr Ferdinand Lamaze of Paris first became aware of natural childbirth or, as it was later termed by him, "painless childbirth."

During the years since 1933, the year my first book appeared, I had lectured upon this obstetric teaching in seventy-one different universities and maternity organisations in the British Isles and at forty-two universities and maternity organisations in different countries on three continents.

On a visit to a certain country in Europe I was shown, rather proudly, a first-stage ward where there were nine patients. When I went in with the professor who was conducting me around, I realized that there was no nurse present. We walked among the patients and I noticed that three of the nine were already in second stage. They all thought their neighbours were suffering the most intense agony, and when kindly spoken to they nearly all expressed sympathy with others. Only one demanded sympathy for herself because of her own personal discomfort. This distressing scene impressed me with the fact that antenatal care was at fault more than labour. Had these women understood labour, learned and practised what to do, and been helped by trained attendants, it would have been so different.

Reports were becoming public by this time of several controlled series of births carried out under the natural childbirth procedures, from as far distant countries as the United States in 1946, by Black-well Sawyer of New Jersey, and Durban, South Africa, in 1947, by the Department of Anesthesia, Addington Hospital.

In 1947 I published *The Birth of a Child* and began compiling material for *Introduction to Motherhood*. At this time the National Health Service was about to be introduced in Britain, so I went to inquire of Sir William Gilliatt, president of the Royal College of Obstetricians and Gynecologists, whether there might not be opportunity to be accepted as a member under the new arrangements. I asked for an assignment to carry out controlled studies in Britain itself, such as those being conducted in other places. He was very charming in manner but offered no hope, and hinted broadly that I should consider leaving the country! On my return home, I wrote him a long letter:

. . . In the absence of any official investigation or indeed recognition of this doctrine by your College, I must ask you to accept my statements as accurate, full of evidence which surrounds me here in my library as I write to you. From all over the world there is a vast fund of evidence that this approach to childbirth has brought safety and happiness to thousands of women. . . .

A frequent request from doctors, matrons and sisters of maternity establishments is: "Where can I come and study these methods?" Doctors in China, America (many), South Africa, Australia, Sweden, Holland and France have all expressed the desire to visit a hospital in England to learn and witness this work.... Books upon this subject are bought and read by thousands in the British Isles and America. They are translated or extracted in ten languages at least, probably more by now. Few editions of medical, obstetric or nursing journals are published without some favourable reference to the benefits of the "new approach to childbirth."...

To me this work is no longer an obstetric practice only, but a mission – no longer a pursuit, but a calling. I am not holy or pious, but I sincerely believe that time has shown clearly that the only justification for my personal existence, now that my family is grown up, is to give up everything to spread this gospel of safe and happy childbirth. I mean everything – my practice and, if need be, my home. I cannot sacrifice wealth as I have not attained it beyond providing for my wife and the future of my children. I want to teach and demonstrate and have a platform where all who wish may listen and learn and, in due course, perfect the technique of which I have evolved the elementary principles. . . .

I must set my course for the future. I hope to have ten years or more of life given to me in active work. I want to use it to good purpose. Can you therefore tell me, in order to assist me in deciding on my disposal: Is there a place for me in this country where practical teaching and demonstration may be given to those who accept these tenets? Do you still consider that my best course is to leave the country and try somewhere else? . . . I know this thing has got to come – and in the near future. The demand for it is growing like a rolling snowball across the face of the earth. Do you wish it to come from within or without?

By November 26th word came that my request was being considered, and on January 25th, 1948, I received word that an eighteen-bed unit at Isleworth was to be placed under my clinical care. It had two labour wards and facilities for an antenatal department. The hospital would provide two obstetric nurses, and one or two of the medical residents who would be trained to carry out my teachings.

It seemed too good to be true! And it was. I discovered that the unit was separate from the main hospital, and had been damaged in the war. The eighteen beds were rickety and old. One of the only two toilets in the unit was out of order. In the room where the babies would be changed and bathed, the washbasin was broken and the baby tub of cracked enamel was covered with a plain wooden board, on which were piled the dressings that were to go into the sterilizer. Shelves in the walls around were stuffed with an assortment of cups and saucers, bedpans, and spare rolls of toilet paper. Paint and plaster were peeling off the walls, and some of the windows were broken and boarded over. The labour wards were tiny, with bare wooden floors. In one of them the only ventilation was through a small window fan, set in a window that would not open. Instruments would have to be boiled in an enamel basin on the kitchen stove.

I inquired if the place could be repaired and brought up to date. The answer was no. I invited the maternity supervisor of a large hospital to take a look at the place the Royal College had offered, in which doctors from all over the country and world would come to witness demonstrations of my teaching. Her reaction was the same as mine. It was impossible.

I was nearly sixty years old. My health was breaking under the strain of opposition. The old World War One injuries were again causing searing headaches and problems with my back and legs. My world seemed shattered around me. Where could I go? What should I do?

Then I remembered what my mother had written to me many years before: "Put your hand in the Hand of God. I have done so in all my troubles and have never failed to find comfort and help." I followed her advice, got down on my knees, and prayed.

A new possibility presented itself to Dr Dick-Read when a group of South Africans proposed building a magnificent hospital for women just outside Johannesburg, and invited him to take full charge of the obstetric section as soon as it opened. On March 27th, 1948, he made a preliminary visit to South Africa, prior to another lecture tour of several countries, with the promise to return to the position in the fall.

But it was not to be. His teaching had caught the attention of the press, and this nearly caused the end of his practicing career. On June 28th, 1948, the following article appeared in the London Daily Mirror:

> I understand that Princess Elizabeth is preparing, by careful study of the nature of childbirth and by doing muscular exercises, to have her baby without an anaesthetic. The Princess has told friends her belief that pain in childbirth can be greatly reduced if a woman has a calm understanding of exactly what is happening when her baby is born. . . .
>
> In all these matters she will, of course, be advised by her obstetrician, Sir William Gilliatt. But I am told that Sir William is not a great believer in natural childbirth. And the Princess will be giving a lead and encouragement to millions of women who fear confinement because they believe it must necessarily be accompanied by dreadful pain.
>
> This "natural childbirth" system was first advocated in modern times by Dr Grantly Dick-Read. Though it is accepted by many doctors all over the world, an early book on it nearly put him out of practice. . . .
>
> Princess Elizabeth has read Dr Dick-Read's book. When it first came out it was almost impossible to sell it. Now it has been translated into five languages, is a best seller in America and is selling at the rate of thousands of copies a month.
>
> Dr Dick-Read is a tall, jovial man with a Cambridge degree, a Harley Street practice and a private clinic in Surrey. . . .

Once that story appeared, the rumour of Princess Elizabeth's proposed natural delivery swept the world. The French newspapers came out with bold headlines such as this: ENGLAND IS DIVIDED INTO TWO CAMPS – FOR OR AGAINST PAIN. *In Australia the* Melbourne Sun *reported:*

> Princess Elizabeth, who is known for her enquiring mind and logical approach to life, has taken an intelligent interest in motherhood. . . . Although it is reported that she is doing regular muscle exercises hoping that she will be able to have her baby without anaesthetics, bushy-eyed, sixty-year-old Sir William (Gilliatt) says that he thinks it most unlikely. . . . But the Princess has read *Revelation of Childbirth* by Dr Dick-Read, first advocator of "natural" childbirth. This book sells over a thousand copies a month in England, has been translated into five languages and is a best seller in America.

Some news reports even rumored that Dr Dick-Read was replacing Sir William Gilliatt as the Princess's obstetrician! Yet at the time the articles appeared he didn't even know she was expecting, or that she had ever heard of his books. The news preceded him to South Africa, where the Natal Daily News *said:*

> South African women, accustomed to having things done for them, will not take too kindly to the advice of Dr Dick-Read, whose theory of painless childbirth has created tremendous interest in the United States. But perhaps the fact that Princess Elizabeth is having her baby the "Dick-Read way" may give a fillip to a revolutionary concept of childbirth which, paradoxically, is as old as woman herself.

Other headlines in South Africa appeared, such as the one in the Johannesburg Sunday Times *on October 31th, 1948:*

JOHANNESBURG TO BE NEW WORLD CENTRE OF PAINLESS CHILDBIRTH

Johannesburg is to become the world centre of "painless childbirth." Dr Grantly Dick-Read, the famous British obstetrician who has taken terror out of childbirth for women all over the world, plans to move his entire organisation from London to Hurlingham, a suburb of Johannesburg. A South African architect has visited Dr Dick-Read in London and discussed with him his plans for the proposed hospital. . . . The building of the hospital in South Africa will mean that students of the new system of obstetrics will have to come to So. Africa for training.

Dr Dick-Read visited Johannesburg in April of this year and demonstrated to doctors and women that normal childbirth can be free from pain. . . .

Thus it was that news items, many of them inaccurate in a number of details, caused him far more harm than anyone could have deliberately planned. The day he left England, December 19th, 1948, millions of Britons read the untrue headlines of the Sunday Pictorial: DOCTOR QUITS IN DISGUST.

The news flashed around the world, in varied and distorted ways, and thus, predictably, on March 26th, 1949, the London Evening News *carried another item:*

HARLEY STREET MAN BANNED IN SOUTH AFRICA
British obstetrician, Dr Grantly Dick-Read, who took fear out of childbirth for women all over the world has been refused registration by the South African Medical and Dental Council.

The council took its decision in committee and later confirmed it in open session. Officials of the Council refused to comment on the decision. . . .

The charges against him by the council were that he had solicited "advertisement" from the lay press, and thus was not a "person of good character," and was unsuitable for registration as a practicing physician in South Africa. Dr Dick-Read hired a lawyer to prepare an appeal. While the legal argument raged he was without income and forbidden to practice, though scores of women wrote or besieged him by telephone begging him to attend their confinements. Scouts were even sent to spy on his home, in case he might be accepting patients secretly.

Finally the Medical Council held a special session to hear the appeal, given by A.J. Israel, one of South Africa's most brilliant lawyers:

According to the evidence before you, Dr Dick-Read is a man whose work is well known. . . . Whether his methods and teachings are correct or not, it is not for me or you to say. This application is not concerned with that aspect. It therefore seems that an unnecessary attempt is being made to prejudice him when one sees that members of this Council wish to indicate that here is a man who is nobody and has done nothing. The type of question put by a member at the meeting of the Executive Committee indicates this. It is wrong to have put that type of question, to belittle a man and his work. It has nothing to do with an application for simple registration. . . .

We have put in letters and evidence from famous obstetricians and gynaecologists and other medical practitioners who have written and read papers on his work.... I handed in today letters from the Lord Chancellor of England and from Dr Thoms, head of the obstetrical department of Yale University; letters from the School of Medicine at Boston; letters from Canada and other places where Dr Dick-Read's work and lectures are known and appreciated and he is treated with consideration because obviously his work is recognised as of some value to the profession.

But here, without any necessity, it is suggested that his lectures and work are, in effect, so bad that an application for him to practice is treated with contempt.

. . . Mr Chairman, I think I am putting the case fairly when I say that, at the Executive Committee, Dr Dick-Read laid himself open to examination and not only to examination but severe cross-examination of himself, where there was no right or even necessity to hold an enquiry. But nevertheless, he answered every question put to him candidly and he must have dispelled any impression that he is not a "person of good character."

Following the appeal, the nineteen members of the council took a vote. One abstained, and eighteen voted against permitting Dr Dick-Read to be registered!

Only one recourse was left – an appeal to the Supreme Court of South Africa for a judgment. Three separate hearings were held, and on June 23th, 1949, the Supreme Court ruled that he was to be issued a certificate of registration without further delay.

In the meantime, the plans to build the new hospital had long since been abandoned. But once he was entitled to practice in South Africa, a small but beautifully equipped maternity hospital, the Marymount, run by nuns of a Dominican order, invited him to come, promising to co-operate fully with his teaching. He had not been there many weeks before he said to them, "In another eighteen months it will not be a question of keeping the beds full, but of building to provide double the number, so that we can cope with all the demands for our services." His prediction was correct.

African Journey

My wife Jessica immediately organised a series of antenatal classes for expectant mothers. The classes were held once every two weeks for women who could attend. Usually ten was the maximum number taken in any one class, which started about the eighteenth week of pregnancy. It was fascinating to watch the difference between these organised classes conducted by my wife and my early efforts at trying to teach women myself. The clumsiness and misunderstanding of men – I don't mean to derogate my sex – but the advantage of women being taught by women is that they understand the mysteries of a woman's mind, as man cannot.

The women were taught many things at these classes, including all the principles of postnatal care from the day the baby was born. It was soon found that these classes became gatherings of friendly women, even though they were very mixed in terms of social position or deprivation. They had a common interest and a common desire to learn the truth and apply it.

I slipped into the antenatal classes one day while the women were relaxing, to see if I could discover to what extent the relaxed women showed any sign of residual tension. The room was darkened and quiet; I entered without any unnecessary noise, the instructress greeted me, and although speaking quietly she used her normal voice. I walked around the women, some of whom were in the left lateral and some in the right lateral position. They had been relaxing for about ten to fifteen minutes. I sat in a chair and watched them individually, and although several had obvious evidence of incomplete relaxation, which was not unreasonable since they had only attended four classes, I was astonished at the sleepiness of all these women, who were not actually asleep. As I sat there in the peace of the room it came to my mind how easily anyone who was not initiated might have presumed that these women were being subjected to some form of hypnosis. When given instruction they reacted slowly but accurately, and it reminded me of the dictum of Edmund Jacobson, referring to relaxation: "No university subject and no patient ever considered it a suggested, hypnoidal or trance state, or anything but a perfectly natural condition. It is only the person who has merely read a description who might question this point." I talked for a short time with the instructress and left the room. I learned afterward that only two of the class had known of my visit.

What was the result of this preparation of women? The result has been that all over the world today the tenets that emerged from that relatively small school are the basic foundation for the organisation of antenatal care of women in universities, teaching colleges, and maternity homes. They are not yet as common as I would wish, but that time will come.

The actual time I practised in Johannesburg was just under four years. In that cosmopolitan community all sorts and conditions of people came under my care. I saw about six hundred babies into the world, of almost every European nationality under the sun. For simple enjoyment it was too many, but for the privilege of attending different types it was unique – English, American, Belgian, Czechoslovakian, French, Latvian, Norwegian, Italian, Spanish, Greek, Yugoslavian, German, Armenian, and Jewish women who had lived in or been born in Russia, Poland, Bulgaria, and Austria. I mention this at length because the physical and psychological characteristics of these people differed considerably. The mental background of the refugees, those who had been in concentration camps, differed from any I had previously met. Some had witnessed the indescribable horrors of slaughter and torture, and others had seen friends and parents walk away from them forever, to be deported to a distant country or to death in the gas chamber.

There were also the women of old Boer stock, physically fit and strong, mentally imperturbable, without fear or frustration. These were women of families of the gold rush whose grandparents had farmed the grasslands, and whose cattle had grazed upon pastures with millions and millions of dollars' worth of gold beneath their feet. These people demanded my books and translated them into Afrikaans.

Here indeed was a heaven-sent opportunity to observe the influence of the new approach to childbirth; call it natural, educated, or physiological, what you will, the result was the same. Physically, in the mass, all women are the same – good, bad, and indifferent anatomical structure. Disproportions between foetus and the maternal pelvis occurred much as they do in England and probably all over the world. But psychologically the picture was different and, in my opinion, more difficult: I attended women with neuroses, psychoneuroses, hysteria, and anxiety states, with real terrors of death and conflicts at diverse psychic levels and intensities. Some had emotional struggles and the mental suffering of ambivalence – for and against children, husbands, marriage, motherhood, homes, social life, and sexual desires. All these came to learn to the best of their ability, at the magnificent antenatal school organised and superintended by my wife.

Of all these, except for those few who required, through disease or disproportion, some operative interference, 96 to 97 per cent, of their own free will, refused the analgesia within their reach, preferring to be fully conscious and watch the birth of their babies.

It was possible during these years to make a sixteen-millimeter sound and colour film of three natural births, as well as a sound recording. It was not possible to pick and choose "ideal" cases, but when the cameraman was hired, the film was made of the next women who came in to have their babies.

But I still had one lifelong dream unfulfilled, that of investigating the childbirth customs of the people who lived closest to nature and furthest from both the advantages and disadvantages of modern science. For weeks and months my wife and I talked about such a project. There were still villages where tribes of Africans were living, in the jungles and on the mountains, in the swamps and on the sand-swept plains, where white men seldom went and never stayed. We decided to go and see for ourselves what the customs of these people were.

For over forty years I had held the beliefs of my medical colleagues as suspect, feeling that they were misinterpreting the laws of nature. I felt that they had used modern scientific methods, not only to hide the pain of childbirth, but also to hide their own failure to understand its cause. I had satisfied myself that the physiological and anatomical apparatus the Creator had evolved for childbearing women was a magnificent manifestation of Divine genius. No further observations were necessary to uphold the belief in my contentions. But the years were telling on me. Night work took toll of my vitality, and tiredness such as I had never known brought home to me the fact that many of my contemporaries had already reached retiring age from hospitals and medical schools.

So the plans were made, and we sold home and practice, had a mobile home built on a bus chassis, and set off into the unknown, hoping to visit not just a few tribes but a hundred, two hundred if possible, to learn of normal childbirth in its natural environment. We wanted to prove or disprove the reports we had heard of the horrors of childbirth among the unwesternised people, the sufferings of women, and the enormously high rate of neonatal deaths. In our hearts we would not believe these stories without a closer examination of the facts.

During our journey through Africa we found doctors, priests, and others keenly interested in helping this project with personal experiences of their life among the African tribes. They brought Africans in to add their information on tribal lore and custom, and interpreted for me. It was generally agreed that childbirth had earned a bad name because of the relatively few complicated cases that were seen by medical people, who never saw the normal. And, further, I discovered that difficult labour cases were only brought in after a long wait in the villages, so that women who could have been successfully treated without any danger were much worse when finally brought in than those with similar complications among Europeans. This was due either to the distances involved, or to the ignorance and delay caused by the witch doctors.

One of my first visits was to the Moffatt Mission, where Dr Manson from Scotland was in charge. He was certainly typical of the best of the doctor missionaries we came across. It was a strange coincidence to find that I was no stranger to him, although I must say I did not remember him myself. He had been present at my lectures in Scotland during the days when I lectured at the university there, bringing to the attention of the students the physiological approach to childbirth. He told me a lot about childbirth among these people. He was a keen obstetrician, and made me realize how much we had to learn.

From there we went a short distance north and called on a Canadian doctor at the Seventh-Day Adventist Mission Hospital, Dr Jack Hay. When I told him my name he said, "This is nothing short of a miracle! My wife has had three babies, and studied your books very carefully with each one. She had not the slightest trouble or difficulty. In fact, she was so enthusiastic about the method that she started antenatal classes for the African women." After a year she found the numbers to have increased so much that seven hundred women attended in that one year. And it was the old women who usually insisted on the girls coming to learn.

I learned that the law of the jungle has two main branches. The Africans told me of the manner of the *maintenance* of individuals and their tribes, their systems and organizations, religions, food and drink, victories and defeats, drought, flood, fire, and disease. But they always expressed surprise that a white man should want to know the other branch of jungle law: the *reproduction* of the people, the marriage customs, and the girlhood of the women who bore children to reinforce the manpower of the tribe.

For this information I had to speak to the women, old and past the years of shyness and reticence, those who were chosen to guide and care for mothers when their babies were born. "Why do you want to know?" they asked me, and I said, "Do you not want to hear the ways of white women?" It was an exchange of confidences freely given, and I believe most of these ancient midwives with whom I talked were honest in their replies, for so many answers to my questions were the same, although from different tribes who lived thousands of miles apart, and spoke totally different languages.

But even if they did not tell the truth it was only to be kind. Dear old Bwalya Kalunda, whose interpreter was a lady of a Protestant mission, replied to me in her own language, although she spoke reasonably good English. "Bwalya Kalunda," I said, "how many children have you had?" Miss X translated that she had had twelve.

"Was it easy to have babies?" The question was put to her very sternly as if to say, "You know the answer to this one." In English the old lady replied in a monotone, "For my sin I suffer the torture of damn."

But, choosing her moment, she gave me a naughty wink. I understood and said, "Bwalya Kalunda, you like having babies?" She smiled, and through Miss X she said, "I love it, and did not want to stop!" Miss X told me Bwalya Kalunda was an ardent Christian. My obvious rejoinder was, "A grand old lady, and very loyal!"

She was one of so many with whom we talked. The young women were difficult to talk to, for most of them are coy and proud of their feminine assets, a fairly general trait throughout the world. They are taught it is a woman's business to be attractive to a male and on her best behaviour before strangers.

But when we talked to the old dames, those who had been "through the mill," had seen life and looked after others, I found them not only charming and polite, but quiet, kindly women and surprisingly knowledgeable. They spoke of the one great experience, motherhood, not only of having their own children and all it meant to them, but of the young women they looked after. They told me, freely, so much that I came to the conclusion that white people have a lot to learn from black people, who should receive our greatest respect.

Until people have been to Africa, they are inclined to think of jungle women as subhuman types. This is entirely wrong! Within the edicts of their own laws and customs they are dignified, and many of them are beautiful people. They are essentially feminine, and there seemed to us to be very little difference between "woman" whether she is European, Asiatic, or African. The African women desire to be attractive, and spend a large part of their time beautifying themselves, particularly their hair. This is done in many different styles among the various tribes.

Black African women are people of amazing character. First and foremost we were impressed by their beauty, and when I say beauty I mean it. It isn't necessarily that they have the same outline of features you would expect to see in a London street or in New York, but they carry with them a personality that is astonishing. As we passed them sitting in groups at the edge of the forests, we stopped and laughed with them often, making signs and getting in touch with them in the different ways we had learned, because none of them spoke any language we understood. We got along well in the towns with our French and English, but in the jungle had to go back to the old primitive method of enjoying each other's company by signs, hands, eyes, and smiles. And there is nothing that gets one further with the African woman than a smile.

Among the majority of the tribes we visited the women in the villages were looked after by the older women in the families, not necessarily relatives but old people especially chosen for this purpose. Very few African women attended a hospital for birth unless there was some definite complication and delay during labour. The more urbanized Africans who lived in the town brought their wives into the hospital, and we were told that they had more discomfort and made more noise than the village women at home.

While customs differed, the following procedures were the most common: The babies are born with the mother squatting on the floor, leaning against the side of the hut. Usually there is someone behind to support them during the later stages of labour, when the midwife takes up her position in front. The village labour is conducted in silence. There appears to be very little discomfort though sometimes considerable hard work on the part of the mother.

The woman who is attended in the village is never left alone. Most of them are well instructed in the course of labour by old women in whom they have complete confidence. And while their errors are tragedies, for they do not have the knowledge or ability to treat the 4 or 5 per cent of irregularities that occur, their customs do not allow the acts and interferences that account for over 60 per cent of maternal morbidity in the Western countries. There will always be abnormalities in all forms of reproduction throughout the realms of nature, but the complications of pathological childbirth are few compared with the man-made troubles that emerge in civilised countries, when there is failure to understand the simple physiological mechanism and its demands. A mission doctor reported that 18 per cent of his patients had abnormal labours *after* admission to the hospital. This I am willing to believe, but I found no evidence to support such a high percentage of abnormal labours in the villages.

A British provincial commissioner told me of one experience he had had when he was carrying an African man and wife on his boat. The wife began labour during the journey, so he stopped. She went into the bush and the husband waited nearby. In a relatively short time the woman emerged with her baby and the journey resumed.

We learned the profound respect that every tribe and village has for the afterbirth, and the manner of its extrusion from the birth canal. They do not interfere with nature's work, and allow no child to be separated from this wonderful structure, which gave it soul and body while it grew within the mother's womb, until it has been born and lies beside the child. Then, and only then, may the cord be cut and the offspring given to its mother to embrace. In many tribes, no one is allowed to touch the placenta, or afterbirth. It is taken away by the woman in attendance and buried. There are many superstitions concerning it, and its burial constitutes an important rite in the birth of a child.

The major cause of difficulty among the nationals, apart from anatomical disproportion or malpresentation, is that often the aged midwives insist on the mother pushing down hard from the beginning and using all her strength. This has resulted in many unnecessary troubles. Prolapse of the uterus occurs, and sometimes the pressure, before the cervix is properly opened, produces swelling and oedema of the outlet, which actually impedes the progress of the oncoming child. I saw a number of fistulas from the vagina into either or both bladder and rectum, rupture of the uterus, and severe exhaustion and shock. When labour is prolonged, the woman might be accused of adultery, adding mental suffering to her physical difficulty. These were the chief complications of labour, and although compared with the normal cases they were only a small number, even these troubles could have been prevented, for the African can also learn from us.

The Africans are intelligent people, but it must be remembered they have a different culture from ours. Their way of life is that which one could expect from those who live nearest to nature, the nature from which they come and upon which they survive. In this journey of ours we found that the simple biological law of all life has stood immutable since the creation of the first living soul, and in a word it is – survival!

As we travelled through strange places among people whose manners and customs were new to us, we were conscious of the power of this fundamental principle. We found it everywhere; human beings, animals, insects, the trees of the great forests and the creatures of the rivers and lakes survive in a ruthless war one against the other, but man in many ways has a higher intelligence than other living creatures, and from the earliest records of his existence we have reason to believe that he has been aware of an all-powerful influence that rules over his destiny.

At one place we had come upon a deserted, hidden temple. It was an awe-inspiring spectacle for me, for when one has lived for over sixty years one seeks some association with our own experience, and recalls analogies from memories past. What can any sensible human being say when he sees, thrown on the canvas of today, the genius of a people long lost in an oblivion that has destroyed their entity, and the brilliance of whose work is secreted beneath a shroud of rampant vegetation? All archaeologists must feel the futility of our existence in terms of man's estimate of success.

It must be accepted that greatness up to a certain standard is attained by acquisition, discovery, and organizing ability, but we very rarely hear anyone say "thank you" to the powers that placed the substance there and gave man the faculties to utilise it for the development of the human race.

I can only say there are some things the black man knows that would be of tremendous benefit to us, though other things are best left where they are, gradually dying out in the hidden places of the jungle. The African is a proud, spiritually minded but essentially practical man. He has for generations been brought up to use his physical prowess as well as his wits for the survival and the maintenance of his people.

In an international medical magazine recently I read: "…When modern science has said its last word, and the patient is still no better, we are not justified in saying that the case is necessarily hopeless. There are still spiritual values to be considered, and spiritual resources of prayer…." We are swinging around once more to the practices of the African over the centuries, in his awareness of spiritual forces in the universe.

In the scorching brilliance of a cloudless sky and in the damp of forest darkness, when wild turmoil bent and frayed the treetops of the valley, and again in the stillness and peace of tropic night, we heard the echo of a Voice in harmony with every discord of the jungle world: "I am Alpha and Omega, the beginning and the ending, the first and the last."

Why is it that the enslavement of the body appeals more to our sympathies than the more destructive slavery of the spirit, which is the ruling force of survival in the modern civilised or cultured world? Soon this glorious array of bounties, which until recently was known as "Darkest Africa," will have been dissolved by the torrent of the white man's infiltration. I give it ten years – until the early 1960s – and then all will be commerce. The destructive hand of Western influence will take so much that is good and replace it with the crumbs that fall from the rich man's table.

Don't look too far ahead. It will give no pleasure and no reward. Go now, not to kill beasts or to find minerals, not to grow cotton, coffee, or bananas, but to open, while there is yet time, the windows of your own souls. Let in the light that floods the forest of the valleys and the hills, the light that is the law of the jungle, the law of nature, and the law of God.

And try to understand.

Some Misunderstandings

During my years in South Africa, experiments in natural childbirth procedures continued to be carried out in all parts of the globe and the results made public. Among the most notable of these was that conducted by Professors Thorns and Goodrich[1] at the Yale University School of Medicine in 1948, and in 1951 by Lawrence D. Roth of Rochester, New York. Since then each year there have been one or more records and publications of controlled experiments in the use of these principles.

Shortly after arriving in South Africa, I completed writing *Introduction to Motherhood*. My books already published or in progress in several foreign languages were: *Mutter Verden ohne Vrees*, in Dutch; *Die naturlige Fødsels*, in Danish; *Mutter Werden ohne Schmerz*, in German; *Att Foda utan Fruktan*, in Swedish; *Rivelazioni sul Parto*, in Italian; and editions were also appearing in French, Spanish, Portuguese, Japanese, and Norwegian. It can safely be said that this teaching was known all over the Western world before my years in Africa began.

Painless deliveries have been of interest to Russian physicians for many years. In 1936 I read of the methods of painless childbirth in Russian papers; at that time it was spinal analgesia. In 1946 a Leningrad doctor reported on the use of vitamin B_1. In 1945 Dr Velvovsky of the Ukraine, who had been studying methods of painless childbirth, first using hypnosis and then trying a variety of other methods, reached for the Pavlovian physiology to assist him in obtaining his design. In 1948 the Russians carefully investigated the benefits of the natural childbirth approach, which was then known all over the world. These natural childbirth experiments found favour among them. They were quick to appreciate its benefits for the health of their nation, but omitted any reference to factors not purely mechanistic.

At the Fourth International Congress of Catholic Doctors on September 29, 1949, the Pope gave an address, outlining the principles and practice of childbirth without fear. He compared it to the procedure in certain hospitals where the mother was plunged into deep hypnosis, stating that this procedure resulted in emotional indifference to the child, and was thus not recommended, but that natural childbirth did not entail this danger. He went on to relate the recent Soviet researches in obstetrics along these same lines, but implied criticism of the Russians for their neglect of the spiritual aspects. He said:

> The Englishman Grantly Dick Read has perfected a theory and technique which are analogous in a certain number of points; in his philosophical and metaphysical postulates, however, he differs substantially because his are not based, like theirs, on a materialistic concept.
>
> The laws, the theory and the technique of natural childbirth, without pain, are undoubtedly valid, but they have been elaborated by scholars who, to a great extent, profess an ideology belonging to a materialistic culture.

By late 1949 and 1950 the Russian experiments in natural childbirth were successful enough for them to call a conference on this subject at Leningrad in 1951. It was sponsored by the Clinical Department of the USSR. Academy of Medical Science and the Scientific Council of the USSR Ministry of Public Health. Here Velvovsky, Platonov, and Nicolayev read papers on the results of a *new* method of obstetric pain relief now being practiced in a number of institutions in Moscow, Kharkov, and Leningrad. It is difficult to know why this approach was called new, since it had been in English textbooks and used in many countries for twenty years! It can be said that this work was known practically all over the civilised world by 1951.

In September of that same year (1951), Dr Pierre Vellay of France wrote me a very kind letter, saying that both he and Dr Lamaze had considered it a privilege to read the last edition of my book, *Childbirth Without Fear*. I remembered Dr Lamaze from my lectures at the Clinique Tarnier in Paris in 1947. Dr Lamaze was now the resident accoucheur of the Ironworkers Policlinic in Paris, and Vellay had been his assistant for the previous three years. Dr Vellay stated that he appreciated the help my book might bring to pregnant women, and requested the right to translate it into French.

I replied, thanking him very much for his letter but informing him that the work was already translated into French, and that my publishers had informed me that it would appear on the market shortly. However, in spite of all our efforts to get it through, it was not until eighteen months later that the book finally appeared on the French market. This was always a mystery to us, but eventually my book *L'Accouchement sans Douleur* was published.

Early in 1952, while still in South Africa, I received information from

Switzerland and other countries that Russian gynaecologists had described a new approach to childbirth called "psychoprophylaxis," based on the work of a Russian named Ivan Pavlov. Those who sent the information stated that there was a striking similarity of what they were claiming to have discovered to what I had been writing, lecturing, and teaching for so long in so many parts of the world, even to the use of the term "psychoprophylaxis" in relation to childbirth, which I first used in 1933. So I visited the Consulate of the USSR in Pretoria, South Africa, to discuss the matter.

The consul invited me to send copies of my book, in English and translated into German, to Dr Lurye of Kiev. These were dispatched by diplomatic bag along with a friendly letter asking to exchange observations:

Dear Professor Lurye:

Medical friends who have written to me from Switzerland and England inform me that you are using a method of natural childbirth based, from some of its aspects, upon the work of the great Russian physiologist, Ivan Pavlov.

I feel therefore that you will be interested to read a book that I published in 1942, *Childbirth Without Fear,* which has sold just under a quarter of a million copies. It has been translated into eight different languages and has been enthusiastically received wherever it has been adopted. And my investigations upon this subject were carried out for twenty years before my first book, *Natural Childbirth,* was published in 1933.

I enclose an English copy and a German translation together with a small practical manual, *Introduction to Motherhood,* that has been published in four countries. I have no doubt that most of your colleagues will be familiar with one or both of these languages.

It seems that there is still in this world one common denominator for all humanity – motherhood. Motherhood has occupied my attention for the last forty years of my professional life and this alone allows me the presumption of writing to you and sending you a work that may prove interesting to those about you.

I shall deem it a great honour if you will read these books and send me some literature published in Russia on modern obstetrics. Please accept as from one colleague in this great work to another my cordial greetings.

Yours sincerely.

I received neither thanks for the books nor acknowledgement of the letter, although it is certain that they arrived safely in Kiev, since they were dispatched through official diplomatic channels. When I inquired at the Russian Consulate they expressed surprise, but offered no explanation.

There is no doubt that those who heard the Russian exposition of their "new" work were struck first and foremost by the resemblance of the speeches at the 1951 Conference in Leningrad to previous published papers of my own, even to the measures adopted for the preparation of women for childbirth, which in the earlier stages of my work had no relation whatever to Pavlovian conditioning. In fact, Pavlov's book on conditioning did not appear until nearly fifteen years (1928) after my own work had begun, at which time I incorporated his explanation of conditioned reflexes, with due credit, as descriptive of what takes place through mental imagery.

Two years later, in 1953, I read a Russian claim that my work had been inspired by Ivan Pavlov but had not been a success! The only successful system of natural childbirth, it was asserted, had been evolved by Soviet scientists from the teachings of Ivan Pavlov.

In 1953 Dr Lamaze, who had been in Russia for six months to study their methods, started widespread publicity from the Metallurgic Hospital in Paris, claiming that the work he was doing was Pavlovian psychoprophylactic method. Visitors to his hospital again recognized the similarity in almost every way to the teaching that had been carried on in America and Britain for many years.

The truth is that the psychoprophylaxis of fear and pain in childbirth had already been discovered, published, taught, and used for nearly twenty years before the Soviet doctors realized its value and began to examine its principles. The Fear-Tension-Pain Syndrome has been the foundation of psychoprophylaxis and has proved its value in countries all over the world. Many have made small changes to suit their people and their climate, but only one country has claimed it as their own.

It is no concern of mine whether this general principle is applied with a hundred different variations, neither can I be concerned with the academic arguments of neurologists or neurophysiologists upon the functions of the brain. There is no end to their opinions. It has been my privilege to work with some of the greatest neurophysiologists of the last fifty years, but I have only come to the conclusion that they are uncertain of all the applied doctrines concerning the reception, integration, and interpretation of the afferent stimuli to the brain and the efferent messages from the brain to the periphery of the body. I speak of *human beings,* not machines made from *cerebrocentric reflex arcs.*

So long as the Fear-Tension-Pain Syndrome is broken down by safe and simple teaching and training, our purpose is served. It is a fact that a series of events takes place that, if disturbed at any level, results in the abnormality of severe pain. I look upon the claim, therefore, of the Communists to be one of ideological rather than medical importance. My sphere is to reduce the pains of labour, to take fear from childbirth, and to bring untarnished love into the homes of the people. My concern is for the betterment of childbirth, parenthood, and marriage, for happy families within the framework of our society, regardless of individual race, religion, or political creed.

This was made clear in my original publication in 1933 and has not changed since. Hundreds of thousands of women of all nationalities have breathed gratitude for the comfort and happiness this teaching brought to them. In 1951 the Russian physicians accepted the advantages of this principle, after two or three years of testing it in practice, and in 1953 it was propagated by Frenchmen, to whom I give all honour for their determination. In the *Revue de la Nouvelle Médécine* A. Bourrel writes of the "new" preparation of women, all the details of which had been used for years by others. Lamaze, Vellay, and Hersilie write on a technique of childbirth without pain that was an imitation so similar to that already published that in its initial stages visitors who observed it in practice saw nothing new. Angelergues, in seventeen hundred words, states that I don't know anything about childbirth, that I don't understand Pavlov's work, in fact that this man Read knows nothing about anything! He forgot to add, "That is why his work has revolutionised childbirth throughout the world, and also why the Communists have rescued him from the risk of his own ignorance."

But there is a serious aspect of this work as it is used in Russia. There are still great scientists who value, before all things, *truth*. This requires a freedom not always available. I am told that in the Soviet states a scientist must say and do what he is ordered to do by officials in high places. I also understand that there is another sort of scientific worker in the USSR, he who, in full knowledge of the truth, adheres to the universal principle of academic honesty and who, for his love of science, desires neither to deceive himself nor his colleagues. The true scientist will always exist, and he must be recognised as different from the one whose work is primarily designed to support, by all available means, the ideology of Communism. If this is compatible with truth, I have no quarrel. But if ideology is upheld at the expense of truth, work loses at once its scientific value and the workers are degraded.

The claims of original production and possession of innovations are effective means of establishing the greatness of an ideology and its leaders only where ignorance and fear prevent contradiction. For instance, we believe that Signor Marconi was an Italian and that Shakespeare was an Englishman and that Columbus discovered America. When, however, we learn that the discoverers were Russians, we cease to be surprised that Pavlov, without realising it, disclosed that psychoprophylaxis in childbirth is a means of relieving the pains of labour. Such nonsense is not taken seriously by educated people, and neither is it worthy of our attention. I have followed the writings of Pavlov for fifty years and, so far as it has been of value to physiology, I have admired it. But this hysterical effort to found a philosophy on his physiology is pathetic, particularly when much of his physiological concept is out of date.

But there is one basic principle of natural childbirth that Communism does not imitate, and in this way the Russians differ entirely from my teaching. They treat childbirth and motherhood as a *materialistic* and *mechanistic* performance with no spiritual association. The miracle of reproduction is distorted to become a means of demonstrating the absence of God and the omnipotence of the Communist leaders. Their teaching stops abruptly at that point where the spiritual associations of parenthood play such an important part. The benefits of their teaching on childbirth will be limited by the atheism and materialism of their ideology.

My teaching is exactly the opposite. I believe in the law of nature and a God-force. I do not accept man's limited understanding as all powerful; in fact, I am very conscious of the small fraction of total knowledge that is within the comprehension of man. To me, childbirth is a sacred event and brings humanity nearest to the spiritual and metaphysical world around it. It is a moment of emergence of new life with unknown potentialities.

When I see a baby born to a happy, healthy mother and witness the superhuman radiance that carries her to a new world of mystery and possession, I say to myself, "What sort of an idiot thinks he can make anything of this life without the hand of God to guide him?"

So, finally, there is no clinical difference between my teaching of natural childbirth and that claimed by the Russians in the early 1950s because there was no "new" Russian method, but only a Communist adaptation of a twenty-year-old teaching, distorted for atheistic, ideological purposes. That is where we differ. They teach antispiritual parenthood and the doctrine of mechanistic materialism. I teach the sacredness of childbirth as a spiritual event, the spiritual power of a mother's love, and faith in the truth of the law of nature, which to me is one of the great laws of God.

Ninety per cent of all civilized countries profess to some form of religious persuasion. Religious teaching calls for obedience to its codes, homage to the Creator, and loyalty to its spiritual and material purposes in the mother-child relationship. This factor knits in a common bond all the people of the world. I am not persuaded that the Communist ideology can destroy in so short a time the inborn devotion of a vast people to generations of religious faith. I believe that in time these naturally devout peoples who constitute the worker masses of the USSR will turn once more to the fervent faith of their forefathers.

Professor A.P. Nicolayev ends his lecture with the words of a Soviet woman after her labour: "I have no fear, I am happy, thanks to Soviet knowledge, thanks to Soviet doctors, thanks to the great friend of knowledge, our own comrade, Stalin."

I end my lecture: "Childbirth is a sacred subject, and I cannot be concerned with any who use it as merchandise to exploit it for personal gain, whether it be for money, social prestige, or political propaganda. I am neither the arbiter of your opinions nor partisan to your persuasions. I endeavour to raise before you the high level of loving homes and families through happy childbearing, for in the end it is the homes of the people that become the standard of a civilization."

United States Tour

When I returned to London from Africa, I no longer practiced medicine. I had passed the age when appointments on hospital staffs could be obtained, even had they been available. Under the present organisation of the medical health services in the British Isles, an age is fixed for retirement of physicians in order to make room for younger men.

During my years of practice and research in Africa it was not possible to accept lecture tours elsewhere, but on my return I began writing and lecturing again, in response to invitations throughout Europe. In the three years after my return from Africa I received a large number of invitations to speak in the United States again. So, at the beginning of October 1957, after completing a lecture tour in Germany, we made our way to the United States once more.

I had been invited by the Academy of Psychosomatic Medicine to speak at their Fourth Annual Meeting in Chicago, October 17th to 19th. This was a great occasion, for we learned in a short time what was taking place in the United States in regard to understanding the mind of women in childbirth, much of which had not been published in English medical journals.

Our host at the congress, Dr William Kroger, who was secretary of this occasion, met us as we arrived. We soon had a taste of the hospitality that was to be heaped upon us for the next three and a half months. During those months I was entertained by seventy different groups in the large cities and towns of the United States, as well as in several cities in Canada.

It was nearly eleven years since I had been in the United States. Everywhere we discovered some organisation flourishing for the education of women in natural childbirth. The interest extended to great universities as well. Preparation for childbirth has come to stay, and although it had still not been accepted by all the large hospitals, the demand of women for knowledge, and for more personal, humane care, is not to be denied. I had found the same rapidly improving conditions in Germany, Italy, France, the Scandinavian countries, Spain, Portugal, and the great countries of South America.

While here I was fortunate in having some extremely interesting conversations with the doctors of large hospitals. I remember one staff especially, where there were environmental differences in practice, but whose fundamental approach to childbirth was as near to the natural law as was possible under their present circumstances. I was taken into ward after ward and introduced to the women whose babies had recently arrived. I was greeted like an old friend and told without inhibition the details of their labours. My wife and I agreed it was a wonderful thing to happen to complete strangers.

One of our warmest memories is of our arrival in Seattle. It was, to say the least, unusual! Our seats were near the end of the train, so we were the last to follow the luggage cart down toward the station. These platforms are very long. After we had walked about a hundred yards toward the station we thought there must be some kind of school picnic, for a very large number of small children were waiting with some adults at the end of the platform. To our surprise, one of the ladies in charge walked toward us and stretched out her hand in greeting. She was the mother of four of the children. The other women were mothers of the other children.

Two very small girls carried a banner that said: "Welcome to Seattle," with my name printed underneath. As we approached, they set up a cheerleaders' shout: "We are Dick-Read babies!" I found it very difficult to know quite what expression to wear, but the spontaneous one was an amused smile, which crept over my face. Then, very solemnly, two other charming little girls walked forward to my wife and presented her with a beautiful bouquet. Then we all gathered around and had a good look at each other, with a lot of laughter. I told them it was the nicest thing I had ever seen.

On another part of our journey, while in Dallas, Texas, my eyes could hardly take in all that I saw in the great Neiman Marcus store. Although appreciating the elegance and art that was so obviously and beautifully displayed, I found myself wondering how long I could live in comfort, without working, for the amount it would cost me to buy my wife just those things I felt sure she would enjoy wearing.

The morning went all too quickly. As we left, our taxi driver threw away three inches of a Havana cigar, which smelled excellent to me. Then he opened the box on the seat beside him and produced another one, a good six inches long, which he lit as though it were his duty rather than his pleasure. Again I began, in a very English way, to wonder how much it would cost me at home to buy a box of fifty of those cigars. Although I had given up smoking some time ago, I used to be a cigar smoker, and Havana cigars are really good. For a moment I dreamed and, in the clouds, so tender to my nostrils, worlds long forgotten formed. I sighed and my wife said, "Isn't it beautiful?" "Indeed it is,"

I replied. She was referring to an expensive coat, and I to an aroma!

We were in Las Vegas only a short time, fortunately, just long enough to see a little of its gaudy illuminations and mechanical decorations, and people standing for hours pulling handles. It seemed to be a place where nakedness was in great demand – postcards, boxes of chocolates, flags, toys, books, and even chocolate bars all seemed to come as close as possible to presenting a naked man or woman. I suppose it is reasonable that a doctor in his late sixties should look upon this approach to life as rather unnecessary and not a little boring, and we were not sorry to get back on the plane.

Another experience that left an unpleasant memory occurred as our hostess drove us through a beautiful mountain range. Although the trees on its slopes had no leaves on them, we could envision them covered with foliage all the way down to the river below. But there we saw vast booms of logs, like enormous water lilies on phantom lakes, gradually moving downstream, on their way to finish life in a pulp factory.

Since I was a small boy, I have never been pleased to see trees cut down, which may be associated with the respect I have always had for anything that lives. To see a tree falling to the axe seemed like murder to me, and I wondered how the pain it must have suffered was interpreted. I was told there was still enough wood to go on cutting more than man could need for a hundred years, by which time the new wood itself would have grown up to continue the supply, yet I could not help being reminded of an occasion when my wife and I were in East Africa. We had been down the Crocodile River, more sightseeing than anything else, when we came upon two large trucks pulled up by the roadside. In a variety of uniforms and weird outfits, about a dozen or more young men were strolling along carrying rifles. We looked at the trucks and saw they were piled high with impala deer, beautiful little creatures that had apparently been herded up, driven together, then shot and carted off in that way. Little white tails, or beautiful antlers, hung over the end of the trucks. Somehow it was a shock to me that men could go out and kill hundreds on one safari and then take them back to be skinned, their flesh dried and sold. It isn't for one moment that I would suggest this wasn't reasonable, because life very largely lives upon life, and yet we need to be more careful not to entirely destroy our associations with all that is beautiful.

During one of my lectures I was asked to tell about my experiences while on safari in the Central Congo, Northern Uganda, and other places where the white man has not yet exerted any influence upon the childbirth customs of the tribes. I gave a short outline of the information we had gleaned and, so far as possible, the factors common to the two hundred-odd tribes and subtribes we had visited. I tried to put these observations in terms of physiology, and the manner in which the birth function was carried out both emotionally and physically in terms of the religious and social rites of the various peoples. In terms of pagan religions, the laws of the gods saw childbirth as the greatest gift of woman, and her happiest accomplishment.

I drew attention to the fact that I was not discussing the abnormalities that arose in 2, 3, or 4 per cent of the women – who died unless they were rushed to some European hospital maybe a hundred, two hundred, or three hundred miles through the jungle – but was giving my observations upon normal and uncomplicated labour, which represented well over 90 per cent of all births.

This we had seen when we were given the privilege of studying the analogy of the white races and the black in the minds and hearts of women. In Africa we often witnessed the natural law of reproduction with its love and its magnificence.

I was surprised when a man who was not even on the staff of the hospital where I was speaking stood up, looking very angry, for this was unusual in my discussions in America. He firmly exclaimed to me that I had no right whatever to compare them – that is, the people of his area – with these "goddamned savages," for, he said, "We are not animals!"

That was, of course, a challenging remark, for whatever else the human being may be, he does remain an animal, par excellence, and his primarily biological reactions, whatever his colour, are those of reproduction and maintenance. For my own part, I can discover no satisfactory evidence of alteration of forces or function in the reproductive equipment of *genus homo,* whether red, brown, black, white, yellow, or American.

The doctor's remark surprised me because, speaking generally, I had not heard these views expressed in public since I had been in the United States of America. This was obviously a sore point, upon which I had inadvertently trodden for the first time, but I did not feel either the person or his dogmatic assertions demanded a serious reception upon this occasion.

I replied, "You have me at a disadvantage, sir, for I would not dream of comparing my hosts and the people of this state with either 'goddamned savages' or human beings who are *not* animals, because I do not know of such specimens. I have never, in all my travels, come across any goddamned savages. In fact, I doubt if they exist, even in the most pagan tribes. I know only too well the white-damned blacks. Perhaps you refer to them? If so, I agree with you. Our lot in life is not comparable to theirs any more than mine is comparable to yours, if you are not animal."

One of the greatest joys during our long tour of America was the opportunity, on occasions like this, to gather as medical people and colleagues for discussion over a drink or at lunch, or after touring a hospital. There was no asperity in our discussions, or an absence of humour. We were earnest and thoughtful; we agreed and differed. I would not have missed one moment of that three and a half months that enabled us to exchange opinions and expose our respective ideas to analysis and dissection.

Any English doctor making a tour of the American hospitals will be struck by the luxury and magnificence of these modern buildings. I became more and more impressed with the meticulous care that had been taken to provide every possible accessory to comfort and convenience in the newer structures. The organization and equipment for the feeding of patients and staff would have left nothing to be desired in a most expensive first-class hotel. I found it difficult to decide whether I was ashamed of the English hospitals or whether I felt sympathy for the people of England that they did not have enough money to supply them with buildings adequately equipped and comfortable.

On the other hand, I often felt that the English women were much better off, particularly in regard to obstetrics. In one magnificent new hospital I was brought into a ward of twenty beds in the obstetric unit called the recovery room. It was here that women who had had their babies were put until they recovered consciousness or had settled down safely from the unnatural interferences to which the majority had been subjected at the deliveries of their normal, healthy babies. There was a special nursing staff for this recovery room, and it was not unnatural that I wondered what they were recovering from, and why there should be such a large place organised for that particular purpose. Did American women, having borne a baby, have to go through a stage of recovery requiring so much specialised attention? It was certainly not so in other countries, except in rare and complicated cases.

I noticed that over each of the beds there was a tap that supplied oxygen, this gas being available through tubes and pipes just as gas for a stove might be, or the electrical wiring for a building. I was directed to notice its proximity to the blood bank; every new mother was as near as possible to grouped blood, stored ready for transfusion should it be required. I was interested to hear that quite a number of patients did have blood transfusions, the number varying considerably in different hospitals, depending on the obstetric routine and the clinical opinion of the attendants.

We went on to a special ward for newborn babies, where they were immediately put into an oxygen tent for one hour, whether they were healthy or not, whether they were born with interference or without. Their first duty of life, impressed on them by the hospital authorities, was that they should spend their first hour of extrauterine existence in an oxygen tent. They were not allowed the security of mother's arms or the warmth of her body, but were placed all alone in an unnatural gas, water, and air mixture (40 per cent oxygen, 75-80° Fahrenheit, approximately 70 per cent humidity), as a psychological boost into a new life! I wondered why one hour in an oxygen tent, with a higher percentage of oxygen in the breathed air than they had been accustomed to in the placental blood, was more advantageous than lying in the arms of a healthy mother, experiencing from the moment of birth the security and warmth that are the natural heritages of a newborn child.

I passed on to a laboratory near to the babies' nurseries whose function, at first, I did not understand. Then I was told it was the milk bank, where the paediatricians came to write the formulas for the milk of each baby, because it was unusual for a woman to feed her baby from the breast. The organisation of the milk bank was made quite clear to me – it was magnificently done, and had women not been born with breasts at all, I can't imagine anything that would have been more efficient.

I learned that when a woman was admitted to the hospital, she was put into a labour room and prepared for the birth by being washed and given an enema and a shave, and was then immediately given a "shot." I asked what the "shot" was and was told it was an injection given as routine when women came into the hospital. They were usually rather anxious, and this helped to calm them down before labour progressed too far. A nurse was in attendance and, from time to time, made the rounds of the labour rooms to see how the women were getting on. The nurses were advised not to answer any questions a woman asked, but simply to tell her to be patient. She was given medicine, usually atropine by injection and 100 to 150 milligrams of Demerol, when the stresses increased, usually at about three-fifths dilatation of the cervix. Some of the staff preferred to give Demerol and hyacine, sometimes combined with a dose of nembutol. It was impressed upon me that no patient who did not wish for medication was forced to have it. It was pointed out, however, that it was highly unlikely that a woman would refuse, even though she was not having much physical pain.

The difficulty is that if she is given 100 to 150 milligrams of Demerol she will react, like so many women, in a manner that *lowers her discretion and intensifies,* to a large extent, *a negative emotional attitude* toward her labour activities. If she is given hyacine, there is no doubt her discretional sense will be partly or entirely destroyed.

As we passed the labour ward, I heard two women cry out. How well I knew that horrifying noise. One woman was particularly uncontrolled; she was terrified, and only in pain because she was trying to overcome her discomfort by resisting it. The thought went through my mind, 'Can't she be told how to stop making it painful for herself? Hasn't she been told how to breathe?' Similar thoughts always pass through my mind when I hear a woman distressed in early labour. But I knew these women were only semiconscious; a routine sedative had already been given, and they could not help themselves.

We moved on into the most immaculate changing room, where I was told the patients' attendants put on sterile garments before they delivered a woman. Nearby was a room where obstetricians rested while waiting for a child to be born. This was fitted with cupboards and closets for clothes, with a beautifully tiled and decorated washroom and shower.

I was then shown into an anteroom that contained a vast supply of instruments in glass cases, visible to all who might pass by, including the patients. There were hoards of drugs in capsules, vials, and bottles, in test tubes and mysterious boxes, all ready for immediate exhibition should occasion be deemed to have arisen. There were syringes and needles for all manner of analgesic and anesthetic injections; some were given to desensitize the whole woman and others for different areas and parts of the woman. Some robbed her of consciousness and others of discretion. It seemed there was no possibility of an emergency arising that could not be dealt with immediately, but there was *no provision for the absence of emergency or abnormality.* I was told it did not happen!

I felt that I was in the general atmosphere of a great nation, *so efficiently equipped for war under the pious persuasion of self-preservation and peace that war became almost inevitable.* In fact, the thinking seemed to be that it would be a shame to have had so much money spent without putting the equipment to use, even though this meant misusing it. Those of us who have seen three wars no longer think of that. We find the mind of man today has so reached a comprehension of the physical world that it gives him power to destroy the human race. Man tends to shrink from the belief that there is a force greater than he. There is a trend in American obstetrics toward an element of servitude to mechanisation and the materialisation of childbirth and motherhood. But man, however brilliant, has no right to assume command of the ship of human destiny before he even knows its purpose.

I believe there is an Omnipotence that makes our presence here purposeful. I cannot understand it, but I have only to look at the ordered brilliance of natural phenomena to seek some explanation of these mysteries in creative genius which are still beyond the comprehension of man. I am never without a sense of awe, no matter how many hundreds, thousands of babies now, I have seen into the world. I experience a sense of awe at the magnificence of the physical and emotional perfection of a woman when she takes her child into her arms and knows at last she has received the gift of God for which she has so earnestly prepared. Surely prevention is better than cure?

Women have written to me of their experiences of being tied down to the table, their limbs fixed, their faces buried in a mask against their wishes, their bodies cut although there was plenty of room for the child to pass, and their infants pulled into the world by instruments in the manner that Soranus of Ephesus said should never be, for force should never be used to empty the womb.

Here in this place I was seeing it for myself. I looked at everything. By this time we had reached the delivery area. The delivery table was an astonishing mechanical contrivance upon which I understood women were pilloried so that, without resistance, all sensations, pleasant and unpleasant, could be taken from them. Consciousness was retained in some cases, but the sensations of birth were thought to be extremely painful and thus deleted.

I found on this stainless-steel and chromium-plated table a variety of pedals and handles that swung, tilted, raised, lifted, and dropped all parts and parcels of the contraption. There were rests in which a woman's legs were fixed so that she could neither move nor use them. Her body lay flat, with her head on the same level as her buttocks, reducing, almost minimizing, the mechanical advantages of the distribution and attachment of the muscles of expulsion. At the sides of the table, just about level with her hipbones, were strong metal fixtures through which saddle-leather straps and buckles passed. I asked if these were still used, having remembered that some obstetricians had discarded them, but learned that strapping down of the hands was routine practice. Every woman's hands were restrained so that she was unable to move her arms while her child was being expelled through the birth canal, or while the surgeon was removing it with instruments from the pelvic outlet, which had been operated on and had to be repaired with stitches. At the upper end of the table there were similar sockets through which straps could pass to fix not only the shoulders but, if necessary, the head of the patient, who might possibly, in her dazed condition, resist complete unconsciousness because she wished to be awake enough to see and greet her baby.

I asked my host whether a woman was conscious of the indignity of giving birth in this way, when she finds herself immobile upon the machine called a bed, fully aware of her position, her immobilisation, and her exposure. My friend replied that he thought women were completely satisfied with the situation, and also commented that it made the job much easier for him. He could desensitise the whole woman or any part of her. Her position on the delivery table had nothing to do with it, so long as she escaped the agonies.

I don't wish to make my comments in any sense a satire. Rather, it is with astonishment that I wonder how such things can still be found as representing the most modern of all advances in childbearing. This vast expenditure, plan, and provision was, to me, a major condemnation of the creative genius. I had a picture of mere man, swathed in green and white masks, caps, gowns, and maybe boots, telling the Almighty it was just too bad He did not know His job. It was a good thing man was there to do it for Him. I had seen all this before, and it hurt.

I was given a gown and mask to put on and taken to observe a delivery. A young and beautiful girl was lying flat on the delivery table, her head resting on a small rubber pillow. Her legs were strapped into deeply guttered supports, and widely opened; her wrists were strapped in padded cuffs, which were attached to the table. She was still and quiet, with her eyes shut, until a contraction came. Then she opened her eyes and looked at the nurse standing beside her. It was an impersonal look received with an impersonal look. I should have preferred a faint smile or a gentle pat on the girl's arm.

The attending doctor sat on the stool between his "victim's" feet, which were on the level of his head. He looked over his shoulder and nodded to a nurse, who wheeled forward a table on which was an array of surgical and obstetric instruments covered by a sterile towel. He looked up at his professor, who was beside him, silently observing.

"She is quite normal, sir, and a pretty quick labour. She is fully dilated now, so I will get the baby. It is not big."

As he said that, he made a deep cut with a pair of scissors, about an inch and a half downward and outward, as if cutting into the centre of the clock face down to seven o'clock on the dial. I turned to follow my host, who led the way out of the delivery room. Perhaps by some strange transference, he felt my feelings and guessed my thoughts correctly.

The day after this exhibition of kindness by incarceration, I happened to see, in a daily paper, a picture presented, along with a number of letters of remonstrance, that was intended to call attention to the dastardly cruelty of the Russians, the most unjustifiable desecration of life, human or otherwise, flaunted under the name of science. It was a picture of the passenger the Russians had the day before sent into space aboard a rocket – a small dog, depicted with a most benign, self-sacrificing expression on its face as it lay there, its hind legs tied down and its forepaws fixed in straps; it was manacled and shackled but supplied with artificial food and adequate oxygen. This, the fear-inducing illustration of ultimate cruelty, was thrust under my nose by a very good obstetrician and personal friend of mine, with the sort of look on his face that said, "Now, how about that?"

I am, above all things, an animal lover, and sometimes would rather see chastisement administered to a naughty teenager than to a helpless animal, but instead of rising up in my wrath I found it very difficult to suppress the most unwelcome grin that threatened to show itself on my face. For when I heard the words "ultimate cruelty," I thought immediately of the woman I had seen the day before, her legs immobilised by straps, her hands strapped down, a band across her forehead so that she could not move her head and so that she could be given an anaesthetic without being allowed to turn away. I saw by her side and all around her oxygen apparatus and food for reinforcement of nutrition, should her metabolism require support. She was helpless, placed there in order to accept the tenets of science in the name of humanity. She had become an experimental piece in the hands of a scientist, and at any moment might be shot in part or in toto into the outer space of unconsciousness.

I could not help seeing a perfectly straightforward simile. I realised the indignity, indeed the cruelty that women should be robbed of the greatest natural achievement, the reward of happiness that has been provided by the physiological law. This experience, if properly prepared and conducted by an understanding attendant, could influence not only her own life but that of her husband and newborn baby, and therefore, in time, the social circle in which we live.

We need to ask again, what is the underlying purpose? What is the biological objective of the reproductive faculty? What are we breeding for at all? Those of us who look after women bearing children must realise that every newborn child may be a potential leader of mankind. Our responsibility goes even further, for we need to be making good mothers while we make babies, in order to make a society worthy of a progressive culture. Are we going to allow our cultural desires to take us down to a level below that of our fathers and forefathers? It is our job to cultivate the stock of tomorrow.

Is the United States willing to accept the long-term results of the substitution of materialism for the metaphysical, the eternal or everlasting? The people of New York reacted strongly when the Russians put their first satellite in orbit. There was a feeling that they had suffered loss of "face," but what went through my mind was, 'Does this great people realize the astuteness of the Russians in adopting the use of procedures of natural childbirth?'

In many of the hospitals I visited, I was confused and baffled by the passion for interference with a healthy natural function. Again and again I heard of: episiotomies, 100 per cent; forceps, 50 to 75 per cent; induction by appointment, up to 70 per cent in some places. The high rate of forceps deliveries came as a shock to me. In most countries the forceps rate is between 5 and 8 per cent. When, therefore, I was told that forceps were used in up to 75 per cent of deliveries in some hospitals, I at once sought justification for this high figure. Such a percentage in a hospital in England or any of the European countries I have visited would call for an inquiry. I soon learned that a school of thought that had considerable following in the United States believed that the only safe method of delivery was by forceps operation. This necessitated some form of general or local anaesthetic and, of course, an episiotomy. Childbirth became a surgical performance.

I looked up statistics published by several hospitals, and found that one of the most famous ones had published tables representing the percentage of forceps deliveries of all cases in the hospital for the years stated:

Year	Clinic	Private
1954	17.5%	50.9%
1955	21.4%	46.0%
1956	18.7%	42.4%

Two questions arose in my mind. Why was the forceps rate of the white, brown, and black clinic population so much lower than for white private patients whose fees were higher? Anatomically and obstetrically, private patients do not present variations that require more help or more interference, unless their "higher intelligence" made it more difficult for them to accept the natural law. The attendant factor seemed to be an influence in this case – what was it? I made some inquiries, but received no satisfactory reply.

The operation of episiotomy is another example of routine interference, without clinical indication, without consideration of its causes or prevention. In many of the hospitals I visited I find that episiotomy is considered to be a necessary routine operation and, what has astonished me even more, that students are taught it is dangerous to deliver a child without cutting the outlet of the birth canal.

Like many other phenomena of childbirth, the cause of the tight outlet has never been carefully investigated. We are told the birth canal is tight, small, or that the head is large, in the wrong position, and so on, but when I asked, "*Why* is this?" the answer has usually been, "Well, because it is." That is all that can be said about the causation of something that is obviously abnormal or pathological.

There are recognised conditions that demand this operation. In England we generally consider there are eight indications, which I need not go into now. They are quite definite, easily diagnosable, and, for one who is not sufficiently experienced to rely entirely upon his or her own judgment, make a very suitable list of the indications upon which to base practical application. But when it comes to results, I must say it is quite extraordinary.

In a large modern textbook I have read that episiotomy is a highly prophylactic operation because it prevents prolapse of the womb, incontinence of urine, undoubtedly prevents stillbirth of the child in some cases, and most certainly prevents the after effects of infantile cerebral haemorrhage.

I suggest that the operation of episiotomy could not possibly prevent all these complications and sequelae of labour! The damage causing these conditions is sustained *before* the head of the baby reaches the perineum. In 90 per cent of healthy women attended by competent obstetricians the mutilation of episiotomy is unnecessary.

At this point in one of my lectures one of the senior members of the hospital staff rose quietly and said, "But have you forgotten so much that must be taken into account? Episiotomy shortens labour, which is good for the baby and the mother. It prevents tears and is a clean incision which is much easier to repair than a tear that may be jagged and rough-edged. We find, too, that it relieves the pressure on the baby's head, and it obviously cannot be good for a child to be pressed down on to that rigid perineum, drawn up and pressed down again, like a battering ram." At this, there were several nods of approval.

I asked him whether he had any idea how often he had seen a truly elastic perineum which stretched easily and large enough to allow the biggest of babies to pass without any trouble or tearing. He said he didn't remember having seen one like that because he never allowed them to get to that stage. I thought this was a very good reply, and I went on:

"May I assure you that episiotomy may shorten labour by five to ten minutes if it is performed at the right moment. But it is not good for the mother, and I am not persuaded it is good for the baby in the absence of obvious tensions. I am surprised you believe tears to be unavoidable because they are not, even in a primipara. Care must be taken and patient delivery understood and performed. The battering ram analogy amuses me. Sometimes it is 'ewe.' "

Then a delightfully suave little man almost leaped to his feet. He said, "But surely, sir, we ought to know. We deliver enough, and there is no doubt about it – in this part of the United States the heads of babies are much bigger than they used to be, and there is no reason to believe that women have grown proportionately larger at the outlet."

I could not resist it, and said, "So you really feel, doctor, that in this particular state some social factor has placed your women in a position of disadvantage in relation to the production of your children and your children's children? How do you account for that? Do you accept the law of Julius Wolfe, 'structure is adapted to function'?"

Then he suggested, "Well, as the brain becomes more developed, I think it is possible that the head gets bigger!"

There was a good, cheerful laugh all around the room at this ambitious concept of development, and I added, "I am not sure I could possibly provide evidence to show that you are wrong, but I have no evidence to persuade me that the youth of this great country become swollen-headed before they are born!" Fortunately this little pleasantry was kindly taken.

Whereupon my friend the professor explained, "Episiotomy is not actually performed 100 per cent of the time, but only about 97 per cent of the time here. About three women in every hundred have their babies before the attendant has time to give the anaesthetic and perform the episiotomy."

As we discussed the condition more seriously, I pointed out that the general rigidity of the birth canal has little to do with the physical condition of the woman, but varies according to her *mental* state. We went into the question of the neurology and the protective resistance and even spasm that could occur in a frightened woman. It was also realised that if a woman had a certain type of anaesthesia she could be unconscious before the influence of fear was entirely absent, so that the perineum would remain tense.

Some forms of local anaesthesia, such as epidural injections, undoubtedly assist in the relaxation of the perineum, and the professor of one large university hospital told me that since he had used that particular measure he found the necessity for episiotomy was not so general. In fact, using the epidural, he was now doing only 65 to 70 per cent episiotomies rather than his routine of 100 per cent with other forms of anesthesia.

We discussed the position in which women were delivered, the details of the delivery of the child, and the behaviour of the mother at that time. I was surprised to find that children were not received from the mother's body in the normal physiological direction, up and over the front of her body. Nature intended every mother to take her own baby and hold it up to herself as soon as it came into the world. I was able to demonstrate easily, on a blackboard, what a large number of unnecessary tears occur because of the baby being pulled straight out from the mother.

"But," I went on, "allowing for all these details of the study of the delivery of the child, there are still a number of factors which must come into it. One is the experience which enables you to know when it is necessary to do an episiotomy in order to prevent a tear."

What impressed me about this delightful conversation was how very little some of the senior men appeared to understand the detailed mechanism of this important part of labour. One oft-repeated notion was that no woman could possibly have a baby pass through the outlet of the birth canal without a terrible pain. They taught this and believed it, so much so that if a woman did have her baby without unbearable discomfort, she was looked upon as a pathological or abnormal person. In fact, when it occurred, students were usually asked to go in and talk to her about it.

I pointed out once more that, from my experience and that of many other obstetricians who followed the antenatal education accurately and delivered according to the procedures of natural childbirth, more than 90 per cent of women did not desire or require any cutting to enlarge the outlet. Occasionally, if the *fourchette*, the little membrane that seems to guard the back of the outlet, bursts early, one must be alert to the possible need of an episiotomy.

But it is not fully realized what a tremendous impact episiotomy has on the minds of a large number of sensitive women. It is not a thing that is discussed freely. But owing to the fact that I have not been a gynaecologist only, or just an obstetrician, but have had the privilege of being a general practitioner of women's ailments of mind and behaviour as well as body, I have become aware of several matters of great interest and importance.

One is that, after episiotomy, quite a definite percentage of women have developed frigidity. I have met many who were perfectly happy in married life until after their first baby was born, when they suddenly felt a deprivation of their virginal perfection. Tumescence ceased to occur and desire became much less importunate. Both husbands and young wives, happy with their babies of six or eight months old, have been to see me to ask why it is that orgasm has deserted the wife. The husband feels that she no longer loves him, and she feels horrified that such a thing could happen when they had been so happy.

If carefully examined, the condition is usually found to be primarily a mixture of physical effects and a psychological sense of deprivation and injury. These young women have suffered birth trauma. This may be a hard thing for gynaecologists to understand, for the episiotomy seems so simple, so effective, so free of danger. Yet many women have told me, "Ever since I found it was sore to sit down for a few days after my baby was born, I felt something had happened to me that could never come right again. I seemed to lose all pride in that part of my body and didn't know whether to be ashamed of myself, angry with the baby, or just apologetic to my husband."

"A dreadful state," one woman told me, "and when I went to see my doctor about it, all he said was, 'Don't be silly!' "

Even if the damage is only in the woman's mind – her self-image as a sexual being – the effect may be as irreparable. That part of her body which, deep down in her consciousness, has meant so much because of its effectiveness and perfection, is now no longer as presentable to her man-lover as it was previously. The most secret gift to her husband's love was tarnished by her baby's arrival.

I emphasise this because it is an example of the repercussions of interference with a physiological function and the normal laws of nature of which we are not always aware. We must bear in mind the possibility of emotional disturbances in a woman's mind, below the levels of rational thought, from events that are commonplace to us. I can't emphasise this enough.

When I got into the car to be driven back to the hotel at which I was staying, my mind turned to the women in the large Dutch hospitals, and in some of the Italian hospitals, and I thought how relatively unusual it is for the doctors there to interfere with a healthy, normal birth. I wondered whether there was a closer understanding of women and their thoughts and feelings in some countries than in others. Naturally I at once thought of the native tribes of the Central Congo, and of that wonderful old midwife in Buganda who came to see me with the local government medical officer. He assured me that to his knowledge she never had tears except in grossly abnormal cases. "How in the world does she do it?" I asked him, and he replied, "She is a child of nature and understands it from A to Z, and she has had fifteen babies herself!"

My visits to other hospitals seemed to be arranged as a salve to my injured obstetric conscience. In Cleveland, Cedar Rapids, Buffalo, Milwaukee, Seattle, New York, Denver, Santa Fe, and many other large towns I found groups or even whole hospitals that had turned away from the mechanistic orgy of sensate materialism. Here women were being educated and trained, made adequate in mind and body to carry out the programmes required by the laws of nature. Everywhere I was told of decreased operative deliveries and a lowered rate of stillbirth and neonatal deaths. There was no maternal morbidity attributable to childbirth, very few blood transfusions were required, and childbirth was approached by women without fear or anxiety for its outcome. A father remarked how everyone at the hospital where his child was born had put him at ease. He described it as a hospital for human, friendly, family-centred care. Another father commented by saying, "I can't say enough about the most loving, kind, and wonderful care." That atmosphere was combined with obviously first-class obstetric work. Thus as I travelled from place to place I found one or the other approach to childbirth, but with the "natural" spreading rapidly.

We learned many things about the Americans that helped us to understand some of their motives and behaviours. When people ask me, "What do you think of Americans?" I say, "Which Americans? From what point of view? Give me a more definite question and I will tell you if I have any experience upon which to give an opinion." We found so little common to all the states, but there were some things that were invariable – the kindliness and thought for its visitors.

Finally my conversations ceased, but I had no desire to leave. There was much I did not want to lose and so many I would miss. And I was conscious of an aching fear that one gets for the safety of a friend in danger! I wanted to stand up and shout: "For goodness sake, look to your production plants! The repair depots will take care of themselves."

In Conclusion

As this imperfect collection of observations is concluded, it may well be asked of me, "Why have you written this book?" There is no more exacting task and no occupation more thankless than the public expression of heretical views. It has been many years since I published my first series of observations and outlined the theory and practice of natural childbirth. That teaching has borne much fruit, and so I write more fully, hoping, not without justification, that more of my medical brethren may be persuaded to give this method fair and prolonged trial. I am not prompted by missionary zeal that seeks to proselytise the obstetric world, but only to invite attention to bare and irrefutable facts.

It is primarily to the youth of our profession that I appeal: to those who have just qualified and to those who are about to qualify. It is for you to join in the battle against pain. Each one of you has it within his or her power to observe carefully the phenomena of labour; each one of you has the birth-right of investigation. Do not accept the conservative teaching of generations past without careful examination. For the most part, such teaching will stand scrutiny and will be proved correct in general principle. But from time to time you will be amazed at the inadequacy of the evidence upon which accepted principles are borne. Be critical of culture; look long and carefully before you accept its tenets; take notice of the subtle way and means by which youth is robbed of its power and its instinctive genius. Be accurate in your deductions, and delve deeply into the details of each succeeding problem. Analyse your observations, and do not be slow to ask: "Why?" Develop an inquiring mind; seek guidance and advice while you have around you those competent and willing to help you. There is no reason to be humble in your questioning, and certainly no justification for aggression in your differing. Learn from your mistakes, for if you seek the truth honestly, the errors that you make will be of service in your search. As you scramble from one pitfall to the next, you will gain strength and experience. The borderlands of the realm of knowledge are shrouded in a mist that is not penetrated by the earliest efforts of the beginner. As each person gains a greater foothold within those realms, so the mist clears, until he or she finds the vista of unending possibility, the existence of which had not previously been envisaged. There is no such thing as knowing all. Cowper wrote:

> *Knowledge is proud that he has learned so much,*
> *Wisdom is humble that he knows no more.*

If, therefore, you feel humble because of your limited accomplishments, recognize that in humility alone lies the true urge and goad to further progress. Let your practice be founded upon the judgment of the intelligent, and your reputation upon the honest opinion of those who are in the best position to judge. Above all, your own personal satisfaction will raise you to a different plane; your work will be in a different cause; you will not be numbered among the "Gehazis who seek only money." Your belief is not in today, but rather in tomorrow and those distant tomorrows which will bring nearer to man his ultimate knowledge. Your faith is in the law of nature; your science is to be an adjuvant and not an impediment in its implementation.

But medicine is a science of opinion, and opinions differ, not only in diagnosis and treatment but in philosophy and ideals. In obstetrics you must form your own philosophy without fear, and observe with equanimity the ideals of those about you.

The privilege of attending women in childbirth is far greater than you are taught to realize. The public applauds the genius of skilled surgeons; famous physicians are beloved and respected for their healing power; great gynaecologists are both surgeons and physicians within a limited field. Their lives are given up to the noble work of succoring the sick, curing the diseased, and mending the broken.

The casualties of living are the first call of the medical profession. But obstetricians do not work among casualties; their work is primarily among the supremely healthy members of the community. They watch over and improve original models from the great factories of human life; their responsibility is to improve the stock and render it fit to meet the new demands that modern communal existence makes upon each succeeding generation. The health of mothers and their babies should be the first consideration of an obstetrician.

You must make your choice now, and to your innermost self lay down the principles upon which your future will unfold. There are many paths leading to the rock of a physician's calling. Along the well-worn roads thousands pass, blindly following the lead of orthodoxy, pushing and jostling in a throng that steadily advances with the years to a comfortable plateau called Mediocrity. Here people gird themselves with mental and material armor, and search the descent to old age for respectable nooks and crannies where they may rest and watch the sun go down. It is possible to decorate a well-selected niche with an accolade, so that those who pass by may whisper to their friends, "Behold!"

There are also the untrodden paths that require not only youth, but freedom and fortitude. Those of you who seek a new truth must blaze a trail of your own. The jewels of our science lie off the beaten track. Press on in danger; with the risk of failure you have the urge to persevere. You will clamber among landmarks accepted by your forebears as immutable. Accept nothing, for under each established fact is the foundation of a new future. Gold is hidden in the solid vein of quartz. Climb alone up the precipice that leads to no plateau, but only to high peaks from which you can look down and see the truth you have uncovered on your way. You need no social armour in your isolation, need seek no comfortable haven of rest: sharpen your ax, respike your shoes, and struggle on, conscious always of the vision of youth, guided by the hand of experience to a greater reward than public recognition.

Pioneers pass on unheard and unlamented until the trail they blazed is followed by a few who have believed. At the end they are discovered where their life's work finished, mourned only by the wildflowers of the wilderness they loved.

Epilogue: Pioneers Pass On by Jessica Dick-Read

Childbirth Without Fear has had an indelible impact upon the world as far back as 1933, when the subject first appeared in England under the title *Natural Childbirth*. In 1942 *The Revelation of Childbirth* brought a "gleam" of sanity to a country locked in the deadly combat of World War Two. With so many dying in warfare, Dick's work brought promise of a happier rebirth.

In 1944, born of "The House of Harper," *Childbirth Without Fear* was offered to the women of America, still in a period when our very future as a human race was so sadly blurred by man's inhumanity to man. Dick's poignant message gave courage to those women who believed they were being denied their right – the right to fulfill their proudly cherished heritage of giving birth in surroundings of kindness, dignity, and peace.

The war ended, and with its passing women the world over heard that "call from out of the wilderness," and responded. Now, mainly through Dick's freeing childbirth from ugly and ignorant concepts, once again women everywhere can give birth more wisely, with their personal dignity restored.

To all potential mothers I can but simply say, he was *great*. I am proud not only to have been a beloved wife but also to have been at his side as, in the face of many conflicts, he introduced many through his teaching and guidance to the loveliness and truth that is childbirth.

To me, *Childbirth Without Fear* still remains Dick's "living" work. Some have asked whether he died a disappointed man. No, he certainly did not, though he was very tired due to the strain imposed by many tours and his determination, in writings and lectures, to exert all efforts in behalf of safer, kinder obstetrics. But he strongly believed that a light was beginning to glimmer among many of his profession who were at least attempting to put into practice the efficacy of natural childbirth. From my heart I say that I know that, though he never lived to see the full flowering of his great work, he died content in the knowledge of having tendered and nourished a "late" budding.

During mid-1955 Dick suffered his first fairly serious heart attack, and another during a tour in Europe the following year. But he continued his work, and came ahead to the United States and Canada in late 1957 for a lecture tour. A third heart attack occurred on this tour, while he was lecturing in Toronto in 1958.

Ironically, it was not a heart attack, as we feared might happen, that took his life. In January of 1959 a different kind of attack, a cerebral haemorrhage, occurred. After a few days' rest Dick again made one of his vital recoveries, and, quite truly, one could not believe that he had suffered in any way. But the second attack of that kind came soon after Easter. Dick was hospitalised for observation, in his old hospital, the London, in Whitechapel. Fortunately, his illness was short lived. When the end was considered by his doctor to be but a matter of hours, Dick looked up at me and said, "Home, Lovey."

With all speed I made arrangements to get him back to our home in Norfolk, and he lived for another nine days, happy, conscious, and content in the knowledge of being among those who loved him so. Toward the end his speech was gone, but through his eyes he continued to register and express that wonderful humanity and intelligence which I am unable to find words to define. His passing was peaceful, and as in 1942 when he held his beloved mother's hand as she crossed the threshold, I held his, and so the link remains unbroken.

Index

19th century impact on today's childbirth experiences 4–5

abdominal supporting belts 229
abnormal labours
  emergency childbirth 179–184
  obstetrics focuses on 86, 131, 172, 217
  as one of Dick-Reads three categories 133–34, 173
Abraham, Dr Johnston 292, 294
Adler, H. 79
African tribes, birth in 308–12
alcohol in pregnancy 105
all-fours, human physiology based on 198, 226
amnesiac state/ dulled consciousness in second stage labour 119–120, 176, 182
anaemia 40–41, 110
anaesthesia and analgesia *see also specific analgesics/ anaesthetics*
  'anaesthesia for all' (failed UK parliamentary bill) 8, 141, 143
  availability for all women (Dick-Read's principle of) 132, 133, 137–39, 147–48
  cannot overcome effects of fear 38
  and Christianity 5, 76
  contra-indications, summary of 147
  and crowning 124
  an educated and controlled mind is the best anaesthetic 146
  education about 146, 225, 227, 260–61
  effect on breastfeeding 191–92
  fear of pain drives women to 90, 94, 121
  history of 4–5, 131–32
  humanitarianism and the anaesthesia issue 141–49
  indications for the use of 134–35
  less work for doctors than Dick-Read's methods 138
  light analgesia for mental relaxation 38
  and the mental imagery of birth 60
  and missing baby's first cry 136–37

natural anaesthesia of the perineum 124
  and natural childbirth 137–39, 148–150
  not given when needed vs giving against woman's wishes 134–35
  often used in place of companionship and sympathetic instruction 42
  principles of relief of pain in labour (Dick-Read's) 148–150
  as a public interest issue 141–49
  routine use of 131–32, 135–37, 146, 322
  should be available for all women 132, 137–39
  for stitching perineal tears 124
  women refusing 15, 114, 130, 135, 147, 282
anatomy and physiology 24–31
Anderson, Professor 38
antenatal education/ classes
  objectives of 217–19
  purpose of 219–225
  style and content of instruction 225–29
  antenatal schools 258–262
  class organisation 259–260
  definition of 'education' 114
  Dick-Read's ideas for preparation for labour 238–257
  history of 12, 86, 117
  how *not* to teach relaxation (witch story) 240
  importance of quality of teacher 247
  improved between early and last editions of the book 98–99
  physical fitness/ exercise 247–257
  senior medics often disagree with 13
  in South Africa 307–8
  unteachable women 236
anti-lactation injections 188
antiseptics, history of 5
anus, and pelvic floor exercises 255
anxiety
  acute fear vs chronic anxiety 52–53
  anxious husbands 208–9, 212

post-war experiences in obstetrics
287–88
marriage and birth of first child
289
writes first book 288–89
starts teaching relaxation 291
lecture tours 300–302, 318–330
death 333
babies arriving during his holidays
162, 297
at Blue Sisters Convent, Malta 41,
284
charged with unprofessional
conduct 293
collecting evidence of successful
application of method 35, 176,
291, 299
colour-blindness 58, 281
on contraception 270
controlled studies 303–4
developing awareness of need
to look after woman's mind in
childbirth 287–89
Dick-Read Method summarised
152–53
finding beauty in the minutiae of
Norfolk marshes 173–74
inaccurately portrayed as against
pain relief 138–39
interest in natural history 280
invention of a maternity belt 229
learning about muscular relaxation
286–87
letters (mothers') sent to Dick-Read
20–21, 61, 241, 300
letters from his own mother 274
loneliness, personal experience 41,
168–171, 282–83
passion for spreading his message
303, 330–32, 333
philosophy of childbirth 6, 15–23,
263–276, 316
possessing qualities of kindness
296
publishes *Introduction to
Motherhood* 313
publishes *Natural Childbirth*
292–93, 332
publishes *Revelation of Childbirth*
299
publishes *The Birth of a Child*
(1947) 302
reasons for publishing this book
263, 330–32

religious beliefs 19, 128, 317
research in African tribes 308–12
in South Africa 304, 305–6, 320–21
in the United States 300, 318–330
unorthodox approach unpopular
with colleagues 101, 263–65,
288–292, 296
war injuries 41, 284, 287
wartime experiences (WWI) 16,
41, 168–171, 282–87
wartime experiences (WWII)
298–99
Dick-Read, Jessica (Grantly's wife)
on her husband and his work
332–33
as organiser of antenatal school
246, 247, 260, 307
rescuing manuscript 299
diet, in pregnancy (recommended)
102–11
dilatation of cervix
impeded by fear-stimulated muscle
contraction 37
and the need for good support 166
in a normal labour 117–18
in normal labour 160
disabilities caused by birth trauma
13–14
disabled women giving birth 123–24,
249
disappointment 42, 92
disassociation 117
discretion and discrimination,
diminishing of 120–21, 323
doctors *see also* obstetrics
academic specialisation 10, 13–14
busy and impatient 162
can learn from watching normal
labours 132
Dick-Read's thoughts for rising
generation 263–276
don't see full labours from start to
finish 88, 115
example of poor care of a doctor's
wife 87
female doctors 11
focusing mainly on the physical 86
forcing women to use chloroform
15, 87, 95, 136
indifference of senior medics to
natural childbirth 262
need to find out women's attitudes
to childbirth early in pregnancy
223

gardener, obstetricians likened to 151, 155
Gardiner, Professor 280
gas and air 135, 142, 225, 241
Gauss, Carl 139
General Practitioners (GPs) 10–11, 194
Genesis 3:16 quote 24, 75, 80
genetics 25, 61
Gilliatt, Sir William 142, 302, 304–5
Glass, Rev BD 76
'God,' definitions of 19, 22 *see also* religion; spirituality
Goethe 128, 273
'good' babies 238, 261
Goodrich, Professor 313
gramophone recordings of natural births 260, 308
Grantly Dick-Read Correlation Chart 259
grunts and moans not necessarily indicating pain 94, 122

Haggard, Howard 4, 273
hand-washing 5
happiness
    husband's role in bringing about 216
    post-birth 23, 59–60, 91, 125, 127–28
hard work, labour as 81, 94, 114, 121, 122, 170
Hartridge, Professor H. 35
Hay, Dr Jack 309
Head, Sir Henry 36, 41, 42, 206, 288
head size (of babies) 327–28
heartburn 105
Hebrew words actually used in the Bible 76, 79
Hellmann, Dr Rudolf 78–79
Hemingway, Ernest 71
heredity (genetics) 25, 61
heroin (morphine) 148
Hingson, Robert H 145
Hippocrates 4, 131, 217
history of obstetrics 3–6
hospital facilities
    do not take account of the mind of the women 13
    not an economic priority 8–9
    organised for convenience of medical professions 13
    in United States 318–330
housework, sharing of 206

humanitarianism and the anaesthesia issue 141–49
husbands
    and antenatal education 259, 261–62
    attitudes towards birth 68–69, 207–8
    benefits of breastfeeding to 195–96
    and childbirth generally 205–16
    men's understanding of women 206–7
    presence or otherwise at birth 213–14
Huxley, Julian 22
hypnosis
    dulled consciousness of second stage not a hypnotic state 120
    not the same as hypnosis 296
    not the same as relaxation 233–34, 246
    as pain relief 151–55

ignorance
    about childbirth 219–225
    of carers, as pain intensifier for women 42
    obstetricians prefer women's 13, 301
immune-boosting properties of breastmilk 189–190
inborn reflexes 61
individual care, essentiality of
    in care of labouring woman 90, 121, 165–171, 173–74
    in supporting breastfeeding 194
induction of labour 297
instrumental deliveries
    and anaesthesia 147
    and cerebral palsy 13–14
    needed less in natural childbirth 177
    obstetricians' need to 'do something' 172
    obstetricians proud of 13, 137, 301
    rates in US 326
    and spinal cord anaesthesia 145
interference, the temptation of 163, 182
Introduction to Motherhood (Dick-Read, 1950) 313
inverted nipples 199–200
iodine in pregnancy diet 106
iron
    anaemia 40–41, 110

massage
  breast massage 199
  postnatal massage not
    recommended 256
  sacral pressure as pain relief
    117–18
materialism 18–19, 22, 273, 317, 326
maternal mortality 145, 311, 330
maternity belts 229
maternity hospitals *see* hospital
  facilities
Mayo, Kathleen 71
McCall Anderson, Thomas 280
media portrayals of birth 70–71,
  73–75
membrane rupture (waters breaking)
  94, 159, 180, 228
memory, and auto-suggestion and
  pain 44
men *see* husbands
menstruation and its effect on women
  206
mental imagery
  colour-music associations 58, 281
  importance of 58–64
  and pain 44
Mesmer, Franz Anton 154
metabolites 38, 54
midwifery
  history of 4
  midwives less likely to force
    anaesthesia 136, 142
  and the need for quiet calm 88
  and understanding about fear 88,
    89
  use of the term 72–73
milk in pregnancy diet 104, 106
milk production, physiology of 189
milk supply (mother's), inadequate
  186
milking (expressing milk) 199
mind, importance of *see* emotions/
  mind
minerals and vitamins in pregnancy
  104, 106
Minnitt's Apparatus 135, 142, 225
Moffatt, Dr James 80
Moffatt Mission 309
morning sickness 56, 85, 105, 209
mother love
  breastfeeding as embodiment of
    190–91
  ecstasy of birthing new life 127–28
  and the first minutes after birth

    125, 127–28
  and peace and happiness 17
  should be the centre of all obstetric
    work 11
  as spiritual gift 21
motherhood
  the baby makes the mother 261
  and beauty (of life) 16–18
  chosen by painters to depict beauty
    16–17
  importance of motherhood for
    society 191, 271–72
  importance of the first 48 hours
    203–4
  importance of the maternal mind
    11
  nature of mother's influence on the
    baby's brain development 56
  not taught in schools (and should
    be) 9, 11–12, 180, 181, 221–23,
    272, 294–95
  not valued by society 7, 9, 273–74
  as part of progression of
    womanhood 17–18
  and peace and happiness 17
  political views of 8–10
  religious views of 7–8
  so strongly associated with fear/
    pain that word is tainted 72
  as spiritual gift 21, 31
  warred over by man and woman
    7, 13
mothers (pregnant woman's own) -
  attitudes of 67–68, 69, 164, 289–290
  Mother's Letters, from 1915-1941 274,
    277
muscle contraction *see* contractions
muscular relaxation 232–33
music-colour associations 58, 281

Naish, Frances Charlotte 194
National Birthday Trust Fund 132, 141
National Health Service, introduction
  of 302
natural childbirth
  Mrs D example (peacefulness) 44
  natural childbirth methods 156–
    178
  natural childbirth teaching 99–101
  a normal labour 112–129
  proven success of 265, 267
  Whitechapel woman example
    15–16

how pain is felt 34–37
how to make a uterine contraction
hurt through suggestive
behaviour 43
'It didn't hurt. It wasn't meant to,
was it doctor?' 15–16, 19, 282
low pain thresholds, factors
predisposing 40
and muscle contractions 29–31
no natural law justifying pain in
childbirth 16, 19, 33, 34–35, 221
not the intention of a creator God
19, 79, 82
only true pains are final dilatory
contractions 118
pain intensifiers 40–46
pain interpretation heightened
as woman drifts to dulled
consciousness in second stage
120
and restricted blood circulation 38
as a subject of great medical interest
32
and suggestion/ auto-suggestion
43–45
and tiredness (mental) 41–42
and tiredness (physical) 41
Pain (Behan, 1915) 32, 44
pain relief *see also* anaesthesia and
analgesia
history of 3–4
hypnosis 151–55
in labour (general discussion)
130–150
not a sign of failure 92
principles of relief of pain in labour
(Dick-Read's) 138–39, 148–150
panting 231
paraldehyde 145
paraplegic woman story 123–24
partners *see* husbands; labour
supporters/ attendants
patience, peacefulness and personal
interest (three P's) 161–171
Patten, Professor Bradley M. 61
Pavlov, Ivan Petrovitch 62, 315–16,
317
peacefulness
in first stage of labour 117
importance of peace in reducing
mental weariness in labour 41–42
Mrs D example (peacefulness in
labour) 44
in natural childbirth methods 161

as one of the three P's 164–65
in painless labour 16, 95
in paintings of motherhood 17
post-birth 23
pelvic floor exercises 254
pentothal 145
Perfect Confinement 161
perineal tearing 124
personalised care, essentiality of 90,
121, 165–171, 173–74
pethidine (demerol) 38, 135, 148, 149,
322–23
phosphorus in pregnancy diet 106
physical fitness/ exercise 247–257
physiology of pregnancy 24–31
physiotherapist's exemplary labour
247
physiotherapy 247
pica 106
piles (haemorrhoids) 255
pillars of labour (elation, relaxation,
amnesia and exultation) 157
'pity' feeds 200
placenta
expulsion of in natural childbirth
127, 183–84, 286
formation of 26
respected in African tribes 311
women wishing to see 227
PMT (pre-menstrual tension) 206
politics
and the anaesthesia issue 142–43
views of motherhood 8–10
Pope Pius XII on natural childbirth
314
positions for labour
in African tribes 311
Dick-Read prefers lying down 160
in emergencies 181–82
exercises to prepare for 252
positions for relaxation 242–45
post-natal depression 193
post-natal exercises 254–57
prayer, alternative, in gratitude for the
gift of the child 82
Prayer books as source of fear about
childbirth 81–83
precipitate labour 181
pregnancy
conditioned fear of 63
physiology of 24–31
pregnancy complaints as indication
of fear/ tension 56, 85, 127

Simpson, James Young 5, 76, 131, 140–41
sleep in labour 42, 119–120
sleeping draughts 148
Smellie, W. 131
Snow, John 5
sodium prophy-methyl-carbinyl-allyl barbiturate 145
Soranus of Ephesus 4, 78, 324
South Africa
  baby rearing practices 195
  Dick-Read in 304, 305–6, 320–21
spasm, muscular 30
spermatozoa 24, 25–26
sphincters 30, 255
spinal cord anaesthesia 135, 145
spirituality
  birth as spiritual experience 21–23, 126, 127–28, 273
  cycle of life 128–29
  death as a spiritual experience 128
  motherhood as spiritual gift 21, 31
stimulus of fixed magnitude 36–37
stitching 124
stockings (hosiery), suspending 228–29
student doctors, Dick-Read's thoughts for 263–276
suckling, physiology of 189
suggestion, influence of
  vs hypnosis 151–55
  and pain 43–44, 45–46, 94
  vs relaxation 233–34
supplementary feeds ('pity' feeds) 200
supporters/ attendants at birth see also doctors; husbands; midwifery
  benefits to, of concentrated observation 173–74
  and the mental state of labouring woman 116
  motor men vs inhibitory men 296–97
  need for positive emotional support 93–94
  role in natural childbirth methods 160–61
  and suggestion (of pain) 45–46, 67–68
  woman needs confidence in her labour supporters 93–94, 95
'surgeons,' use of term and suggestion of pain 46
suspenders (hosiery) 228–29
sympathy, not over-sympathy 175

tense woman:tense cervix 112, 233, 290
tension see also Fear-Tension-Pain Syndrome; relaxation
  in physical strain 122
  residual tension 245–46
  tense woman:tense cervix 112, 233, 290
thalamus 36, 37, 226
thioethamyl 145
third stage 127, 183, 286
Thoms, Professor Herbert 143, 306, 313
three C's (confidence, concentrated observation and cheerfulness) 161, 171–78
three P's (patience, peacefulness and personal interest) 161–171
tiredness
  caused by anaemia 41
  and pain in labour 41
  in pregnancy 210
translation issues with the Bible 77–80
trichlorethylene (Trilene) 135, 148, 225
'twilight sleep' 137

unassisted births 182
unconditioned reflexes 61
Undset, Sigrid 71
United States, childbirth in 318–330
urination in labour 184
uterus
  blood circulation 38, 55
  can only register pain stimulus of excessive tension 34
  circular muscle fibres (of uterus) 28, 29, 30, 37, 117, 127, 233
  involution/ restitution 192
  longitudinal muscle fibres (of uterus) 28, 29, 30, 37
  muscle layers of 27
  nerves of 29–31
  pain receptors 34–35
  size of 27
  teaching about antenatally 226
  will get on by itself in first stage 160–61
  work of uterus assisted by breathing techniques 230

Vellay, Dr Pierre 314, 316
Velvovsky, Dr 313